PRAISE FOR VIBRANT

"Dr. Stacie Stephenson is a lifestyle medicine doctor who understands that health begins with the basics you control: eating good food in small portions, moving every day, and connecting with the people you love. Anyone can do it, but not everyone knows how. This book contains everything you need to know to get started and stick with healthy habits for life."
—Goldie Hawn, actress and founder of MindUP

"In *Vibrant*, Dr. Stacie Stephenson delivers on how we can achieve the goal of her book's title. We all want to age and live vibrantly, and this book tells you how. Elevate your health by reading *Vibrant*!"
—Dr. William Li, *New York Times* bestselling author of *Eat To Beat Disease*

"Life is like a great banquet, at which each person is only well if everyone is well. This is how Dr. Stacie Stephenson sees her mission. Her energy is boundless and this book is an amazing achievement, with the admirable goal of bringing physical and mental wellness to all, so life can be the ultimate celebration for everyone. We don't know how she does it, but she keeps on working to bring good into the world."
—Andrea & Veronica Bocelli, The Andrea Bocelli Foundation

"The idea that health comes from lifestyle, rather than drugs and doctors, should be common sense, but somehow, it's not. That's why we need books like *Vibrant*. This colorful, warm, and energetic book can help anyone build (or rebuild) a foundation for vibrant health. Dr. Stephenson walks you through the essentials, while dipping into health wisdom from the wide variety of integrative fields she's studied. Whether you are a beginner or you just need a refresher, this book can set you on the path to enjoy vibrant health for the rest of your long and happy life."
—Dr. Will Cole, leading functional medicine expert and author of *Ketotarian, The Inflammation Spectrum* and *Intuitive Fasting*

"What an inspiring, exciting, vibrant book from my friend Dr. Stacie! I love how she combines accessible science, inspirational wisdom, deeply personal stories, and actionable strategies for individual health empowerment. We are on the same page all the way with our commitment to lifestyle as the primary path to health. We will always need doctors, but what you do for yourself right now is what will determine your health in the future, and that's something you get to control! I love how this book walks you through the steps to make that happen."
—Samantha Harris TV host, certified health coach, and author

"This book really struck a chord for me. Music is my arena, and music is all about vibration. The root of the word 'vibrant' is the same as the root of the word 'vibration,' and vibration has been used for centuries as a form of healing as well as inspiration. I can feel the positive, healing, inspirational vibrations emanating from these pages. My dear friend Dr. Stacie Stephenson has proven herself a master of vibrancy! This book is pure gold. Its straight—forward information, understandable for the layman, provides the key to unlock the secrets of vibrant health for all those who desire it but aren't sure how to get there. I've learned so much and I'm so thankful that Dr. Stephenson was willing to put in the time and investigative work to create a roadmap for this wonderful and important journey. I'm truly impressed and I feel lucky to have this gem in my hands. I recommend it for anyone who wants to feel better, enjoy their lives more, and experience the profound vibration of deep inner health."

—David Foster, producer, songwriter, and artist

"I am completely inspired to be vibrant! I consider myself a healthy person, but after reading this delightful and illuminating book, I've got a whole list of new habits to incorporate into my life. I want energy, glow, and joy for many years to come, and this book is a path to get and keep that amazing feeling of vibrant health. Brava, my friend! I am forever inspired by you and your heart to help others. Keep sharing your beautiful light."

—Pia Toscano, singer and contestant on *American Idol* season 10

"Dr. Stacie Stephenson's book *Vibrant* does exactly what the title implies. It provides an uplifting, can-do program for all of us trying to get the most out of the rest of our lives. It represents a road map for the achievement of vibrant health."

—Jeffrey Bland, PhD, FACN, FACB, president of The Personalized Lifestyle Medicine Institute

"Only 15% of disease is due to genetics. That means your health is under your control. Dr. Stacie shows you how."

—Dr. Joseph Pizzorno, author of *The Toxin Solution* and coauthor of the *Encyclopedia of Natural Medicine*

"Finally! Simple, easy-to-do actions anyone can take to reclaim glorious health. Dr. Stacie's no-nonsense approach will delight you, and if you follow her savvy advice, you'll soon see a vibrantly beautiful new you."

—Lara Pizzorno, MDIC, MA, LMT, author of *Your Bones: How You Can Prevent Osteoporosis and Have Strong Bones for Life*

"VibrantDoc Dr. Stacie Stephenson has seen your future . . . and it is vibrant! In this book, she draws on her deep personal and professional reservoir to journey with you to truly vibrant living. Dr. Stephenson not only embodies the vibrancy she exudes in this book, she is catalyzing a more vibrant world through this message and her work. This book is truly a gift. Open it—and be vibrant!"

—Michael Stroka, JD, MBA, MS, CNS, LDN, CEO of the American Nutrition Association

"I was thrilled to learn that Dr. Stacie Stephenson is finally writing a book. I've long been impressed with her knowledge and natural, integrative approach to healthcare. Health has always been a priority for me, but when I experienced my own health struggles, I became acutely aware of how precious health really is. Read it for you. Read it for your family. Make your health a priority and take care of yourself using the techniques in this book, to lay the foundation for a long and healthy life."

—Cameron Mathison, actor and cohost of *Home and Family*

"Dr. Stacie Stephenson is one of the most vibrant women we know! Part of creating an energetic, effervescent life of health, happiness, and hope is doing for others as you take care of yourself. Through her work with Childhelp, Stacie has shown her loving spirit as an advocate for abused and neglected children. We have seen what good nutrition, recreational therapies, art, and lots of love can do to transform healing hearts. *Vibrant* is a book about cultivating that vitality in your life so it can shine upon the lives of those in need. Find your abundance, joy, and sense of vibrant purpose between these pages."

—Sara O'Meara & Yvonne Fedderson, founders of Childhelp

Finally—a holistic, common-sense approach to overall wellness! In *Vibrant*, Dr. Stacie Stephenson offers a guided tour to optimal health that educates, informs, and empowers you to take control of your daily well—being. As the wife and caregiver of someone who suffered with Parkinson's disease, I witnessed the power of conventional medicine when paired with integrative medicine. *Vibrant* offers a prescription for better health to those battling chronic illness as well as those of us looking to live our best lives."

—Lonnie Ali, philanthropist and Parkinson's advocate

"This indispensable book is your pathway to a happier, healthier, more vibrant you. Your trusted guide on this journey is Dr. Stacie Stephenson, who brings deep wisdom, inspiration, and passion to every page of this must—read work. Take that first step with her and you will soon be living your best life."

—Michael Burton, president and CEO of Gateway for Cancer Research

"So many books to read—some for pure fun and some to improve your knowledge in a specific, defined area. But now, here is *Vibrant*, the book which will give you the knowledge for life itself! No question, *Vibrant* is a must-read if you want the knowledge to improve the quality of your life. Should you meet Dr. Stacie, the author, you would see this knowledge personified—beauty, intellect, grace, and health. Now available by reading and applying—*Vibrant*!"

—Horst Schulze, author of *Excellence Wins* and founding member of the Ritz Carlton

"If I had to recommend just one new book to read this spring, it would be *Vibrant* by my friend Dr. Stacie Stephenson. Full of energy, life, vitality, and *vibrancy*, this book is full of inspiration for how to own your health and live a more healthful life by making better choices. Her nutrition and health information is highly advanced— yet easy to understand and apply to your everyday lifestyle. Full of great advice, interactive assessments, and delicious recipes, this book can set anyone on the right path to a vibrant life! *Brava*, my friend!"

—Christine Avanti, CN, author of *Skinny Chicks Eat Real Food*

"When I was in training to become a physician in the early 1980s we were essentially taught to make a diagnosis, prescribe the right drug or refer them to the right surgeon, and to then quickly move on to see the next patient—the 'sick care' paradigm. We spent almost no time studying or practicing prevention or health promotion. In *Vibrant*, Dr. Stacie Stephenson drives home the concept of integrative medicine which embraces all of the best practices of psychology, regenerative medicine, clinical nutrition, lifestyle medicine, chiropractic care, anti-aging medicine, functional medicine, and more to provide the patient with a truly personalized, holistic approach to healthcare. She lays out a groundbreaking 30-day program to engage patients and their healthcare providers on a path to optimizing their wellness and health. And she does it all in a way that a 'conventionally' trained practitioner can wholeheartedly embrace. Dr. Stephenson's approach embodies the future of healthcare; it places a new emphasis on wellness and health promotion which strives to keep the patient healthy and vibrant and to prevent sickness or injury. This is the direction we must go if we are to create a healthy, resilient, productive, and vibrant society."

—Robert G. Darling, MD, FACEP, FFSEM, former white house physician (1996–1999) and founder and chief medical officer of Patronus Medical, LLC

VIBRANT

A GROUNDBREAKING PROGRAM to GET ENERGIZED, OWN YOUR HEALTH, and GLOW

DR. STACIE STEPHENSON

BenBella Books, Inc.
Dallas, TX

BENBELLA

BenBella Books, Inc.
10440 N. Central Expressway
Suite 800
Dallas, TX 75231
benbellabooks.com
Send feedback to feedback@benbellabooks.com

BenBella is a federally registered trademark.

Printed in the United States of America
10 9 8 7 6 5 4 3 2 1

Library of Congress Cataloging-in-Publication Data is available upon request.
LCCN 2020049059
ISBN 9781950665822 (print)
ISBN 9781953295170 (ebook)

Editing by Laurel Leigh
Copyediting by Michael Fedison
Proofreading by James Fraleigh and Lisa Story
Indexing by WordCo Indexing Services
Insert photography by Bob and Dawn Davis Photography
Interior artwork and illustrations by Commune Communication
Text design and composition by Kit Sweeney
Cover design by Sarah Avinger
Printed by Lake Book Manufacturing

Distributed to the trade by Two Rivers Distribution, an Ingram brand
tworiversdistribution.com

Special discounts for bulk sales are available.
Please contact bulkorders@benbellabooks.com.

To my beloved husband, Richard—the most vibrant man I know.

CONTENTS

INTRODUCTION: *Set Yourself to Glow* 1

PART I: Deep
CHAPTER 1: *Becoming Vibrant* 15
CHAPTER 2: *The Fountain: How to Get More Energy* 41
CHAPTER 3: *The Indicator: How to Cultivate Glow from the Inside Out* 65

PART II: Deeper
CHAPTER 4: *The Communicator: How to Use Food to Feel Better* 85
CHAPTER 5: *The Activator: How to Move More to Live Longer* 117
CHAPTER 6: *The Connector: How Human Connection Supports Physical and Mental Health* 139

PART III: Deepest
CHAPTER 7: *The Mainframe: How to Fine-Tune Your Brain and Nervous System* 167
CHAPTER 8: *The Rejuvenator: How to Detoxify, Inside and Out* 191
CHAPTER 9: *The Sustainer: How to Build a Truly Resilient Immune System* 215

PART IV: Surfacing
CHAPTER 10: *30 Vibrant Habits to Cultivate* 235
CHAPTER 11: *The Vibrant Kitchen: 40 Recipes for Vitality and Glow* 271
CHAPTER 12: *The 50-Year Challenge: Toward a More Vibrant World* 319

APPENDIX: *Integrative Medicine 101* 323

NOTES 329

INDEX 344

ACKNOWLEDGMENTS 352

ABOUT THE AUTHOR 355

Set Yourself to Glow

Imagine you, but better. You, but with enough energy to zip through your day in a good mood without ever thinking about how nice it would be to take a nap. You, but with an immune system that vanquishes the colds and flus everyone else around you seems to suffer from, while you keep feeling amazing. You, but with firmer, clearer, more luminous skin. You, but with an inner glow that radiates outward, so that everyone who sees you wonders what your secret is. You, but at your ideal weight, which you easily maintain. You, but stronger, more resilient, and with less pain. You, but younger looking. You, but more vibrant.

Health is hard to define because it means different things to different people. To most doctors, health means the absence of disease. To others, it may mean not being overweight, or being pain-free, or feeling more energetic, or looking better or younger, or finally overcoming a chronic disease condition. When I assess someone's health, whether it is one of the patients I used to see when I was in private practice, or a friend who comes to visit, or just someone I notice as I'm out and about, I assess their health according to whether or not they are *vibrant.*

The root of the word vibrant is "vibration," and its original meaning was "light." To me, this perfectly describes what it means to be vibrant: to be full of lightness and the vibration of positive energy. But vibrant is also something that I believe can be more objectively assessed. To be vibrant means to have:

- Good muscle tone, and the ability to walk, run, sit down, carry things like groceries, pick up children or pets, and get down on or up off the floor easily and without pain.

- An amount of body fat that helps your body function but does not interfere with organs, movement, or comfort.

- No chronic systemic inflammation (low-grade hidden cellular inflammation that is pervasive and insidious—you can't necessarily feel it or see it, but it puts you at high risk for serious health problems including heart attacks and autoimmune conditions) as measured by advanced laboratory testing.

- Normal blood pressure, blood sugar, and cholesterol levels, as measured by standardized lab tests.

- Good cardiovascular fitness, including a strong heart, flexible arteries, and good lung capacity, as evidenced by the ability to walk a brisk mile or climb a flight of stairs without getting out of breath.

- No daily pain, such as joint pain, headaches, or stomachaches.

- Easy digestion without chronic bloating, gas, reflux, constipation, diarrhea, or nausea.

- A sharp, clear mind that can concentrate, focus, remember, and think quickly and creatively.

- A good sleep on most nights, with sufficient REM (dream) and deep (refreshing and reparative) sleep to regenerate the body and mind and feel awake and alert in the morning and all day long.

- A positive outlook and the capacity to feel a wide range of natural emotions without getting stuck in chronic depression and/or anxiety.

Vibrancy is also somewhat subjective. You likely have your own idea about whether or not you feel vibrant, and that's just what vibrant is: an assessment of how *you feel* every day. How you feel indicates how healthy you are. Do you feel graceful in your movements, strong in your body, energetic and awake during the day, and soundly sleeping at night?

Do you eat and enjoy a diet full of a wide variety of colorful organic whole foods, from berries and fresh greens to wild-caught salmon and cold-pressed olive oil?

Do you move your body every day in ways that feel good and build your cardiovascular fitness, strength, and flexibility?

Do you have healthy relationships that feel supportive and rewarding? Do you love others, and know they love you? Are you involved with other people in your community, through work, personal projects, religious organizations, clubs, or social groups?

Do you feel like you have the brain of a younger you, even as you are getting older? Can you concentrate and remember things the way you always have?

Do you rarely if ever need to take any pain or antacid medications? Do you feel awake without stimulants like coffee, and can you sleep without pharmaceutical sleep aids? Do you choose clean food and clean living most of the time?

Do you stay well when everyone is getting sick, or recover quickly from illness or injury? Do you consider yourself to be resilient, both physically and mentally, in the face of any challenge?

To be vibrant is to have the motivation to do whatever it is you want to do every day, as unencumbered by fatigue and pain as you can possibly be. It means waking up ready to embrace whatever's coming with passion and optimism. If you are slogging through your day, you aren't vibrant. If you move through your day with a feeling of vitality, with a sharp mind and an open heart, that's vibrant. When you feel not just physically but emotionally and mentally strong and stable enough to make good choices and act with empathy and courage, that's vibrant. When you live mostly free of aches and pains and stiffness, as well as anxiety, fear, and over-whelm . . . *that* is what vibrant means to me. To circle back to my first definition, which I hope will mean even more to you now: To be vibrant is to be full of light and vibrating with life from the inside out.

As a doctor and as an individual, I have dedicated the last few decades of my life to the concept of vibrant living. To be vibrant is what I strive for personally, and it's also what I've used as a barometer of health for my patients and associates, friends, and followers. For fourteen years, I was in private practice as an integrative practitioner trained in functional medicine, nutrition, anti-aging medicine, chiropractic care, acupuncture, and more. Today, I am the Chair of Functional Medicine for the Cancer Treatment Centers of America (CTCA), a board member for the American Nutrition Association (ANA), an American Heart Association (AHA) ambassador, and the founder and CEO of VibrantDoc (vibrantdoc.

com), a health media enterprise dedicated to disseminating actionable, cutting-edge information about how to live a vibrant life.

In these capacities, but especially with VibrantDoc, my goal is to bring a meaningful understanding of what health really is to public awareness. This book is my way of reaching out to you, in a world that can be stressful, toxic, and challenging in ways that I believe deeply compromise inner health. I want to help you break free from crippling mainstream ideas of how we are supposed to live, so you can aim higher, with loftier, more empowered goals for health and vibrancy. And I want to help you achieve your goals. The more vibrant we are as a society, the more successful, resilient, happy, and long-lived we all will be.

This isn't easy. We live in a climate where conventional medicine mostly ignores prevention and patient empowerment. Add to that the stress of everyday life along with the stress of big things like global health crises and natural disasters, and being healthy can feel impossible, or at least low on the priority list. The truth, however, is that the more strong, resilient, and vibrant you feel, the better you will be able to speak up for yourself, take your health into your own hands, and deal with the stresses of life in this modern world. Every step in a vibrant direction counts and can make your life feel a little better and a little bit easier, too.

You may have to do this on your own, however (or, with the help of this book!). Chances are, your doctor won't tell you how *not* to get sick or how to *create health*. Most likely, your doctor will only want to see you if you are *already sick*. Doctors are not in the business of preventing illness and injury. They are in the business of managing it, most often with drugs or surgery. I know I'm not the only one who has often been left wondering: *But wait . . . how can I keep from getting sick in the first place? What can I do to* become healthy? In fact, these are the exact questions that got me where I am today.

How I Became VibrantDoc

I grew up training as a competitive figure skater, and throughout my teens and twenties, I assumed that would be my career. I never thought beyond that because I trained intensely and obsessively. It was my life. I was a good athlete. I ate well, I trained hard, but what I didn't do was address my chronic stress. I was always pushing through the pain, the exhaustion, and the minor injuries. I thought I would always have endless access to energy and that I was invincible.

Then, one fateful day, I had a terrible accident and ended up in the hospital. It was the end of my figure skating career. I wasn't invincible, after all, and I was devastated. I became quite depressed, and as I recovered over months, while dealing with chronic pain and mobility issues, one of my biggest disappointments was my medical care. I assumed the doctors could fix everything and get me back on the ice, but all I got were a series of diagnoses as my health deteriorated, and prescriptions to "help." I came down with mononucleosis, rheumatic fever, and recurring strep throat. My immune system was shot. I began to realize that I was going to have to do a much better job of taking care of myself. I always had an intuition that there was more to what was wrong with me than my accident. Why did I have that accident? Was something going on that caused it to happen? I knew there had to be a bigger picture, but my doctors never seemed to acknowledge that I was a whole person, not just an injury. I have always been a competitive and ambitious person, so once I accepted that my Olympic dreams were never going to happen, I shifted gears and decided I could do better than those doctors who hadn't been able to help me. I would go to medical school!

I was a good and serious student, studying hard and doing well in my classes. I was the one who chose not to go out partying because I had a test the next day, and I drove myself just as hard as I had as a figure skater. But medical school didn't give me the opportunities I thought it would. I wanted my chosen career to reflect my values. I needed my work to make sense to me, and inspire me, but I quickly learned that mainstream Western allopathic doctors are trained in a very specific system of diagnosis and prescription—a name-it, blame-it, give-it-a-pill philosophy. I kept asking myself: *Why are we only learning about sickness?* and *When do I get to take the classes about how to be healthy?*

That lesson never came. Those classes weren't part of the curriculum. Medical school is not about maintaining health or preventing disease, I was unhappy to learn. It wasn't what I'd signed up for. I became unsure of where I belonged or what I really wanted to study. I began to search for alternative tracks and switched direction several times, as I tried to escape the "drugs and surgery" model and find a course of learning and practice that felt authentic to me. I knew there had to be a "building health" model out there somewhere. Isn't it common sense to try first to avoid sickness, rather than wait for it to happen and only then try to cure it? Isn't it common sense to optimize wellness so you never have to go to the doctor in the first place? Medical school didn't seem to think so, but I knew the answer had to be out there somewhere. I knew from experience that the body knows what it needs to heal, and I wanted to learn how to support that process, rather than try to interfere with it, with the arrogant attitude that we doctors, with our pills and procedures, are wiser than the body itself.

Then, one day, some of my fellow medical students were attending a convention, and they convinced me to go along. Dr. Jeffrey Bland was speaking about a new field he was developing called functional medicine. At the time, I didn't know what this was (few did), but I tagged along. In the lecture, I listened to Dr. Bland with wonder and amazement. I remember having a revelation: It wasn't a profession I needed to choose. It was a philosophy—and what I was hearing was the closest thing I'd heard to something I could believe in and embrace.

Dr. Bland wasn't talking about fixing health problems. He was asking why they occurred at all. This was a whole new way of thinking about health. Dr. Bland was asking: Why does the body slip from a healthy to a dysfunctional state? Where did things first start to go wrong? Why do some people get diseases, and others don't? Why do some people get injured, and others don't? Can we follow illness and injury back to their root causes?

That got my attention. Why had I gotten injured, when others hadn't? Why was I then plagued with viral illnesses, when others weren't? I went home that day with EPA/DHA supplements and glucosamine supplements and a whole new attitude. I had found a path I actually wanted to follow— one that would let me interact with and help people in a way that felt ethical and true. I passionately embraced the whole concept of lifestyle medicine as an alternative to conventional medicine, and I never looked back.

Since then, I've enthusiastically studied and trained in many different but related fields, including clinical nutrition, regenerative medicine, acupuncture, chiropractic care, psychology, environmental medicine, and anti-aging medicine. I've always chased knowledge with an obsessive curiosity. If it sounds like something that can legitimately help people, then I want to know everything about it, and I want to use that knowledge to help my actual patients.

But modern medicine is a stern and narrow-minded taskmaster, and even those of us who work in integrative medical fields must contend with it. After all, integrative means integrating the best of all approaches, including conventional ones. Candidly, I spent most of my years in private practice pushing the rules as far as I could when conventional medicine resisted an integrative approach. The truth is that when lifestyle medicine clashes with conventional medicine, it's conventional medicine that has the money, influence, and power. However, I have always been (and remain) determined to continue to do what I think is right, for my own health and the health of my patients, family, friends, readers, and followers. When I was in private practice, I never shrank from what I perceived as my duty as a healthcare provider, or what I believed to be the rights of my patients. Have I been controversial? Sure. Have the powers that be always agreed with me? Certainly not. But what is new and empowering is often threatening to the establishment, and that's the line I try to walk. I do it for you.

Eventually, I left private practice to become the Chair of Functional Medicine for the Cancer Treatment Centers of America so I could help to bring an integrative perspective into an arena that tends to rely heavily on conventional medicine. More recently, as I've mentioned, I joined the board of the American Nutrition Association, and have forged a partnership with the American Heart Association. I want to have a hand in those national organizations that I believe work sincerely to empower patients, and I believe that operating at this high level is an effective way for me to trigger changes from the top down.

But I do miss private practice, and lately, I've longed to get back to spreading my message of prevention and health empowerment to people in all walks of life. Working for national organizations can help to gradually change policy, but I hope this book can help to change people's lives in the here and now. That's also why I decided to start VibrantDoc, a unique enterprise dedicated to educating, informing, and empowering all who wish to live a more vibrant life. I want to reach as many people as I can, to help assure that as a society we can begin to see that each of us can build health for ourselves and enjoy more vibrant lives. In doing so, we make our communities, countries, and world stronger, more unified, and more enlightened about what health and wellness are. With every improvement you make to yourself, you have the potential to set an example for how to achieve a vibrant health state, extended youthfulness, vigorous longevity, and a happy, fulfilling life.

We can't rely on anyone else to do this for us. The more we give away our power, the less control we will have over our own quality and length of life. We can make ourselves stronger, better, more vibrant. I want to help you navigate your own path toward that goal. *You* can be stronger, better, more vibrant, and you can start moving in that direction *today*.

Becoming Vibrant Is More Important Than Ever

Those years of helping people with one hand and fighting the system with the other have stayed with me. What I think about most is how ironic that physician's oath really is: "First, do no harm." And yet, what does modern conventional medicine so often do?

Let's look at some statistics.

According to patient safety experts at Johns Hopkins School of Medicine, medical errors are the third leading cause of death after heart disease and cancer, and 10 percent of all deaths in the United States are now due to medical error.[1] Doctors and surgeons are incredibly prone to stress and burnout. According to a study that anonymously surveyed nearly 8,000 surgeons, 700 of them reported they were concerned they had made a major medical error in the past three months, and these were the same participants who had the highest scores for depression and burnout (emotional exhaustion and other signs of severe chronic work stress). Over 70 percent of them said the error was their own fault, not a problem with the system.[2]

Medical errors and other adverse healthcare events not only often lead to injury and expense, but they far too frequently result in fatalities. Deaths due to preventable adverse healthcare events each year exceed deaths from car accidents.[3] Deaths from medication errors exceed deaths from workplace injuries.[4] According to the National Safety Council, drug poisoning is the number one cause of unintentional death in the United States, and many of those drugs were legally prescribed by doctors.[5] About 700,000 people a year visit the emergency room for adverse drug events, and approximately 5 percent of hospitalized patients experience adverse drug events.[6]

I could go on with more scary statistics, but what I see when I look at the current state of modern medicine is not a healthcare system. It's a sick-care system. And with all those drugs, surgeries, and procedures, it's no wonder that modern medicine could literally kill you. How is that doing no harm?

I'm not saying conventional doctors have bad intentions. I know they don't. They dedicate their lives to helping people. The doctors at the CTCA are passionately committed to helping cancer patients in any way they can, using every possible resource and every new technology. When the system doesn't work, it's usually not the doctors who are at fault. The system is driven by special interests who mostly do not have patient-first care as their priority. When you have a heart attack or break a bone, modern medicine is great at swooping in and quickly fixing the problem to save life and limb, but when it comes to chronic health problems, conventional medical practice is often of little to no help. It's just not designed for those medical issues that come from years of neglecting good health practices, living a stressful life, and existing in a toxic environment. Medications, surgeries, and symptom-focus are end-stage patches. They don't do anything about causes and sources.

On the other hand, prevention and health optimization *are* accessible to you. Looking at where health begins and nurturing health and wellness at its source in the human body is the most natural, human-centered, whole-person way of living. It involves taking a close and curious look at what you eat, how you move, how you nurture relationships, how you deal with stress, how you sleep, how you keep your environment, and how you choose to view and respond to your circumstances. That is the journey I'm inviting you to join me on in this book.

We all have many daily opportunities to make poor health choices, but they *are choices*. You are in charge of what you do and how you choose to think about the things that happen to you in your life. If you don't feel vibrant right now, chances are pretty good that you aren't taking charge of how you live. You may feel like you can't do it, or you don't know how. That's not surprising because, for many people, this toxic, stressful world we live in is taking its toll and the messages are numerous and confusing. It's distracting, disillusioning, even debilitating.

Do you remember when, as a child, it felt effortless to run and play and be outside and eat well and sleep soundly and feel joy and delight at the smallest things? Somewhere along the way, we can lose that ease of living we enjoyed as kids, and now, in this time, in this world, most of us (sadly) probably will end up with a chronic disease. Maybe you already have one . . . or more than one. According to the CDC's National Center for Chronic Disease Prevention and Health Promotion, 60 percent of adults in the United States already have a chronic disease such as diabetes, heart disease, cancer, lung disease, kidney disease, or dementia, and 40 percent have two or more chronic conditions.[7] Those statistics are *incredible* to me, and disheartening.

But it's never too late to turn it around, and you are not a statistic. If you assume you will someday suffer from failing health if you choose to remain on your current course, why wouldn't you choose a new trajectory? What have you got to lose? Many of you reading this book don't yet have a major health problem, and you can keep it that way by refusing to be a victim of a culture that glorifies poor health habits. It takes some effort to achieve a vibrant life, but what awesome things are easy?

The secret I offer you in these pages is that achieving vibrant health isn't as hard as you might think! If not quite there, you can achieve your ideal weight. You can get strong. You can become more limber. You can strengthen your immune system and generate all the energy you could ever want. You can glow from the inside out with radiance that comes from profound health at the deepest levels. I want to guide you toward a life in which you feel vibrant every day, live with intention and joyful effort, are able to eat well, move easily, sleep soundly, wake refreshed, cherish your relationships, contribute to your community, and love what you see in the mirror—both the external you and the vibrancy that comes from health and happiness. I want you to have vast inner resources you can draw on when you need them. My wish is for you to love your life!

If this is also what you want for yourself, then let's get started now. With each chapter, we will gradually, incrementally remake you. You will still be you, but with an abundance of energy and excitement about your life. You're going to feel younger, stronger, slimmer, fitter, and have less pain. We're going to steer you away from a future of chronic disease and toward the body and brain you deserve—and that you can continue to have for years to come.

Your health is yours, and nobody can take it from you if you choose to own it. In this book, you will find the knowledge and inspiration to make changes in the way you live, and the guidance to know how to do it. You will experience firsthand real, tangible, visible shifts in your energy and appearance. You will be *vibrant*.

Yours in Vibrancy,
Dr. Stacie J. Stephenson

PART I
Deep

Welcome to your vibrant life! I'm really happy you have decided to begin your quest for optimal health, and I'll be with you at every step. I have a lot in store for you, but we're going to start with the basics and work our way deep, deeper, and to the deepest depths of creating health from your inside out.

But how do I help someone reading a book, without being able to look at them? I can't ask you to stand in front of me so I can assess you. I thought long and hard about this. I am a firm believer in the external as a reflection of the internal, and I also believe that personalized medicine is the imminent and necessary future, so that led me to the obvious conclusion: You are the expert on you.

You know your body better than anyone else in the world, including a doctor. You are always right there, feeling everything that goes on inside of you, and you always have the opportunity to evaluate yourself, inside and out. You may not know all the anatomical terms or be able to tell someone how your endocrine system works, but you have intuition and your body is always telling you what it needs. That means you are the best and most capable person on the planet for evaluating your own health.

So, together, let's take a deep dive into what it means to be vibrant, how to gauge your current health state, and how to achieve more energy and glow by living the vibrant life.

Vibrant = Energy + Glow

CHAPTER 1

Becoming Vibrant

"**Y**ou changed my life!"

I hadn't seen my massage therapist (let's call her Tina) in over a year, but when she came to my house, I had to do a double take. I barely recognized her. The puffy, overweight, blotchy-skinned, forty-something woman I'd first met had been replaced by a fit, curvy, beautiful woman, maybe fifty pounds lighter than she was before, with a sparkle in her eyes, enthusiasm in her voice, and a deep inner glow that radiated outward. That thick layer of toxic fatty fluid I so often see on unhealthy people was gone. She moved with ease, her skin was clear, and I could feel her positive energy—she was vibrant!

"You look fantastic!" I said. "What did you do?"

"I did just what you said!"

I vaguely remembered that she had shyly asked for just five minutes of my time back when she had first come to my house for our massage appointment the past year, but I couldn't remember specifically what we'd talked about. All I could think to say was, "Tell me more!"

She laughed, then reminded me that she had summoned all her courage, knowing I was a health professional, to ask my advice, fearing it might be inappropriate but feeling desperate. She had suffered for years from allergies to "everything," chronic unidentified skin issues, swelling and bloating, and she kept gaining weight, no matter what she did.

She had eliminated so many things from her life, for fear she was allergic to them, that she spent almost all her time trying to keep track and figure out what she could and could not eat, touch, breathe, and do. It was exhausting. She had been obsessing about the materials in her cookware and food storage containers, her indoor air quality, detergents and shampoos, and everything else that touched her skin. She grasped onto every fad, thinking it might finally hold the answer—she'd tried to go gluten-free, dairy-free, keto, vegan, low-carb, and low-fat, but each successive diet was no better than the last, and she was never quite sure she was doing any of them right anyway. Vitamins made her sick, she reacted to every skin cream, and everything she ate seemed to make her condition worse. "Even fruit!" she told me. "Even salad!"

She told me that she'd had her hormones checked, she'd been to multiple doctors, but they all said they couldn't find anything wrong. She knew there must be a missing piece out there—the magic potion that would finally alleviate her suffering—but her world had become small and she was losing hope. She hardly had the energy to work anymore, and the only reason she agreed to take my appointment was that she knew I was a natural medicine doctor. She thought maybe I could tell her something all the other doctors hadn't.

I was already thinking about what I would tell such a person now, but asked, "So what did I tell you to do?"

"All you said to do was eat a lower-carb Mediterranean diet with no gluten or dairy," she said. "And you told me what actually had gluten and what actually counted as a dairy product, because I'm embarrassed to admit that I didn't know! And . . ." She paused dramatically, as if saving the best part for last. "You told me to forget about everything else I was trying to do until I got my food right!"

That's exactly what I would have told her today because, in my experience, with chronic health problems, especially those mysterious ones that seem to deny a diagnosis because the symptoms are so variable and vague, the number one problem is usually food—and the number one intervention is also usually food. People tend to want to focus on everything else around them because they think food is the hardest thing to change, but food is actually the easiest thing to change because you have the most control over it. It takes a lot more effort to overhaul your entire environment than to stop eating bread and cheese. You may really like bread and cheese (I certainly do—I think it's my Francophile proclivities), but it's not complicated or expensive to say no to it, especially when you aren't feeling well. You have more control over what you choose to put in your mouth than you do over your air quality, water quality, the toxins in the environment, or even how much time and opportunity you might have to exercise, especially if you have a sedentary job. Get the food right, and the other pieces will begin to fall in place: You'll have more energy to exercise, more motivation to detox what you can, more clarity for making smart decisions, more calm for better sleep quality, and more optimism for a better quality of life. That's not to say food is the only health influence. Far from it. But it is job one.

Tina continued, "So I went totally gluten- and dairy-free and started eating a lot more vegetables, fruits, and olive oil, and cutting out my two favorite foods, bread and pasta. I started choosing fish over beef and had nuts and seeds for a snack instead of something sweet. And, Dr. Stephenson . . ." She put a hand on my arm. "It was like a miracle! All my skin problems resolved, the blotchiness and hives went away, the bloating and swelling went down, and then I started losing weight so easily. I couldn't believe it!"

If my memory serves, the massage I got that day from my vibrant massage therapist was a lot better than the one I'd had a year previous. This woman was remade. She was focused, she had energy and strength, and she was tuned in to exactly what my body needed during our massage. She was not only vibrant; she was better at her job! That's just the start of what can happen when you tune in to what your own body needs and answer its call.

Was Tina's core issue a gluten intolerance? Likely. A dairy allergy? Also likely, as these two often go hand in hand. Was it too many carbs, or too little healthful fat? Or just too many calories, exceeding her energy needs? These may all have played a role. Was it just a lack of knowledge? That certainly didn't help, since she (and she's not alone in this) didn't know what foods contained gluten and which foods were dairy products. All I can say for certain, however, since she was not officially my patient and I didn't do any testing on her, is that she found a way to live that was both sustainable and turned her health and her life around. Today, she runs a busy massage therapy practice with great success, and she feels and looks fantastic.

So what did she do that you could do?

You aren't Tina (unless you are Tina, and happen to be reading this book). If you aren't feeling your best, if you aren't feeling vibrant, you may have a different set of issues, or more likely, a slightly different version of the same issues, since most people's health problems have at least something to do with what they are eating. You could be inadvertently sabotaging your wellness, but the good news is that, for the most part, you get to decide how you live. With a little know-how, and the willingness to begin at the beginning and start paying attention to your body's messages, you could (like Tina) turn it all around.

INTEGRATIVE MEDICINE 101

I fall into the integrative medicine camp because I believe in taking the best, most effective, most natural, and least harmful elements from all healthcare systems, therapies, and techniques, both holistic and allopathic, ancient and modern. Modern medicine does some things very well, but there are also wise and useful therapies and strategies in many other, more holistically oriented approaches to health, both ancient and new.

My "secret sauce" has always been a willingness to invest all my time (and, in the early days, most of my money) into learning, practicing, and getting certified or licensed in many different disciplines. My goal is to come at health from diverse angles, so I'll be referencing some of these perspectives in this book. You may also hear about others as you read health information out there in the world, so in case you aren't sure what some of them are, or need a refresher, you can find a quick-start guide to some of the more common integrative terms in the appendix at the back of this book.

HOW TO START DIAGNOSING YOURSELF

There is a lot I can tell just by looking at someone, before they even say a word. When I assess a patient (or a friend), there are a few things I look for that almost without exception indicate that person's health status. I can tell at a glance if someone has energy or not. Energy might be the most obvious and most powerful indicator of vibrancy. It is ethereal and intangible, but you can see it in someone, and you can see when they don't have enough.

I also look at external features that indicate internal health or the lack of it, like skin tone and color, nail length and quality (unless this is obscured by a manicure), the brightness and animation in someone's eyes that can indicate both physical and mental health, how freely and easily someone moves, what their posture is like, how clear and easy their voice is, and the general shape of their body. All body types can be beautiful, but if your natural healthy body shape is hidden due to excess weight, you will feel more vibrant if you set it free.

Each of these seemingly superficial aspects of the body is actually a deep indicator of health, and is very telling. Your health is evident through these internal and external, subjective and objective indicators. In other words:

Vibrant = Energy + Glow

A NOTE ABOUT DOCTORS

I've amassed quite a lot of knowledge over the years about what it takes to regenerate vitality and restore health. There is an amazing intuition that exists within each of us. If you let people talk long enough, they will tell you what's wrong with them, even if they don't realize that's what they've done. Sometimes it only takes a few minutes for me to see what's going on with someone, but I always give people enough time to talk. I have always allotted at least a full hour for appointments.

As I've said, you are the best person to tell whether you are healthy or whether something is wrong, but sometimes you really do need to go to the doctor. If you do, you will have the best and most productive experience if you find one who takes the time to really get to know you. This is much more likely with an integrative practitioner, such as a functional medicine doctor.

I may sound like I'm getting on my soapbox here (and I guess I am), but one of my criticisms of today's conventional medicine is that doctors typically only spend a few minutes with patients before rushing on to the next exam room. (This is often because of pressure from hospitals or large practice requirements, not the doctor's choice.) This isn't nearly long enough to figure out what's really going on. I was always fully prepped for a patient, and the entire office was focused on what that patient needed. I believe doctors should already know the patient's name, all lab information, all reports, and should not waste the patient's time looking over all of that in the exam room.

You should not have to wait in a waiting room longer than a minute or two, either. I believe your experience at your doctor's office should be like pressing the pause button on the hectic doctor's office environment. The entire appointment should be about digging into the things about your life, and your health, that may not be evident from the paperwork. It should be about understanding how you live, and about building the doctor-patient relationship.

If you don't have a personal relationship and rapport with your doctor, how can they help you? How can they ever see the big picture of your health story without taking some time to listen to you, look you in the eye, touch your skin, and assess your color, movement, energy, expression, skin quality, hair quality, the brightness or dullness in your eyes, and the presence or absence of that inner glow that reveals health at the deepest level? Maybe your doctor will even hug you— you probably need it! A doctor can't know your context if they don't find out about how you live, where you came from, and what health issues other relatives have. This is the essence of lifestyle or holistic medicine. Doctors should take the time necessary to understand the big picture.

And one more thing—I want to say something about telemedicine. Seeing your doctor over video certainly has its benefits. People may have greater access to doctors and waste less time traveling to appointments and sitting in waiting rooms. Doctors may be able to quickly alleviate anxiety about minor problems, and there may be better follow-up frequency. However, on the side of the healers, there is a price. We get a lot from our patients just by being in physical proximity to them and feeling their energy. We can read their emotions and get unspoken information about how they are doing, and this is a lot harder to do through a screen. Also, when patients don't have to make as much of an effort to see a doctor, they may be less motivated to follow the doctor's advice. It's a trade-off and I certainly understand the need for it in many situations, but I do hope we won't ever lose that genuine physical connection between doctors and patients that tells us so much about what is wrong and how to help.

Throughout this book, I'm going to keep reminding you and giving you guidance for self-assessment, body awareness, and internally directed intuition. Your goal is to be more observant of, sensitive to, and in tune with your own body. Everyone does this to some extent. You know when you get a rash. You know when you are bloated or constipated. You know when you look pale, or feel exhausted. But you can fine-tune this natural awareness to the point where you can tell when you are vibrant, and when you aren't. You will soon be equipped to detect much more subtle signals. And as for a diagnosis, every single one of the indicators of health in the above list is something you can assess independently. All you have to do is look in the mirror.

One of the first pieces of advice I have for you is to begin each day with a mirror assessment. Strip down (or wear close-fitting clothing, like leggings and a tank top) and take a good hard look at yourself in a full-length mirror with an eye for diagnosis rather than criticism. Many of my women patients tend to be appearance-conscious anyway (our culture is so fixated on female appearance), but women also tend to be self-critical. Or, they are in denial, only glancing at parts of themselves at a time—face, shoulder, calf—so they don't have to see the big picture. It's time to let that go. I want you to look at yourself every morning, head to toe, not with criticism, but with curiosity. You are getting to know yourself and your fluctuations better. You are fine-tuning your awareness. Imagine you are a compassionate and caring doctor, and the woman in the mirror is your patient. What do you see?

- **ENERGY.** Do you look energized, alive, bright, or do you look tired and dull? Energy is perhaps the most obvious and most powerful indicator of vibrancy.

- **SKIN.** Skin is an obvious indicator of health. Does it glow? Does it have tone? What is the texture?

- **NAILS.** Are they thin, splitting, curving up; are there dents, pitting, ridges, lines; or are they thick and strong? If you can't tell due to a manicure, consider taking a break and letting your nails heal so you can fully assess them.

- **EYES.** When I look into someone's eyes, I'm looking for animation, light, excitement, and joy as well as clear irises and white whites that are not bloodshot or yellowing. What do you see in your eyes? They reveal much about physical as well as mental health.

- **GUMS.** Are they pink and full or pale and receding?

- **TONGUE.** Is it pink and textured or swollen and coated?

- **POSTURE.** Note how you are standing—or how you were standing before you read this line! Are you upright, with your ears, shoulders, hips, and knees in line with the arches of your feet? Or are you slumped with a bowed back, your head jutting forward, or throwing all your weight over to one hip?

- **MOVEMENT.** Walk back and forth in front of the mirror. Do you move freely, easily, with supple joints and supportive muscles, or can you tell you are stiff, in pain, or that your body is hindering your movements? Does your movement look strong and energetic or weak and frail?

- **VOICE.** Say hello to yourself. Is your voice lively, animated, and expressive, or does it sound sluggish, distracted, hoarse, or congested?

- **SILHOUETTE.** Can you see the natural shape of your muscles and bones, or is your silhouette expanded beyond its natural boundaries due to excess fat?

- **TAKE A PHOTO.** Your very first mirror assessment is a great opportunity to take a photo of yourself. This is your "before" shot. (You probably don't want to do this naked—you might want to show your "before and afters" one day.) We'll be doing some other initial assessments in this chapter, but this is your visual record. Keep this for inspiration, and as you work through this book, you will begin to see changes. A month or two from now, you might not recognize how far you've come until you compare your mirror image with this Vibrant Day One photo.

Make a note of which aspects of you looked (and felt) strong and vibrant, and where the weaker spots are today. Most people find that when they do this exercise, there is room for improvement. Nobody's perfect, and how boring if they were!

When I do a mirror assessment, I always recognize fluctuations because I do it regularly. People often ask me what my secret is to looking young and having so much energy, but I have plenty of mornings where I recognize, in my self-assessment, that I'm puffy, or that I look tired, or move without as much energy as I would like, or that a few extra pounds are creeping up on me. When I get dressed, sometimes I notice that my shoes feel tighter than usual, or my clothes don't fit quite the same way as they did the day before—or the year before. I always take those cues as messages from my body to get back to basics and take better care of myself.

YOUR BODY'S BUILT-IN FEEDBACK MECHANISMS

Your body is wise, and it's also communicative. You may not be accustomed to noticing, but your body is giving you constant feedback about what you are doing and how it is affecting your ability to function, not to mention build health. Some of the primary feedback mechanisms you already have "onboard" include:

Your five senses: You have vision, hearing, smelling, tasting, and touch to inform you. Use them purposefully to experience and understand your external and internal environments. Notice when any of your senses seem to be perceiving things differently than usual. This is your primary feedback system. It allows you to pay attention to the signs your body is sending you about the internal effects of how you are interacting with your environment.

Your "sixth sense": You also have a sixth sense, which is your intuition. You may not always be able to pin down exactly why you feel like something isn't right, either in the world around you or inside of you, but trust that feeling because it is another way your body tells you that you need to be doing something different, or that you need to intervene when something is going wrong.

Your digestive system: Stomach pain, bloating, gas, constipation, and diarrhea are all signs that you aren't giving your digestive system something it needs. Smooth, easy digestion without pain (and with a daily bowel movement) is a sign that you are eating and moving in a way that is allowing your body to eliminate waste effectively.

Your nervous system: Signs that your nervous system isn't working well include brain fog, inability to concentrate, forgetfulness, anxiety, depression, panic attacks, mood swings, and irritability. These can also indicate gut microbiome imbalance since your gut microbiome and your nervous system constantly communicate with each other through biochemical signaling along the vagus nerve, aka the gut-brain axis (I'll talk more about that in chapter four).

Your endocrine system: Your endocrine system is composed of all the glands that produce hormones, so every hormonal symptom you get, from irregular periods to depressed thyroid hormone production to exhausted adrenal glands, is a sign that your endocrine system isn't getting what it needs. This can be due to a poor diet, high stress, or often both.

Your lymphatic system: This network of lymph nodes and vessels just under the skin is an important immune system component and waste removal system. Your muscles function like a "pump" that pushes lymph through the vessels and nodes. If you are retaining water, feel swollen, or have an uncomfortable, vague feeling of being "toxic," your lymphatic system is probably slow or stagnating. This is often a sign that you are not getting enough exercise and not drinking enough water. Practicing even, deep breathing helps to activate your lymphatic system.

Your connective tissue: Tendons, ligaments, and other connective tissue hold you together and facilitate smooth, easy, graceful movement, but if you have constant injuries, joint pain, or all-over soreness, your connective tissue is likely letting you know that you have a higher-than-normal level of inflammation. Connective tissue pain can also be a sign of an autoimmune disease such as rheumatoid arthritis.

Every single one of us changes in subtle and not-so-subtle ways from year to year, as well as from day to day, morning to morning—even minute to minute. We are complex and intricate biochemistry experiments and engineering marvels, and our bodies are always giving us feedback about what we've been doing. In turn, what we do will change how our bodies react, feel, and look. It's a conversation. When you eat wholesome, clean, organic, nutritionally dense whole food, the way nature intended, or when you eat processed, salty, or sugary junk food, that will show in the mirror. When you get eight hours of high-quality sleep, or when you are awake all night with some physical or mental discomfort, that will show in the mirror. When you exercise your heart, lungs, and muscles with cardiovascular exercise, resistance training, and flexibility training, or when you spend twelve hours a day sitting at a desk, that will show in the mirror, too.

When you have a really tough, stressful day full of anxiety and worry, you will not look the same the next morning as you will after a relaxing, fun day full of positive human connection. You can even learn to notice, in your own reflection, the effects of different kinds of supplements, different kinds of stress, and different moods. The changes may be subtle, but you're going to learn to see them. Remember, the mirror is your first tool for assessing and making positive changes in your health. It is your feedback mechanism for assessing your level of vibrancy. With a little practice, you won't need a doctor to tell you how you feel, and, in fact, no doctor could ever know as much about your body's feedback as you do. A doctor can help you interpret negative feedback, especially if you have already progressed to the stage of a diagnosable condition or disease. But let's not get ahead of ourselves. Let's get you moving away from that avoidable event, rather than thoughtlessly allowing yourself to become a little less healthy every day.

To begin moving in the right direction—toward vibrant, and away from disease—let's get granular about where you are right now.

IT'S NEVER ALL OR NOTHING

You may not want to do all the things I recommend in this book, but I'll give you lots of ideas so you can choose the ones that feel right to you. Not every change is for every person. There is no need to put pressure on yourself to do everything perfectly. Health is never an all-or-nothing proposition. I'm going to give you ample opportunity to experiment, and I will always encourage you to listen to your body's feedback. Keep up that daily mirror self-assessment, and tune in to the changes, because they are coming! Most importantly, never, ever give up on yourself, your health, your wellness, and your potential to be vibrant. There is always more you can do to bring vibrancy into your body and energy into your life if you so choose.

YOUR HABIT PROFILE

We all have some good habits and some not-so-good habits. Even the healthiest of health gurus slip up sometimes, and probably have some things they could be doing better, so remember—no judgment. Let's assess your lifestyle with curiosity, not criticism. To help get you in the right frame of mind, let's start with the positive. What are you doing right that we can build on? Of these 30 good health habits, check all the things that apply to you right now:

○ I eat at least three to four servings of non-starchy vegetables every day.

○ I eat at least one serving of berries or citrus.

○ I eat fish or seafood at least a few times a week.

○ I eat more real, whole food than processed or junk food.

○ When I use oil for cooking or for salads, it's usually olive oil or avocado oil.

○ When I need a sweetener, I usually choose something natural like real maple syrup, raw honey, agave, or coconut sugar. Or I don't usually use sweeteners.

○ I don't eat gluten.

○ I avoid dairy products.

○ I buy fresh organic food whenever I can.

○ I have some nuts and/or seeds on most days.

○ I have one or fewer alcoholic beverages each day (or I don't drink alcohol at all).

○ I take vitamins and minerals and/or other supplements (such as probiotics or herbs) to be sure I get everything I need.

○ I exercise for at least a total of 150 minutes a week (that's about 30 minutes, five times per week).

○ I go on walks at least a few times a week.

○ I lift weights or do bodyweight exercises once or twice a week.

○ I do some kind of stretching or yoga at least once or twice a week.

○ I consciously work on improving my relationships with my partner, family, and/or friends.

○ I am happily married or otherwise partnered with someone who is loving and supportive, and/or I have a close friend or small group of friends I can always confide in and rely on.

○ I do something social at least once a week—even if it's a "virtual" social gathering.

○ I take at least 20 minutes for myself on most days to meditate, pray, breathe, or just relax.

○ I sleep seven to nine hours every night.

○ I can tell when I get stressed, and I try to do something about it.

○ When I'm stressed out, worried, anxious, or sad, I talk to somebody about it, formally or informally.

○ I only take medications when it's absolutely necessary.

○ I use mostly natural cleaning and personal care products.

○ I don't catch colds or get the flu very often.

○ I don't have any serious allergies.

○ I often think about what my purpose in life might be, and I try to fulfill it.

○ I believe in something greater than myself.

○ I have my faults, sure, but I have compassion for myself.

Every check mark on the above list is a piece of good news! Take a moment to celebrate everything you are already doing to become vibrant.

Now let's take a look at those habits you probably already know are not so great for you. Out of these 30 bad health habits, which ones do you have that you would like to do something about? Check all that apply right now:

○ I eat fast food or take-out food and/or eat in restaurants more than once a week.

○ I don't cook.

○ I eat or drink something containing sugar or artificial sweetener on most days (soda, diet soda, loaded coffee, sweet tea, fruity drinks like lemonade or fruit punch including the "zero calorie" kinds, cocktails with sweet mixers).

○ I have a serious caffeine habit! I have more than two caffeinated beverages on most days (like coffee, black tea, or cola).

○ I love fried food! Mmmm, French fries!

○ I'm addicted to cheese (and/or ice cream).

○ I eat a lot of saturated fat, like steak, pork chops, burgers, bacon, eggs, ham, and deli meats.

○ I eat a lot of refined grain products on most days, like bread, pasta, pizza crust, tortillas, crackers, bagels, white rice, and baked goods.

○ I have red meat or processed meat (like bacon, sausage, or deli meats) on most days.

○ I don't eat vegetables very often.

○ I don't eat fruit.

○ I'm a chocoholic. I can't control myself!

○ Sure, I eat gluten. Gluten-free is just hype.

○ I rarely drink water.

○ I don't exercise on most days.

○ I never lift weights.

○ I'm very inflexible and don't stretch.

○ I sit for eight or more hours per day.

○ I don't sleep very well, waking a lot during the night.

○ I get less than seven hours of sleep on most nights.

○ I don't feel supported by the people in my life.

○ I don't have anyone I can easily confide in.

○ I don't have a life partner or truly close and supportive friends, and I feel incomplete because of it.

○ I drink more than one alcoholic drink on most days.

○ I take over-the-counter medications, like ibuprofen, antacids, or allergy medications, more than twice a month.

○ I am more than a little overweight.

○ I admit that I complain a lot.

○ I know I spend too much time on my phone.

○ I have a stressful job.

○ I let stress, anger, or other unresolved negative feelings build up because I don't want to deal with them.

Visit vibrantdoc.com for a printable checklist to keep with you.

After going through these lists, you might already be feeling inspired and thinking about what you can change, but let's narrow it down. Just for now, pick three things on the first list that you are not doing, but that you think you can start doing. Then, pick three things on the second list that you are doing that you think you can stop doing. Write them down here. Later, you can look back and see how much progress you've made. (Of course, you are not limited to these six items, but it's usually a good idea not to take on too much at once. Slow and steady wins the race!)

I'm going to start doing these three things, so I can be more vibrant:

1. _____

_____

2. _____

_____

3. _____

_____

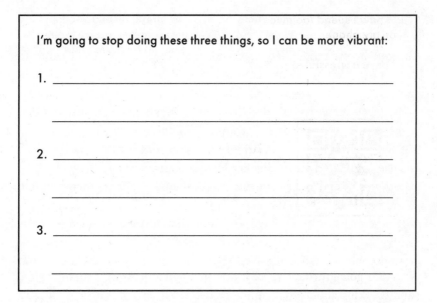

I'm going to stop doing these three things, so I can be more vibrant:

1. _____

_____

2. _____

_____

3. _____

_____

Next, let's rate your energy, based on how you feel at this moment. I'll ask you to do this again throughout the 14-day plan in chapter four, and again at the end of the book, and so this is your baseline. Sit still for a moment. Take a few deep breaths. Close your eyes. Focus on how you feel. Notice your level of fatigue. Are you tired? Could you go for a brisk walk right now? How is your mental clarity? Does your brain feel sharp, or a little foggy? Take all these things into consideration and then score your overall energy. It doesn't have to be precise. This is just your subjective feeling in this moment, but on a scale of 1 to 10, with 1 being "exhausted" and 10 being "I feel like I could do anything right now!" circle the number that best describes your energy level:

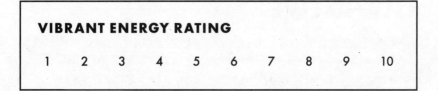

VIBRANT ENERGY RATING

1   2   3   4   5   6   7   8   9   10

Wonderful. Now that you've got a picture of where you are now, and some initial goals for yourself, let's see if, step by step, we can shift that balance, increasing your energy, your glow, your habits, and your health. Ideally, by the time you finish this book, you will be able to check many more items on the first list, many fewer items on the second list, and have a higher energy score. If you're really ambitious, maybe you can shoot for 30 good habits and no bad ones, and an energy score of 10—it's great to have lofty goals! Just remember that you have to start where you are right now, and you can only do what you can do in a way that is sustainable for you and works with your lifestyle. It's more important to do three things consistently over time than 30 things every once in a while.

But don't short yourself, either. You are capable of more than you may realize. You can do this! Chapter by chapter, we're going to tackle those habits (and some other ones) just a few at a time, and let them settle in to become part of who you are. If you try to do too much, you could get overwhelmed and give up. We don't want that! Just stay with me, progress with a steady consistency, and you will see results. They might not be the results you expect. The number on your scale may not change, but your body composition and shape may shift. Maybe the number on the scale will change, even dramatically, but you'll realize you're even more excited about the changes in your skin or endurance or strength or how happy and confident you feel.

In the rest of these chapters, I'm going to walk you through a lot of different aspects of health, and give you action steps all along the way to help create a transformed lifestyle that you can maintain for life. Even with incremental changes, it won't take long at all to start feeling better, and those changes will create a ripple effect of vibrant health as you build on your successes, step by step. Just imagine where you could be and how you could feel by next week, next month, or this time next year!

SUPPLEMENTS 101: MY DESERT ISLAND FIVE

Like most integrative doctors, I am a firm believer that most of your nutrients should come from your food, which is the most bioavailable form of nutrition. I am also fully aware that our industrial food system, food processing, practice of shipping food to every corner of the globe, and depleted, chemically laced soil have all impacted the nutritional quality of what we eat. Neither animals nor plants are quite as nutritious as they once were. This alone justifies the insurance policy of a few high-quality, pure dietary supplements.

I have also studied and worked with practitioners in functional medicine, holistic nutrition, Chinese medicine, anti-aging medicine, and other fields, and I can assure you that we know more now about optimizing human health than we ever have. You can give your health a boost by targeting certain areas and issues with many different kinds of supplements, from herbs to probiotics. While study results are mixed, many have shown that supplements really can reduce the risk of chronic health issues like heart disease and many kinds of cancer.[1]

In each chapter, you will find supplement recommendations relevant to the subject at hand. Not all supplements are right for all people. It depends on what your health issues are. However, right now, I want to get you started feeling better ASAP with five basic supplements I recommend for everyone. I call these my "desert island" supplements because if I could bring just five supplements with me to a remote location, these would be the ones:

- **VITAMIN C.** This is far and away my favorite vitamin. It will do you many favors, from stronger immunity to better skin. Start by taking 1,000 milligrams (mg) per day, preferably divided between two or three doses, since your body processes and eliminates vitamin C quickly. You can work up gradually to 3,000 to 5,000 mg per day, for maximum support, but even 1,000 mg per day will support your immune system and help to reduce inflammation. Don't go up too quickly or you could experience some gastrointestinal issues. Let your body adjust.

- **VITAMIN D3.** After vitamin C, I would say that vitamin D is the most critical supplement. Your nervous system function depends on it. Vitamin D may be one of our most pervasive deficiencies.[2] According to the former director of the Centers for Disease Control, approximately 40 percent of Americans don't get enough, but I believe this number is actually quite a bit higher. Conventional medicine doesn't consider someone to be vitamin D deficient unless they have less than 20 ng/mL (nanograms per milliliter) of vitamin D in their blood. Some even say you are not deficient unless you have less than 12 ng/mL. Those of us trained in functional medicine, however, believe that everyone should have a vitamin D level of at least 50 ng/mL, and optimally as high as 80 ng/mL. I can assure you that most people in the United

States, with our indoor lives and seasonal climates and sunscreen use (the body manufactures vitamin D in response to sunlight on the skin), are well below that number. Vitamin D and other fat-soluble vitamins are measured in IUs, or International Units. Calculate 1,000 IUs (25 mcg) per 50 pounds of body weight. (I recommend taking at least 1,000 IUs for anyone, as a minimum dose.) Although people often recommend more sun exposure to get enough vitamin D, most people simply can't get enough that way, and the cancer risks outweigh the benefit. If you want to build immunity right now as well as far into your future, take a D3 supplement daily all year round.

- **VITAMIN B COMPLEX.** This is one of the few instances where it's okay to take several vitamins in one supplement, because the B vitamins work together. Choose methylated B vitamins if you can; these are more bioactive and don't require your body to convert them into usable forms. Look for a formula that includes all eight essential B vitamins: thiamine (B1), riboflavin (B2), niacin (B3), pantothenic acid (B5), pyridoxine (B6), biotin (B7), folate (B9), and cobalamin (B12). The B vitamins have many important functions, including energy, growth, digestion, organ function, and hormone production. Vitamin B12 in particular will give you a boost of morning energy. Most B-complex formulas contain appropriate dosages, which are normally formulated for a 150-pound person. (Note that B vitamin formulas can turn your urine a brighter yellow and add a particular odor—this is nothing to be concerned about.)

- **MAGNESIUM WITH OR WITHOUT CALCIUM.** These are minerals with many important functions. Magnesium is important for nervous system regulation, and blood sugar and blood pressure regulation, just to name a few of its many functions in the human body. It also helps with constipation, keeping you regular (especially magnesium citrate), and eases anxiety, helping you to relax and sleep (especially magnesium glycinate). Magnesium oxide is the least expensive and most elemental form of magnesium salt and is absorbed more slowly, which may mean you will utilize more of it. Calcium is also important, especially for building strong bones and teeth. The ratio of magnesium and calcium should be about 1:2. Women who take approximately 1200 to 1500 mg of calcium daily should pair that with with 600 to 750 mg of magnesium. Calcium citrate and calcium carbonate are both acceptable forms of calcium. (I also recommend calcium for men, to prevent osteopenia.)

- **EPA AND DHA** (eicosapentaenoic acid and docosahexaenoic acid) are omega-3 fatty acids from supplements made from fish oil or krill oil. Look for supplements that give you EPA and DHA amounts, not just fish oil amount. I recommend getting up to 4,000 mg of combined EPA and DHA per day for maximum benefit. EPA protects your heart and is anti-inflammatory, while DHA protects your brain and can help to fight off depression and reduce your risk of dementia. Both EPA and DHA also help maintain the health of the cell membrane. Be sure to get a purified, mercury-free version, so you can get your omega-3s without toxic exposure. Even if you are taking these supplements, I still recommend eating cold-water fatty fish at least a few times a week. Note that the plant version of omega-3 fatty acids from foods like flaxseeds and walnuts is called ALA (alpha-linolenic acid) and it must be converted into EPA and DHA, so it is a much less efficient form of these essential oils than fish oil. Really, it's like not getting your omega-3s at all. If you are a vegetarian, look for EPA/DHA supplements from algae.

  Vibrant Pro Tip: Some people worry about the fishy aftertaste, or burping fish oil all day. There is a simple way to prevent this—keep your fish oil in the freezer! When you take the pills frozen, you get all the benefits and none of the burps.

Before you run out and buy a supply of supplements, though, a note about quality. Many cheap supplements available in the grocery store are, unfortunately, unreliable because the supplement industry is not well regulated.[3] Many do not contain much or, in some cases, any of the ingredients they say they contain. That's not even considering the common problem of adulteration with substances like lead, highly toxic PCBs, and even prescription drugs—a few years ago, a study scanned the FDA database for reports of supplements that claimed to be natural botanicals, and when testing them, the researchers found that many of them contained pharmaceutical drugs! They found 746 different brands adulterated with prescription medications including things like antidepressants, erectile dysfunction drugs, banned appetite suppressants, and steroids (many of these were herbal formulas, not multivitamins).

Unfortunately, cheaper formulas tend to have the most problems, but any widely available store shelf vitamin may have quality control issues because the FDA can only police supplements after a complaint, not before they are put on the shelves. Others simply contain poor, low-quality ingredients that aren't going to help you.[4] Before you buy supplements from any company, I recommend checking out the company to try to determine what level of quality control they have, and where they source their ingredients. You can call them and get a good idea of how reputable they are (and how much they care about their customers) just by how much information you are, or are not, able to get over the phone.

Although they are expensive, your best bet is medical-grade supplements available through integrative practitioners, because these supplements have more internal oversight. You can't get them at the grocery store, but you can order some of them online. I recommend doing some research into whatever company you are considering. (I found this frustrating personally, so I am in the process of creating my own line of clean supplements that are at the level I would choose for myself. They are not the only good option, but they will be a good option for those who want to take what I would recommend. As soon as these are available, I'll make an announcement on vibrantdoc.com.)

WHAT ABOUT MULTIVITAMINS?

Should you take a multivitamin as an insurance policy? Actually, I don't recommend multivitamins. They may seem like a better bargain, but many if not most of the multivitamins you see on the shelves don't contain an impactful dosage of everything in there, and they may contain excessive amounts of some things and deficient amounts of others.[5] Many also contain versions of vitamins or minerals that you can't absorb. For instance, many cheap vitamins contain vitamin D2, but you want the more biologically active vitamin D3. Most contain the inactive form of vitamin B12 called cyanocobalamin, but you want the superior active form, methylcobalamin. Some multivitamin pills don't break down in the body, so you never absorb any of the vitamins they contain. Many also contain cheap fillers and binders as well as artificial colors and preservatives, some of which could be allergenic or toxic.

Instead, take individual vitamins and other supplements according to your needs, and take them consistently. Taking them randomly when you remember won't have the same benefit. A daily morning and evening supplement routine that becomes a habit is the key to building a foundation of health support. I also recommend starting small and gradually building more supplements into your routine, as needed. As your system gradually adjusts to regular supplement intake, you'll avoid any stomach discomfort and that gag reflex some people say they get if they take too many supplements.

YOU HAVE THE POWER

What I would like you to do next is to begin visualizing yourself from the inside. Have you ever thought about all that's inside of you? An amazing brain. A beating heart. A liver that keeps you from poisoning yourself. A thyroid that influences just about every biochemical process in your body. Adrenals and a pituitary gland and a pineal gland and a hypothalamus and ovaries or testes, all pumping out hormones to keep you functioning in a complex delicate ripple effect of chemistry. Bones that hold you up and muscles and joints that move you. Eyes that see the world. Ears that hear the world. The ability to smell and taste and appreciate the food that sustains you. A highly evolved sense of touch. It's all a miracle, if you ask me, and it's all going on inside of you, every second of your life on earth. What you see in the mirror is just the tip of the iceberg.

So, let me ask you this: How will you choose to take care of your astonishing internal machinery? Are you caring for your brain? Are you nurturing your heart? Are you giving your hormonal system the nutrients it needs to work for you? Are you supporting your liver as it supports you? Are you appreciating your five senses and the way they are so perfectly integrated into your perceptions of your very existence, inside and out? Life is a great gift and you have the ability to direct it. Why be a passenger on the ride of your life when you can drive?

When you ask your doctor about wellness, it's like asking someone for a screwdriver when all they have is a hammer. It's like bringing your horse to an auto mechanic. Sometimes, you need a hammer. Sometimes you need an auto mechanic. When it comes to your own health and wellness, all you need is an awareness of your own body and the ability to respond to its needs. Sure, doctors have a lot of information and they could probably delegate better. They could probably advocate better to get people to other professionals who can help them with what they need. Some of them have prejudices that preclude them from recommending holistic practitioners. Honestly, people end up wasting a lot of money that they could probably save if doctors were better at guiding them, and your insurance dollars could certainly be put to better use. But, at the end of the day, you are the one personally responsible for your lifestyle. To use yet another metaphor: You are the CEO of your own body. How are you going to run things?

The reality is that being healthy today means being healthy in an unhealthy world. It's easy to criticize doctors for not giving patients wellness tools or advising on lifestyle. I get that, and sometimes I even feel like not doing so borders on malpractice, since lifestyle is so obviously a major factor in health. It makes me angry sometimes that mainstream doctors don't seem to have the courage to work with people to change their lifestyles and hold them to their goals.

On the other hand, how do you do that? Your well-intentioned doctor can't follow you around and police you all day long, and like we all do, you are going to do what you are going to do. I have treated patients who think it's easier to take a pill than to eat a vegetable. How should a doctor change that mindset? The truth is that those of us interested in integrative medicine are fighting an uphill battle when we make lifestyle recommendations. Change can be hard and uncomfortable, and even when seeking health, people often don't want to do it—and won't do it until they're ready to do it. We all sometimes resent being told what to do, even if we're asking for advice, and we may have a hard time following instructions even when we know it's best for us. Habits are hard to break, and we all love what is familiar and common.

Conventional doctors are a bit stuck ethically as well. Their hands are tied by insurance companies and pharmaceutical special interests who dictate what they can and can't prescribe. But even a functional medicine doctor who doesn't take insurance and charges you full price doesn't have the magical ability to make you follow lifestyle advice. We can rail at doctors all we want for not knowing about nutrition or not supporting supplement use or not being open to alternative treatments, but the simple fact is just this: It's not their job. A conventional doctor, especially, has the job of helping people with injuries and illnesses. They are not in the business of wellness. Your wellness is not their priority. But you know whose priority it is, or should be?

Yours.

Only you can decide what you are going to do to feel good. Only you can decide what you put in your mouth, how much you are going to move your body, how well you are going to get along with others, and how well you are going to treat yourself and take care of yourself. To a larger extent than you might realize, you and only you have the power to choose to be healthy, or to choose to be at the mercy of the sick-care system when you get sick.

I suggest, with all due respect, that you stop looking outside for approval from your doctors, from your family, from your friends. The status quo isn't working, and it doesn't matter what anyone else is doing. The average person isn't doing very well, health-wise, so why be average? To be average in this world means to keep getting sicker. In this book, I'm offering you information. What you do with it is up to you. You can use it, or not. I can't force you to change your habits. I can't force you to adopt any particular lifestyle. But I can try to inspire you and guide you to take back the reins of your life.

If you decide to embrace wellness and a vibrant life, you're going to have to stand up for yourself and take care of yourself. Some people won't get it. Other people will try to steer you away from your goals. Be ready. Most of the world doesn't know how to advocate for their own wellness. They know how to be sick, and the culture responds. You broke your leg? You can have time off. You have a disease diagnosis? We're all so sorry. What can we do to help? But try taking a stand to be well. You don't want to eat that? Come on, just a little. You don't want to skip your workout? Just this once! Let's go get ice cream.

It's socially acceptable to stand for your sickness, to get your T-shirt and punch your ticket. You need to go home early today? Why, are you sick? If you're sick, go home. But if you need a mental health day, or a nap, or you just need to take some time for yourself, that's often too bad. You have work to do. It is our social convention to give sick-care excuses for not being able to perform because we have a sick-care culture. If you are going to break out of that mold, it's going to take some courage and confidence, but I say you can do it. What good is life if you don't feel good in your own skin? If you don't have energy and a clear mind and a purpose? Your health is worth it. Right at this moment, start thinking about what matters to you and what you want out of your life. Would you rather be a sick person who gets sympathy, or a strong, glowing, gorgeous, vibrant person who doesn't need it?

If you are reading this and starting to feel excited that you can make a change, then your healing has already begun. The physical tools are in this book and, candidly, they are also out there everywhere. Health information isn't new, and it's widely available. It's the psychological part you have to contend with. It's in you. It's your vision. You have agency. You can own your choices, and in doing so, make better ones.

You have the power.

. . .

VIBRANT BEGINNER WINS

Are you ready to start winning? At the end of each chapter, I have three small things you can do to leave bad health habits behind and establish a lifestyle that supports and optimizes your health and wellness. I call these your "wins." For this first set of wins, choose the one that sounds the most doable to you, or go for it and do them all. These habit nudges will shift you gradually and easily toward better health, greater vitality, and a more vibrant life. Make a note for each win that you try, so you can remember your first impressions.

LOOK IN THE MIRROR. Each morning, spend just five minutes in front of the mirror, assessing your vibrancy. Look for clues and feedback about your health. How are you standing? What is your expression like? How does your skin look? Do you look energetic or tired, strong or unsteady, happy or sad? If it helps, keep a record by writing down the date and your basic impressions in a journal.

○ *I tried it! Here's how it felt:* _____

_____

_____

AFFIRM. Hand in hand with your morning self-assessment, get in a mindset of self-love and compassion. Your body is doing the best it can for you. As you look for clues about your health, repeat this very important affirmation often: I am always curious, never critical.

○ *I tried it! Here's how it felt:* _____

_____

_____

LISTEN TO YOUR BODY. Throughout the day, practice tuning in to your body's signals. Notice when you feel tired or energetic, when something hurts or feels good, when you are in a good mood or get irritable, and see if there are any obvious links. Was it something you did or didn't eat, how much you were moving around, how stressful your workday was, where you are in your cycle if that's relevant, or anything else you notice? If you make brief notes about your observations, you'll likely begin to see patterns, such as feeling tired every time you eat something sweet for breakfast, or feeling more cheerful in the evening on the days you have a good workout, or that your skin looks better when you drink more water. The more you get in the habit of tuning in to your body's signals, the more you will know, without anyone else's guidance, what you need to feel, look, and perform better.

○ *I tried it! Here's how it felt:* _____

_____

_____

CHAPTER 2

The Fountain: How to Get More Energy

When you think about what it means to be vibrant, the first thing that might come to mind is energy. To be vibrant is to have energy that animates you and propels you through the day. But energy is more than just a perk of health. It is fundamental to life.

Energy is the subterranean river that underlies everything we do and everything we are, and it bubbles up into your daily life like a fountain. It is what distinguishes life from death. It influences motivation, drive, ambition, memory, competence, and the ability to get things done. It's also responsible for your beating heart, your breathing lungs, your hormone production, your digestion, and your detoxification. Everything that happens inside you runs on energy, and while it's always there, the degree to which your fountain is turned on varies according to how you live. Is your fountain stopped up, turned on low, turned off? Or is it wide open and spouting vitality?

To be vibrant is to have a well-maintained and free-flowing energy fountain that is accessible to you whenever you need it. In this chapter, we're going to continue the habit of assessing your energy level and give you some tools for clearing the debris from your energy fountain.

WHAT IS ENERGY?

Energy sounds like something definable, but it actually has many definitions. It's hard to pin it down. If you ask a Western-trained scientist or doctor what energy is, they might tell you that you get it from the food you eat, but to get even more granular about it, organelles inside your cells called mitochondria transform the components of the food you eat—primarily carbohydrates and fats—through a complex multi-step process that yields adenosine triphosphate (ATP), which is a kind of energy currency the body uses to fuel life.

ATP isn't the only way we get energy, but it is the main way we get energy within cells, which is then further processed and converted in ways that allow it to be taken up by your muscles and other systems all over your body, wherever it's needed. You will remember from the last chapter that one of the fundamental principles of functional medicine is to follow symptoms back to their root causes and treat the root causes, rather than attempting to merely patch up the symptoms. If we follow the fountain of energy upstream to its origins, we can trace it back to this cellular level. Since most of your cells contain mitochondria, most of your cells are capable of producing energy, so the mitochondria in muscle cells (for example) produce energy for your muscles to move your body, while the mitochondria in your adrenal or thyroid glands (for example) produce energy for those endocrine glands to manufacture hormones, which in turn put that energy to use to keep you healthy and functioning.

If you were a car, your mitochondria would be a bit like a gas tank (if gas tanks actually created the gas) and the ATP would be the fuel. Your endocrine system would be like the engine with its many parts, transforming the energy into movement, and the rest of you would be like the chassis and the wheels and the lights and the windshield wipers, using the energy for the functions that allow you to drive down the road of life, so to speak. You are far more complex than a car, but you get the idea.

Of course, a lot happens between putting gas in the tank and driving away. It may seem simple: Get in the car, turn the key, put it in gear, and drive. But just as there is a lot more going on under the hood than you experience directly when driving, there are a lot of steps between eating an apple and actually using the energy you get from it to go for a walk or do your work or even to think hard about something. Complex as it is,

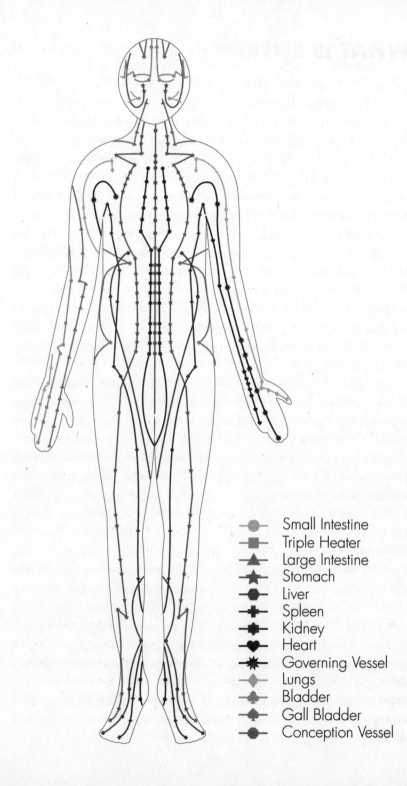

- ● Small Intestine
- ■ Triple Heater
- ▲ Large Intestine
- ★ Stomach
- ⬣ Liver
- ✚ Spleen
- ✦ Kidney
- ♥ Heart
- ✳ Governing Vessel
- ◆ Lungs
- ◆ Bladder
- ♠ Gall Bladder
- ⬢ Conception Vessel

from the Western medicine perspective, the process of energy production, assimilation, and usage is relatively linear. We have mostly figured out how it works and can explain it.

But that's not all there is to the energy picture. An integrative medicine perspective takes a more global view. In Eastern traditions, such as Chinese medicine and Ayurveda, energy is something different (although not all that different, in my opinion). In Traditional Chinese Medicine (often called TCM, or sometimes just Chinese medicine), qi or chi (ki in Japan) can be loosely translated as energy. To put it in very simple terms, this energy runs along meridians within the body (which you can see on any Chinese medicine or acupuncture chart) named for organs and structures, such as the stomach, liver, spleen, kidney, heart, and lung meridians, as well as some others such as "triple heater" and "governing vessel." Each of these organs also has its own unique energy or essence (for example, Kidney Essence is considered a specific kind of energy). Along the meridians are points where an acupuncturist would insert needles to move stagnant energy and correct energy imbalances, blocks, and deficiencies.

In Ayurveda, an ancient Indian system of health, prana can be loosely translated as energy, and is essentially equivalent to chi. Prana runs through the body along channels called nadis. Again, to put it very simply, energy pools in points along the nadis, called chakras, and therapies such as yoga exercises and breathwork can help to release stuck energy, moving it through the nadis and balancing clogged or deficient chakras. A Reiki practitioner might use some of this terminology when doing energy work on someone, working to clear their chakras and move stuck energy.

This Eastern view of energy might seem quite different from the Western view, but if you study these various systems, you can see that the meridians and nadis loosely correspond with the network of nerves in the body, and the points or chakras loosely correspond with certain organs and glands. For example, in Chinese medicine, the kidneys are an important center of energy production, but guess what rests on top of the kidneys? The adrenal glands, which from a Western perspective play an integral role in energy management. In my view, the Western view of energy is a detailed, biophysiological, profound, and accurate explanation of energy, but the Eastern perspective on energy is deep, precise, and equally profound as well as equally accurate.

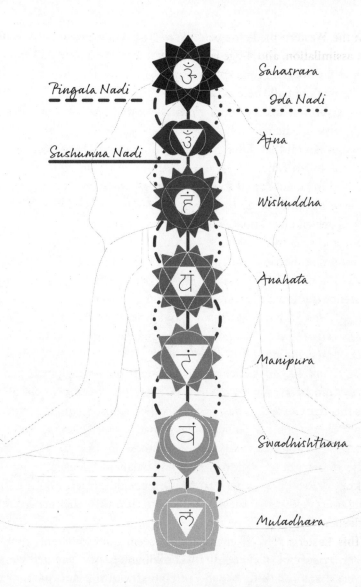

And finally, there is a third type of energy: a spiritual energy I sometimes call the netherspace energy. This is that ineffable energy that
connects us to something higher. You could call it God or spirit or the
universe or you may not know what it is, but it distinguishes something
that is alive from something that is dead, and it is the thing that weaves us
into the web of life. Neither the Western nor the Eastern interpretations
of energy quite encompass this spiritual aspect. It is not a part of any
culture or religion—it is the big picture of energy.

None of these energy viewpoints contradicts the other. I see them as a three-legged stool, or a triad, with you at the center. Here's a Venn diagram to illustrate:

When you look at energy in this broad, integrative perspective, you can see that it is a thing beyond you but within you. It is part of your individual imprint and your consciousness. It is bigger than any one person, but it is also a gift for each person. You cannot destroy universal energy, but you can choose to partake in it and engage with it, or to inhibit and block it. Your decisions throughout the day directly impact whether your body is making more energy or making less. So, let's explore how you can maximize your energy flow, because how you live determines how much energy you will have to do everything you want to do.

HOW TO TURN UP YOUR ENERGY FOUNTAIN

Now that you have a big-picture view of the complexities of energy, let's look at how you can begin to perceive it, direct it, and optimize it within you, so you can have all you need to live the life you want. First, let's look at the Western view.

Your cells (via the mitochondria) are always churning out energy, but how you live will directly impact how well they can do this job. Cells don't make energy in a vacuum. They need cofactors from the nutrients you eat in order to have the raw materials to make energy as well as to support the systems that make energy.

They also need input from you. When you don't use the energy they make, your cells respond by making less energy. When you use the energy they make, and demand more, the cells respond by producing more energy. This is all part of the conversation your body is always having, or trying to have, with you. It talks to you, and you also talk to it via your lifestyle. If you are low on energy, lying around on the couch will make it worse, both physically and psychologically, because you are telling your body, "Hey, it's okay, I don't need energy. I'm just lying here." But if you make yourself get up and do something, you are saying to your body, "Okay, let's get going here. I'm moving, see? I'm going for a walk, so you're going to have to generate some more energy in there." It might seem counterintuitive—to solve that feeling of not having enough energy to exercise by exercising—but that is how the body works. In other words:

> THE MOST IMPORTANT THING YOU CAN DO TO INCREASE YOUR ENERGY IS TO USE MORE ENERGY.

For most people, that is most easily accomplished by exercising more. We'll dive deeper into exercise in chapter five, but in terms of energy, many research studies have shown that exercise leads to increased feelings of energy,[1] and this process of your body listening to your lifestyle cues is the reason why. The energy you get in response to the energy you demand is also the way your body talks back to you. If you exercise and feel great afterwards, your body is saying: "I liked that! That is good for us! Let's do it again tomorrow!" If you spend the day lying on the couch eating junk food and you feel sluggish and guilty, your body is saying, "That did not make me feel any better."

Of course, you can take this too far. If you are highly active and you begin to feel overstressed, sometimes a day of relaxation can be a good idea. How will you know? Your body will tell you by making you feel calm, relaxed, and replenished. Using energy makes more energy, but you also need recovery time, so the body can translate that information into generating more mitochondria, to produce more ATP. You need rest days for this purpose. You can't go hard all the time. Remember, your body is always giving you feedback.

Now let's consider the Eastern perspective, which is similar but does not recognize structures like mitochondria or chemicals like ATP. Instead, it is more movement-based in its perspective. The energy flow through your body can, in many different ways and depending on which perspective you are looking at (such as Chinese medicine or Ayurveda), become stagnant or depleted. Movement is good and stasis is bad. The ideal is to have an even, free-flowing, balanced energy presence in all parts of your body as needed. You could compare this to a river that flows freely across a landscape without dams or blockages like fallen trees or rockslides, but that also stays within its banks, not flooding the landscape around it.

As with the Western point of view, the Eastern solutions for energy imbalances are lifestyle-related and involve certain kinds of remedies, often movement-based or herbal, depending on the source or area of the energy flow disruption. Herbal medicine is very important in Chinese medicine and also in Ayurvedic medicine. Other lifestyle remedies tend to focus more on stress relief than fitness, with more common emphasis on meditation, yoga, tai chi, massage, and other meditative and therapeutic practices. This is likely due in large part to cultural differences.

EXERCISE AND CULTURE: LET'S GET PERSONAL

Traditional life in both the East and the West involved a lot of walking and physical labor, but in this modern era of automation and digitization, life has become much more sedentary everywhere. Everyone knows exercise is good for you and likely necessary at least to some degree in a world where movement is less and less required. However, while Western cultures (especially in the United States) tend to have a "the more the better" idea about exercise (whether people actually do it or not), and we tend to glorify athletes and people who do things like run marathons or triathlons, or who spend a lot of time doing cardio or weightlifting at the gym, "exercise" per se in Eastern cultures tends to be more gentle and aimed at optimizing energy flow—think qi gong, tai chi, and yoga.

For example, in Chinese medicine, qi gong is considered therapeutic, but there is a concept that certain more intense exercises can cause stagnation of qi (aka chi): for instance, that weightlifting can cause qi stagnation in the lower back, jogging can cause stagnation in the knees, and tennis can cause stagnation in the elbows.[2] The idea behind this is that the overuse of a particular area can cause the energy to stall there. This may sound like a uniquely Eastern perspective—you could hardly call qi gong or tai chi "cardio," and only in the United States do we do things like "power yoga"—but we do know that excessive exercise can certainly be a stressor, even an addiction, that leads to energy depletion.[3] The stressful effects of over-exercising are in fact well documented.

It is my belief, and my experience, that the ideal view of exercise in terms of energy (and in fact the ideal view of all health practices) is that personalization is key. The level of exercise any one person needs to generate more energy rather than depleting energy is highly individual and depends on many factors, including the obvious, like age, condition, health, and fitness, but also the less obvious, like genetics, family history, psychological state, resilience to stress, and maybe even microbiome profile, or the specific makeup of the microbes in the digestive tract. One could argue that, in the West, we overdo it, and in the East, they underdo it, but as modern medicine moves ever closer to the realization that the treatments for illness as well as the strategies for wellness are not one-size-fits-all, I believe the answers to these questions will have to be personalized and the amount of exercise any one person needs will likely vary quite a bit, not based on culture but based on who that person is.

And what about that third type of energy, the netherspace energy? We can't measure it, but we can feel it. It offers a powerful way to turn up your energy fountain. This may not feel relevant to everyone reading this book, but I believe we all have a spirit that requires nurturing and that can connect to something bigger than ourselves. The best way to generate more netherspace energy is to nurture that spirit. How you do that depends on your beliefs, but prayer, meditation, study of spiritual texts, attending religious services, giving to others, looking at the stars at night and contemplating humbly how big the universe is, and spending quiet time each morning reflecting on the things that matter most to you really will fill you up with netherspace energy. Whether your focus is on God or nature or love or your own inner light or something else that feels spiritual to you, give it some of your energy and your energy will grow. When you feel connected to something larger than yourself, whatever you perceive that to be, you take energy from that source, and that energy is boundless and infinite. It will never run out and it is always available to you, if you open yourself up to it.

LESS STRESS = MORE ENERGY

To take the Traditional Chinese Medicine concept of overexertion back into the realm of Western medicine, energy certainly is directly tied to the stress response. A little stress can increase your energy, but too much stress can deplete it. Stress is a response to a perceived threat, and when someone is threatened, their survival could depend on having enough energy to fight or flee. This is why the release of stress hormones is often called the "fight or flight" response. Energy is great when you actually need to fight or flee, but if you are chronically stressed, over time this will drain your energy reserves and you can end up feeling chronically fatigued. You can't fight or flee all day every day.

Your nervous system has two modes. When you are calm and relaxed, your parasympathetic nervous system is in charge, and your body uses your energy stores for growth, repair, digestion, reproduction, and all the other things bodies do to maintain themselves. It also stores energy for emergencies. When your brain perceives a threat, the sympathetic nervous system takes over. This triggers the coordinated efforts of the endocrine glands to release stress hormones (such as cortisol and adrenaline/

epinephrine) that divert energy away from those "peacetime" functions. In other words, you can ovulate later.

You'll have more energy activation in the muscles of your extremities (so you can run faster and lift heavier things) and an increase in blood sugar to your brain so you can think more quickly. That's great in an emergency (or if you have to do something stressful, like give a speech or be charming on a first date), but you can't divert energy away from important functions like digestion, repair, and reproduction for very long. Your essential systems need most of your energy most of the time. If you deprive them of what they need to operate, you could eventually develop dysfunctions that begin to cause symptoms like high blood sugar, high blood pressure, high cholesterol, impaired digestive function, eventual muscle weakness, rapid weight gain, anxiety, or depression.

This is why stress management is so important. "Management" doesn't mean you never let yourself experience stress. Stress can be necessary and beneficial for building strength, endurance, knowledge, and making more energy. But for maximum health, you also need enough time with the parasympathetic nervous system in charge, so you can recover from the stress and give your body a chance to respond and get stronger.

Stress management is also important when you aren't overly stressed, to help you maintain your baseline. Sending your body "calm down" signals can help to build up your energy reserves so that when the stress comes, you have the energy to get through it without breaking down your health. Later in this book, we'll dive into some targeted stress management exercises and strategies, but for now, just know that every poor health habit, from junk food to sedentary life to unhealthy relationships to isolation to poor sleep to over-exercising, can cause stress, and nothing will work as well in your life if stress becomes chronic. Practicing stress-reducing techniques like deep breathing (see page 79), yoga (see pages 182 and 205), meditation (see pages 183–186), or gentle exercise (see chapter four) helps your body to more accurately perceive when you are actually in an emergency situation and when it's okay to relax and redirect energy back to where you really need it most of the time. Stress management makes your body smarter at energy management.

The truth is, my life is consistently stressful and overscheduled, and I have to mindfully practice a lot of stress management. During times of high stress, exercise is huge for me, and I do more yoga when I'm feeling overextended. Meditation is another important remedy for me, and, being an introvert, sometimes all I need is some alone time to recharge. I get regular massages (especially lymphatic massage, which is very effective for detoxification and moving excess fluid out of the body) and regular acupuncture even when I'm not stressed. I consider it an insurance policy for my adrenals, which is where I always feel my stress first.

When I need a stronger intervention, I will get IV vitamin infusions, and sometimes I do ozone therapy and use the hyperbaric chamber in the clinic where I get my vitamin infusions. I'm always looking for new, interesting ways to deal with stress and improve my health, and if it's new and sounds promising, I'll try it. I also like guidance. I know how to exercise, but a trainer helps me make it happen, and my life coach helps me figure things out when stress threatens to overwhelm me. I freely admit one of the things I'm not very good at is enforcing downtime for myself. I'll get the apps, I'll get the devices, I'll get the fitness trinkets, and then I don't use them. But I always check in with myself when I don't feel right, to try to figure out what I need to do. I'm not too hard on myself when I don't do everything I wanted to do every single day. And I rely on the Vibrant Triad, a powerful tool I'm excited to share with you in the coming pages.

CAN YOU BANK ON YOUR ORGAN RESERVES?

Think of your organs like bank accounts. If you make too many withdrawals (stress) and not enough deposits (nutritional support and rest), eventually you can deplete your reserves and exhaust your organs. I think it's human nature to use up energy as soon as you feel it, but it's better not to use it all up every time. Build your reserves. If the depletion becomes severe enough, it can be quite difficult to repair, so start investing now! The two best ways to invest in your organ reserve, which can extend your life span as well as your health span, are nutritional support, so organs can stay both nourished and detoxified, and rest, so organs aren't working overtime.

Nutritional support for your organs doesn't have to be organ-specific. The supplements mentioned later in this chapter and the Desert Island Five covered in chapter one will go a long way toward giving your organs the support they need, but I am personally an enthusiastic supplement user because I don't believe we can get optimal amounts of nutrients from food alone. I recommend many other supplements throughout this book, and I take them all. They each contribute to organ reserve in their own way, especially those in chapter eight, which covers detoxification. Herbs that naturally detoxify your organs, like milk thistle and dandelion root, help lighten the load of the organs that are mainly responsible for detoxification—i.e., your liver and your kidneys.

Rest is about stress management to some extent, and sleep to a larger extent, when the body repairs and the brain consolidates memories and purges toxins. Rest is also about giving your body a break from digestion. When you eat every two to three hours (as some suggest you should), you are always in digesting mode, so your organs never get to relax and focus on repair and restoration. In anti-aging circles and in some Eastern traditions, there is a belief that we only have so much capacity in our organs, so resting them contributes to longevity.

There is a reason breakfast is called breakfast—it is meant to break the fast you were on all night while sleeping. The body expects and needs that time, and if you extend it a bit, you give it even more time off. Wait at least twelve hours between the end of dinner and the beginning of breakfast the next morning, so your body has ample time to clean house, make repairs, and fill up with energy again. Today we call this "intermittent fasting," but really, it's not a trick. It's what we've always been meant to do. We aren't supposed to be sitting up until past midnight eating potato chips and drinking wine. Your organs can't rest if you never stop the constant influx of calories. It's like never turning off your car or never turning off your computer. You will reduce their life spans. (Some people take this too far. Longer fasts release cortisol and cause more organ stress. I'll talk more about fasting on page 208.)

LOW ENERGY AS CAUSE OR SYMPTOM?

Conventional medicine is not oriented around energy the way other alternative medicine methods are, and it doesn't consider lack of energy as a root-cause problem. Instead, it views lack of energy as a symptom, downstream from some other problem. Medical doctors are trained to diagnose problems in a specific way. They look for symptoms that bother the patient or impede quality of life, and then they do tests to see what things in the body aren't working. If you complain to your doctor about low energy, they will use that as part of their symptom list, or what conventional doctors term your "complaint."

Take thyroid dysfunction, for example. The conventional medicine view is that if your thyroid isn't producing enough thyroid hormone, one of the symptoms of this problem is fatigue. Low energy is a symptom of hypothyroidism. But from an integrative medicine perspective, if you don't have enough energy production in your thyroid gland, the output of thyroid hormones will be compromised, leading to thyroid destruction and, eventually, hypothyroidism. Do you see the difference? Conventional: Organ destruction leads to fatigue. Alternative: Insufficient energy leads to organ destruction.

The problem with the conventional view is that it doesn't intervene soon enough. Until the thyroid gland is significantly destroyed to the point that it shows up on a test and warrants a diagnosis of hypothyroidism, to a conventional medicine doctor, everything is "normal." Yet long before your thyroid gland is destroyed, you will feel a lack of energy. It's a sign from your body that something is wrong. If you feel it, your thyroid is probably feeling it, too. If you intervene into the energy problem before you experience organ destruction, you could prevent the problem from ever advancing to that point.

In integrative (and Eastern) traditions, you can detect subclinical dysfunction (i.e., low energy) in areas of the body prior to the disease state. Doctors don't like to recognize subclinical conditions because they don't have solutions or remedies for these undiagnosable issues, but since normal-but-decreasing thyroid hormone production is a warning that something is going wrong in the thyroid, and normal-but-increasing cortisol production is a sign that something is wrong in the adrenals (these are just two examples), why wouldn't you want to intervene before you have a serious problem that requires medication?

You can. Your doctor might tell you that your lifestyle won't affect whether you get a chronic disease, but it is becoming more and more obvious to everyone (conventional doctors included) that this simply isn't true. Of course lifestyle influences health. What you eat and how you move and how happy and fulfilled you are determine how well your body is able to produce energy to respond to your body's needs. Even if you have a genetic propensity for a disease, something has to turn those genes on. And what turns genes on or off? Mostly lifestyle: food, movement, connection, sleep, toxic exposure, mood, and stress.

THE BIG SIX

A century ago, you were much more likely to die from an infectious disease than a chronic disease, but today, chronic diseases have surpassed infectious diseases as the leading cause of death. Even if they don't kill you, chronic diseases can severely compromise your quality of life, and the dysfunction almost always begins with energy depletion. Some are so common that most people have a pretty good chance of developing one or more of them eventually. I call them the Big Six:

1. Heart disease
2. Cancer
3. Type 2 diabetes (including pre-diabetes and metabolic syndrome)
4. Obesity
5. Autoimmune diseases (there are hundreds, but these include such things as rheumatoid arthritis, lupus, multiple sclerosis, celiac disease, Crohn's disease, and Hashimoto's thyroiditis)
6. Dementia and other neurodegenerative diseases, including Alzheimer's and Parkinson's

If I had to round out the list to ten, I would probably add severe depression, liver disease such as nonalcoholic fatty liver disease, lung disease such as COPD, and kidney disease, all of which are on the rise. The program in this book can drastically reduce your risk of developing any of the Big Six, or any chronic disease at all, at least until very old age.

So, don't wait for a diagnosis. You can start filling your energy tank now, so you always have enough in your energy fountain for when you need it, no matter what life throws at you. Your doctor probably isn't going to tell you how to put energy deposits into your thyroid, adrenal, pituitary, hypothalamus, and other endocrine glands. Your doctor isn't going to tell you how to put energy deposits into your heart, your liver, your kidneys, or your lungs. Your doctor isn't going to warn you about caring for the lining in your gastrointestinal system or your veins and arteries, all in the name of protection against future health dysfunction. But I'm going to tell you, because having energy reserves is what makes you glow from the inside out. It's what building health is all about. It's what makes you vibrant.

KEY SIGNS AND SYMPTOMS OF ENERGY DEPLETION

A trendy word for energy depletion these days is "burnout," and it's an apt term. Are you burned out? Let's assess your current energy level in more detailed fashion. If you consider that energy depletion is at the root of most health dysfunction, this could be the focus for your wellness efforts. How many of these describe how you feel today, or how you have felt in the last month?

○ I have trouble waking up. I feel groggy and grumpy in the morning.

○ I dread getting out of bed. I feel stressed about the day ahead.

○ By midafternoon, I feel like I desperately need a nap.

○ By midafternoon, I crave sugar or refined carbs. I can't make it to dinner without eating junk.

○ I do pretty well at breakfast and lunch, but I can't help overeating at dinner or after dinner, despite my best intentions.

○ At night, I often doze off in front of the television.

○ Once I sit down in the evening, I find it very difficult to get up and do anything.

○ I want to get things done but I feel like there is just no way I can do it all. It's too much.

○ I have dark circles or puffiness under my eyes.

○ I have trouble falling asleep, or I wake up in the middle of the night and can't get back to sleep, even though I feel tired.

○ I have no libido, or less than I want. (Or less than my partner wants.) Intimacy seems like too much trouble.

○ I'm often irritable and annoyed, even at people who don't deserve it. I have a short fuse.

○ I can't seem to walk very quickly. I'm slow and shuffling. Moving takes effort.

○ I can't seem to make a decision to save my life.

○ Personal hygiene feels difficult. Sometimes I can't even get myself to wash my hair or brush my teeth.

○ I know I should exercise, but I dread it. Exercising sounds like the last thing I want to do. I often make excuses not to exercise.

○ Cleaning, ugh! I just can't. The kitchen is messy and I need to vacuum, but I don't have the will.

○ I always seem to catch every cold or virus that's going around.

○ I'm so unmotivated. I must be lazy. Everything feels hard and takes too long.

○ I have joint pain or muscle aches all over, even though I haven't been exercising and I don't have an injury.

○ I'm always cold, or I get hot flashes (or both).

○ Nothing is fun anymore.

○ I'm often nervous, anxious, fearful, or panicky, for no obvious reason.

○ Bottom line: I just know I don't have as much energy as I could or should have.

Checking even one of these boxes means you could use more energy, but if you checked more than three boxes, you need an energy intervention as soon as possible. You are not prepared for a stressful event, and a stress trigger could put you at risk for developing a chronic disease. Your energy reserves are low, and the people with lower energy reserves are the ones most likely to succumb to both infectious diseases (such as viral illnesses) and chronic diseases.

If you are experiencing low energy, you are probably already trying to deal with it in some way. Every chapter throughout the rest of this book has the goal of restoring your energy, in many ways and from many directions, but first let's consider how you are trying to deal with your low energy right now. Are you using energy crutches?

ENERGY CRUTCHES

Energy crutches are things you do to give yourself more energy but that, ironically, cause energy depletion because they stress the body through overstimulation, releasing cortisol and depleting your organ reserve, especially in your adrenal glands. Your brain is not designed for the unnaturally high level of stimulation that these substances can cause, and after an initial "high," will generally respond with an equal "low." Over time, your pleasure centers can become dulled, worn out, and exhausted, so that you have an even more difficult time feeling pleasure and deriving energy from anything. Some of these things are okay (although not ideal) every so often. The question is, do you feel that you need them to function? It's okay to want the occasional cup of coffee, but not so great if you can't function without it. That is the sign that something has become a crutch. Here are the six most common energy crutches:

1. **CAFFEINE:** This is most often consumed in coffee, black tea, and caffeinated soda.

2. **SUGAR:** Sugar is everywhere, but is most obvious in sweet drinks, soda, candy, sweetened cereal, cookies, muffins, doughnuts, and pastries. It's also in many other foods, frvom ketchup to soup to bread.

3. **REFINED CARBS:** Anything made with white flour or other refined grains without the bran and germ. This includes most kinds of bread, pasta, white rice, potato chips, corn chips, French fries, bagels, and any of the items in the sugar category above that also contain white flour.

4. **NICOTINE:** Most people get this through smoking and vaping, but some also get it through patches, gum, or lozenges. If these are a method to quit, great! Otherwise, they are energy crutches.

5. **STIMULANTS:** Energy drinks (many also contain caffeine), prescribed (or not) ADHD medications, appetite suppressants, some antidepressants, decongestants, or any pharmaceutical with a stimulant effect are all common forms of stimulants. For some people, this includes marijuana, although it has a more sedating effect on others.

6. **ALCOHOL:** Although technically a depressant, alcohol can initially stimulate an energetic and positive mood in many people.

If you use any of these energy crutches, you are in the majority, but that doesn't mean you are doing what's best for you and your energy stores. Remember that the status quo is not usually acting in the best interest of health. But don't worry too much—I'm not going to tell you that you have to quit using your crutches right this minute. I don't want you to fall over! As you saw in chapter one, we are going to work on minimizing bad habits bit by bit, so you never have to feel like you're doing too much at once. You may not (yet) have the energy for that kind of major lifestyle overhaul. Just keep in mind that these crutches aren't really help-ing you, and get ready to start feeling better and better, until you don't need them anymore. I'm also going to show you how to begin scaling back on your energy crutches using the Rule of Halves. It's not drastic. It's paced just for you.

THE RULE OF HALVES

I've found over the years that "all or nothing" rarely works when people are trying to change their habits. I've had much more success with the Rule of Halves. Use this trick for cutting back on bad habits without telling yourself you have to go cold turkey. The concept is simple: Just cut your bad habit in half. If you drink too much wine, try drinking half your normal amount. If you drink too much coffee, cut it down by half. If it's the candy jar, take half your usual amount. Can you cut back to half the nicotine, half the energy drinks, half the stimulants? You'll be moving in the right direction without feeling like you can't have that thing you (think you) enjoy so much right now. You'll also be giving your body a chance to calibrate down and more gradually adjust to doing without that bad habit.

Instead of energy crutches, I recommend turning to energy boost-ers. Energy boosters give you a boost of energy but without the crash. They contribute to your health, rather than compromising it. As you work on scaling back on the use of your energy crutches, try replacing them with supportive and restorative energy boosters. Here are three of my favorites:

1. **WALKING.** Even a brisk 10-minute walk can give you a burst of energy and reset negative thinking. Make yourself get off the couch or get up from your desk and move. You won't regret it. Remember, using energy creates more energy.

2. **A 20-MINUTE CATNAP.** A longer nap can make you groggy, but 20 minutes seems to be the sweet spot for midday rejuvenation. Set your alarm, lie down, close your eyes, and let the energy resto-ration begin.

3. **YOGA.** My favorite energy-generating yoga pose is Warrior 2. As you hold this pose, breathe deeply and imagine breathing in all the power of a warrior woman!

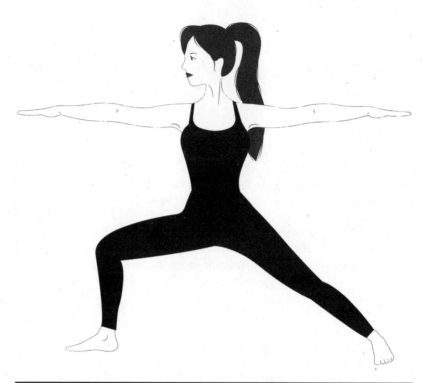

SUPPLEMENTS FOR QUICK ENERGY

These are my favorite supplements for when I need more energy immediately, as recommended by my friend and acupuncturist, Dr. Jing Liu, a practitioner of Traditional Chinese Medicine.

1. **Astragalus.** This herb is called Huáng qí in Chinese, and it's one I rely on frequently. It's also one of the fundamental herbs in Chinese medicine. A daily safe dose is 9 to 15 grams divided in two doses for morning and evening.

2. **Panax Ginseng.** Known as Ren Shen in Chinese medicine, ginseng supports your adrenal glands, which help to regulate energy production and, when under stress, release cortisol. Dr. Liu recommends a daily dose of 3 to 6 grams, divided in two doses for morning and evening. It's also good for better blood sugar control.

3. **Deer Antler Velvet.** Another Chinese medicine remedy, deer antler has been proven in scientific studies to reduce fatigue and increase endurance.[4] I recently started taking this, and I can really tell a difference. A therapeutic dose is 1 to 3 grams, taken as a powder. This one is quite expensive, by the way.

• • •

The ultimate goal of this chapter, as well as the Vibrant lifestyle in general, is to build your energy stores from the deepest cellular level so you always have what you need. To build up this solid reserve of energy over the long term, it is important to keep mindfully shifting your lifestyle. You can work on energy generation at your own pace, and I suggest kicking off your energy generation efforts with the three energy wins in the box at the end of this chapter.

Choose one of these wins to start, or if you are up for it, go for two or even all three. Each one of these shifts is a way to gradually begin dripping more energy into your tank. As an initial intervention, see if you can achieve your chosen win(s) every day for one week. Pay particularly close attention to any differences in your energy level. Remember, you are cultivating body awareness now. Listen for those messages that you are on the right track, or on the wrong track. If you feel better, then keep going. The last thing you need is more on your to-do list, so, for now, I only want you to do what feels good, like a natural nudge in the right direction. You can take as long as you need to establish these habits—a few days, a week, a month. If you are very low on energy, I suggest starting with just one win and really working on it until it begins to feel easier, before moving to the next one. Every step you take toward being more vibrant matters, so go at your own pace. Once you've got your new habit down, keep it and appreciate it! This isn't a temporary fix. This is how you create lifelong energy for the new vibrant you.

ENERGY WINS

Try these today, and keep trying them. There is no reason to ever stop doing any of these three energy wins, so as you integrate these habits, see if you can make them part of the rest of your life.

MOVE IT. Get moving for 10 or 15 minutes today, even if it's just a brisk walk. If you already walk, add 10 to 15 minutes more to your regular walking time. The ideal amount of time to walk each day is 30 to 60 minutes, so if you're not there, see if you can add just a few minutes to your walk each day until you achieve that goal. No rush—every added minute is progress and it's better to go at your own pace than to take on too much and give up. As you add more walking into your days—it is arguably the most natural human activity—pay attention to any changes in your movement, your pain, and your energy levels. (We'll get you moving even more in a few chapters.)

○ *I tried it! Here's how it felt:* _____

_____

_____

CUT IT IN HALF. Let's jump right in with a Rule of Halves exercise. Pick the energy crutch you rely on the most. Is it caffeine? Alcohol? Sugar? Whatever it is, cut the amount you consume each day in half. If it's four cups of coffee, try two. If it's a couple of glasses of wine, try just one. Whatever it is, don't put pressure on yourself to go cold turkey. Cold turkey is stressful and you are trying to build energy right now. Just cut it by half and pay attention to any difference in how you feel. Remind yourself, if you are tempted to pour yourself another, that it's a crutch and there are better ways to get what you need. You may not feel better immediately with less caffeine or sugar—your body may rebel because it wants that addictive "drug"—but any withdrawal symptoms should be much milder than if you were to quit completely. You are simply dialing it down. Give your body a chance to adjust to your new normal, keep that list of energy boosters handy, and see what positive changes you notice.

○ *I tried it! Here's how it felt:* _____

_____

_____

GO DARK. One of the best ways to feel more energetic in the morning is to improve your sleep quality, and a great way to do that is to sleep in total darkness. Remove all ambient lighting from your sleeping area. Turn off all the lights, including electronics, before you go to sleep. Leave your phone in another room, or at least turn it facedown and keep it a few feet from your bed. Consider installing blackout curtains if you have junk light coming through the windows (like from streetlights). This really does make a difference in sleep quality. Try it and notice if you sleep better and have more energy in the morning. (I'll give you more sleep guidance in chapter seven.)

○ *I tried it! Here's how it felt:* _____

_____

_____

CHAPTER 3

The Indicator: How to Cultivate Glow from the Inside Out

You now know that energy is a primary internal manifestation of vibrancy. Glow, or beauty, is a telling external indicator of that internal vibrancy. Glow and beauty that radiate from within indicate deep health, and no matter what your external features are, no matter your age or height or weight or abilities, when you are vibrant, you will glow. You will be beautiful. And if you are over age thirty, you are also quite likely to look much younger than you are.

Life in this modern world, on the other hand, tends to be prematurely aging us. While people statistically live longer nowadays, the stresses and poor health habits so common today have dimmed the glow, blunted the natural beauty, and aged much of our population. I used to be really good at guessing how old people were. Scarily good, in fact. I think most doctors who pay attention and have a lot of experience are good at this. We learn the signs of youth and the signs of aging. But I've noticed something in the past few years: I'm getting fooled more often. It's not that I'm thinking people are younger than they really are. It's the opposite. I'm seeing people who I think look 55 or 60 years old, and finding out they are only in their early 40s.

I tend to pay close attention to the people around me, including passersby I don't know. (Don't worry, I'm not judging you! I'm just health-curious.) I consider myself an observant person. I am always evaluating health based on the external signs. The most telling external indicators of health (as I've previously mentioned) are hair, skin, nails, eyes, expression, muscle tone, movement, silhouette, and posture, and let me tell you, what I'm seeing lately is disturbing.

When I look at the shape of people, or their silhouette, more and more often, the shape does not follow the general lines of their frame, due to excess adipose tissue—i.e., fat. The way some people walk seems to be degrading. I see a lot of lumbering, waddling, even limping. People's necks are looking worse than they used to, which I suspect is due to computer use and hunching over smartphones so often. Most people seem to slump when they stand and hunch over when they sit. I'm seeing a lot of grayish skin, wrinkling, redness, rashy or inflamed areas, and veins in the face as well as puffiness and dark circles under the eyes. I see a lack of color in the face, and overall, I am seeing more and more frequent dull expressions of worry, anxiety, or sadness. Honestly, I want to carry a stack of these books with me and hand them out on the street!

I believe what I am seeing is rapid, degradative aging in the general population due to poor nutrition, sedentary living, insufficient sleep quality, environmental toxicity, and an underlying sense of unhappiness and lack of fulfillment. In other words, lifestyle and environment are sapping our youth and beauty!

Diet has a significant effect on the external indications of internal health. You can't get the rapid cell turnover you need for youthful, glowing skin if you aren't feeding your body the nutrients it needs. You can't build strong muscles and supple joints, not to mention thick, shiny hair and strong, resilient nails, without all the right nutrients. The other two most influential factors that make people look older and less alive are toxicity (see chapter eight) and a lack of exercise (see chapter five), in my opinion. These problems are pervasive and hard to fix, and it's obvious. Just look around. Now, when I guess someone's age, I find that if I adjust for these effects by subtracting about 15 years from the age I think someone looks, my guesses are getting more accurate again.

You don't have to be one of those people who looks 15 years older than you are. Wouldn't you rather look 15 years younger? Wouldn't you rather have the energy and animation and movement of a young person? No matter how old you are, you can glow. An unhealthy young person can look older, grayer, and less vital than their years would suggest, but you can have the freshness and vigor that comes from vibrant health, no matter your age. Everyone will want to know your secret.

THE ANATOMY OF BEAUTY

You know it when you see it—that glow radiating from someone in a way that makes it difficult to stop staring. In the same way your body is sending messages to you about things that are going wrong, it's also sending you messages about things that are going right, in the form of beauty indicators.

Let's look at how this works.

Glowing Skin

Skin is one of the things I look at first. It's your largest organ, and most adults carry about eight pounds of skin. It is what separates you from the outside world, but it's not an impermeable barrier. It lets things in and it lets things out. When it is in good condition—smooth, supple, well hydrated, evenly colored—that is a major sign of internal health. Your skin is a detoxification organ, so when you have problems with toxicity, you'll see them manifested on the skin in the form of rashes as well as acne, redness, dry scaly patches, and irregular color.

Toxicity can come from the outside, such as when you put products on your skin that contain chemicals your body absorbs, or you encounter allergens or pollution; or from the inside, when your body attempts to get rid of toxins through the skin, produces excess hormones, or when your body's natural detoxification process isn't working like it should. (You'll learn more about detoxification in chapter eight.)

Some of the common skin problems I see are eczema, psoriasis (an autoimmune condition), scaly flaky skin, rosacea (an inflammatory condition), white papules like gooseflesh, and darkening velvety skin around the creases in the neck, which is a sign of diabetes called Acanthosis Nigricans.

A likely reason for unexplained rashes and conditions like eczema and rosacea and other skin issues is food sensitivities, especially to gluten but also to dairy. People often don't think of food as related to the skin, but when you are sensitive to a food, it becomes a toxin for you. You might think that sensitivity to gluten or dairy will manifest as gastrointestinal problems, and it often does, but in some people, the only indication of a food sensitivity is on the skin. There is one form of celiac disease that only shows up as a skin rash, but even non-celiac gluten sensitivity can have skin manifestations—it's a classic example of how an internal problem can cause an external symptom.

Skin is also indicative of circulation. Your lymphatic system lies just under the skin, moving fluids through your body, attacking viruses and bacteria and eliminating waste via the lymph nodes. When the lymphatic system is sluggish or stagnant, you can develop puffiness and a swollen appearance. Blood vessels under the skin also contribute to color. If your blood is well oxygenated and you have good blood circulation, your skin will have a healthy color. If the circulation is slow or blocked, or if your blood is low in oxygen, your skin can take on a dull, grayish color. If you are pale, that can also indicate anemia (insufficient iron), a low red blood cell count, or a problem with the thyroid, kidneys, or blood pressure.

And, of course, skin reveals damage from ultraviolet light—i.e., sun damage—which can cause discoloration, fine lines, and premature aging. I am all for getting some sun for a little vitamin D production, but I'll reiterate that most of us can't possibly get enough to generate sufficient vitamin D without putting ourselves at serious risk for skin cancer. It's just not worth it, when you can take a vitamin D3 supplement and save your skin from cancer as well as premature aging.

When I see smooth, supple skin with good, even color, without puffiness or sagging, I know that person is getting good nutrition, exercise, sleep, and isn't suffering from excessive toxic exposure—or their natural detoxification systems are working to keep toxins down.

THE NOTORIOUS EARLOBE CREASE

Just to the right and left of your beautiful face are your ears, and they can also show signs of health, for better or for worse. You may have heard that a crease in the earlobe is a sign of heart disease. Technically known as Frank's sign, a diagonal crease along the earlobe really has been associated with heart disease in many (but not all) scientific studies,[1] some quite recent and quite large. People with earlobe creases may be almost twice as likely to have coronary disease as people without earlobe creases. There are some theories, such as that some of the coronary arteries end at the earlobe so their degeneration shows on the earlobe (another external sign of an internal condition).

Don't assume if you have an earlobe crease that you have heart disease. There are better ways to test for heart disease, such as angiograms. But do take an earlobe crease as a suggestion from your body that your heart health may be something you should be paying more attention to, and that a heart-healthy diet and exercise are important to keep your coronary arteries in good condition. The good news is that lifestyle changes have been proven to actually reverse some of the damage to the arteries caused by a poor diet, lack of exercise, and inflammation. With the Vibrant lifestyle, you can foil that earlobe crease!

Hair

Hair is another obvious indicator of health. It doesn't respond as quickly to internal changes as the skin, but eventually, health or the lack of it will show up in the hair. Hair holds a record of what's going on inside—it can indicate toxins like heavy metals, drugs from marijuana to opiates and amphetamines, and its condition can indicate your nutrition status. It can also fall out if you are not getting sufficient nutrition, or if you have certain types of autoimmune conditions (see chapter nine).

Graying, in particular, is a sign of aging. Recently, I was having a conversation with a colleague who is also a friend of my husband's, and since I'm always secretly evaluating everybody's health and guessing their age, after this colleague was gone, I said to my husband, "So he and his wife are in their sixties, right?"

My husband said, "Oh no, their kids just graduated from high school. They're in their forties."

I was surprised! Both this man and his wife were completely white-haired. In Chinese medicine, gray hair indicates a lack of chi, which, as you may remember from the energy chapter, is a word for life-force energy. As energy drains from the body with age, the hair goes gray, but this shouldn't happen until very old age. And yet, in our culture, we think nothing of the fact that thirty-year-olds are getting gray hair. That is far too young to have your chi draining away! While there is a genetic component to when you begin to go gray, how you live can determine when those gray-hair genes get activated. Graying hair is just one more sign from your body that you are losing energy.

Another hair-related indicator is facial hair on women. We all have a bit of fuzz, but when women develop prickly chin hairs or thick hair on their upper lips, that may be a sign of hormone disruption, such as with polycystic ovary syndrome (PCOS), a condition that can cause high blood sugar, excess testosterone, and infertility. It can also happen with the drop in estrogen that comes with menopause, in which case the only real solution is to find that pair of tweezers (or see a skin care specialist about the best options for more permanent removal, if it really bothers you).

I'm sure you've noticed that some people have thick, glossy, full, gorgeous hair, and other people have hair that is thinner, duller, limper, finer, or falling out. There are certain hair characteristics with a genetic component, like a tendency to get split ends or frizziness or hair with nodules in it that tend to cause breakage. You can also inherit a tendency toward hair loss. But like most genetics, how you live determines which of these genes get activated. For example, while hair doesn't stop growing at a certain length, it does fall out after a certain amount of time, and how long it takes for each strand to shed is genetically determined. If you don't live a healthy lifestyle and get the nutrients necessary to build healthy hair, it could keep breaking off or falling out before its (genetically determined) time. A healthy head of hair can reach its genetic potential, while an unhealthy head of hair may not.

While there are some obvious ways to abuse your hair, like subjecting it to high heat or treating it roughly, getting chemical treatments like coloring and perms, and exposing it to too much sun, chlorine, or saltwater, what you eat is one of the most instrumental lifestyle elements for healthy, lustrous hair. Hair that splits, breaks, thins, or looks dull is often a sign of nutrient deficiency. Specifically, deficiencies in iron, B vitamins, vitamin E, vitamin D, vitamin A, biotin, and zinc can influence keratin production and the intake of amino acids and omega-3 fatty acids (EPA/DHA specifically). There are also more complex factors, like how well your body is metabolizing protein and how much toxicity you have. You can also lose hair from severe calorie restriction and rapid weight loss as well as stress, likely because you're not eating enough and being stressed often translates into nutrient deficiencies.

Even if you think your genes are against you, you can make the absolute most out of your hair. When I see someone with thick, lustrous, gorgeous hair, I know they are probably eating a nutrient-dense diet with plenty of lean protein and omega-3 fatty acids, reducing their toxic exposure, and managing their stress.

WHAT IS YOUR THYROID TELLING YOU?

An underactive thyroid gland is a common reason for thinning hair, as well as thinning eyebrows (especially the outer third of each eyebrow) and eyelashes. Other signs of a thyroid that isn't producing enough thyroid hormone are pale skin, puffiness, aggressive weight gain, cold sensitivity, depression, and fatigue. Thyroid problems have become too common, especially in women, but fixing your thyroid isn't as simple as getting a prescription for synthetic thyroid hormone, as a conventional doctor might have you believe. The thyroid is in many ways the master hormone, with ripple effects throughout the entire endocrine system and all through the body. It is a reactive gland, and a primary indicator of toxicity. The thyroid needs nutritional support and protection against toxicity. Are you taking care of your thyroid?

One necessary mineral for the thyroid is iodine. Before salt was iodized, goiters were a common but serious health problem. A goiter is a lump in the neck caused by an inflamed and swollen thyroid, due to iodine deficiency. Iodizing salt in the 1920s was one of modern medicine's most brilliant global public health successes, drastically reducing the incidence of goiter. Now, with the more frequent use of gourmet salts that aren't iodized, we may be seeing more iodine deficiencies again, so making sure to get enough iodine is one way to support your thyroid. If you love your gourmet salt, include more iodine-rich foods in your diet. The best sources are seaweed, eggs, shrimp, and tuna. I recommend eating sea vegetables whenever you can get them. Try a seaweed salad when you go out for sushi, or experiment with different culinary seaweeds and kelp granules in your home cooking.

However, more iodine alone isn't the solution to hypothyroidism. Restoring thyroid function is a complex collaborative treatment of lifestyle factors, with or without medication, but definitely with dietary improvements and nutritional supplementation. Remember that healing is never about just one thing because all parts of you are connected. All the health-restoring habits in this book will have an effect on your thyroid because your thyroid is integral to all your systems. When your thyroid function does come back up to normal, it will definitely show on the outside, and you'll also feel it with increased energy and less fatigue.

One thing I like to do for my thyroid is use a seaweed mask, or even an iodine paste, on my neck, over the area where my thyroid is (iodine can be absorbed through the skin). To make your own seaweed mask for your neck and/or face, not just for iodine replenishment but for an infusion of nutrients into your skin, try this DIY recipe. It's like a fancy spa treatment, for a fraction of the time and cost.

DIY SEAWEED MASK

1 cup of plain green tea, cooled to room temperature
4 sheets of nori (the seaweed sheets used to make sushi rolls, widely available in grocery stores)

1 tablespoon extra-virgin coconut oil, at room temperature (you could also use almond oil)
Optional: 2 thick cucumber slices, chilled

1. Put the green tea in a shallow bowl. Tear or cut the nori into strips, about 1 inch wide.
2. Dip a soft cloth or cotton balls in the green tea and moisten your face and neck. Use just enough to dampen your face.
3. Dip the nori strips into the green tea, then apply them to your face—leaving space for your eyes, nose, and mouth—and/or on your neck, from chin to collarbone.
4. Using your fingers, smooth the coconut oil over the nori strips.
5. Lie back in a comfortable position (or in the bathtub). If using the cucumber slices, put one slice over each eye. Relax for 10 minutes.
6. Remove the cucumber slices and discard or compost them. Peel the nori strips from your face and neck, and discard or compost them.
7. Wipe any remaining seaweed and oil from your face. Optionally, you can wash your face with a gentle cleanser, or take a shower.

Strong Nails

As you saw in chapter one, your fingernails and toenails are also good indicators of health. Thin, splitting, flaking, or cracking nails with ridges or that bend upward or have a warped shape might be due to excessive manicures and the wear and tear and chemicals that go along with those, but they can also reveal dehydration or mineral deficiencies, such as low zinc levels. Biotin is an essential nutrient for healthy nails (as well as healthy skin and hair), and if you aren't getting enough, it may show in your nails. Omega-3 fatty acids also influence nail quality. In fact, most of the nutrients that lead to healthy hair and skin also lead to healthy nails because your hair and nails (and the top layer of your skin) all contain keratin, in different configurations. Weak keratin can be due to a deficiency in the minerals that contribute to healthy keratin production.

Your nails can also reveal other health issues, like poor oxygenation or cardiovascular risk. Horizontal lines across the nail, called Beau's lines, can be a sign of diabetes, peripheral vascular disease, any disease that causes a high fever (such as pneumonia), or severe nutritional deficiencies. I often see Beau's lines in people with gluten intolerance, probably because gluten can compromise the ability of your small intestine to absorb nutrients. When I see these lines, gluten is my primary suspect.

When I see strong, well-shaped, smooth fingernails and toenails with hydrated cuticles and good pink color, and strong straight fingers with tapered ends, I know that person probably has a healthful diet with plenty of omega-3 fatty acids, biotin, zinc, and B vitamins, and is staying hydrated.

SUPPLEMENTS FOR GLOW

These supplements will help you glow from the inside out, and they all have scientific support for their anti-aging effects.

1. **Collagen peptides or hydrolyzed collagen.** Collagen is what keeps your skin, bones, and joints together, and is also present in your hair and nails. It has traditionally been used topically in skin cream (and it's naturally concentrated in bone broth, as it melts out of bones and cartilage when boiled), but it is the latest craze in the supplement industry, and taking it internally really can make your skin look younger. Other forms of collagen aren't absorbed as well, but collagen peptides and

hydrolyzed collagen are broken down to be more bio-available. Regular supplement use as well as topical use has been shown to improve droopy, wrinkled skin (or skin laxity).[2] One study showed that collagen supplements improved skin hydration, elasticity, roughness, and density.[3] Several other studies report that hydrolyzed collagen relieves joint pain from injuries in athletes and also from osteoarthritis.[4]

2. **Biotin.** Sometimes referred to as vitamin H even though it is technically one of the B vitamins, biotin is famous for thickening and strengthening hair, skin, and nails. Many people are deficient. For use as a glow supplement, I recommend 50 to 100 micrograms (mcg) daily. Just FYI, high supplemental intake of biotin renders many lab test results inaccurate, so let your doctor know if you are taking biotin.

3. **Vitamin E.** This vitamin is a powerful anti-inflammatory, so it can ease rosacea. It also may have an anti-aging effect. I recommend approximately 400 IU daily. This dose has also been shown to significantly decrease the number and severity of hot flashes,[5] so if you suffer from those, vitamin E is a two-for-one!

Bright Eyes and Expression

The eyes may be windows to the soul, but they are also windows to health. When people look in the mirror, they may avoid a frank examination of their entire bodies, but most of us do look ourselves in the eyes. You can tell by your own eyes when things aren't quite right with you, if your eyes are swollen or red or just don't look happy. It's one of the first signs we recognize in ourselves that we aren't feeling our best.

Physically, eyes should be bright and clear without puffiness or redness around them. If the whites of the eyes (technically called the sclera) are more yellowish, that can be a sign of dehydration or jaundice due to liver issues. I can also tell by the eyes if somebody has high cholesterol. They get a blueish ring around the outside of the cornea that would normally be clear. This is called the arcus senilis, and is a sign that cholesterol is being deposited in the cornea.

Red, bloodshot eyes can be a sign of insufficient sleep, irritation, allergies (which indicate immune system issues), toxicity from pollution, smoke, or too much alcohol. Or, it could be that you are spending too much time staring at screens. Redness can also indicate hormone conditions, especially thyroid conditions, as well as inflammation, food sensitivities, and toxicity. Cloudiness can be a sign of toxicity or developing cataracts. Another sign of toxicity is when the pupils respond more slowly to changes in light.

But eyes also indicate your emotional life. Your expression is mostly about what's going on in your eyes. When I see bright clear eyes without yellowness or redness, without puffiness or sagginess or excessive creping or drooping, and when those eyes look alive and animated, that to me speaks to physical and mental health. When the face looks clear, happy, purposeful, motivated, or engaged, that person looks beautiful to me.

YOGA FOR YOUR FACE

You know you should work out your muscles, but have you thought about the muscles in your face? Exercising your facial muscles can keep your face firmer and reduce the signs of aging. There has been at least one small study out of Northwestern University on the effects of facial muscle exercises on women with sun damage between the ages of 40 and 65. The study subjects performed 30 minutes of daily facial muscle exercises for 8 weeks, then every other day for 12 additional weeks. According to the published results, evaluators estimating the ages of study participants before and after the study did guess lower ages for the participants at the end of the study, which suggests that, objectively, the exercises did work. Also, participants were "highly satisfied," claiming significant improvements in their facial features.[6]

Facial yoga is also trendy, with celebrities trying it on social media. The facial expressions may look funny, but you can't argue with the results. There are yoga teachers who teach yoga for the face, and some very traditional yoga exercises extend to the facial muscles. I've also seen facial muscle exercises in some old fitness books from the 1970s. Many of these exercises involve pushing the skin and muscles of the face upwards. There is an old saying that up is the direction of youth, and down is the direction of age. This may or may not tone the muscles but it should increase circulation in your face, and stretching and strengthening the muscles does seem to make them firmer and more lifted. There are also exercises that tense various facial muscles, then relax them. This likely will tone the facial muscles. These exercises certainly can't hurt and they may help restore blood flow and tone to your face and add glow, so it's worth a try. You can search "yoga for the face" or "facial muscle exercises" online and find videos that you can follow. Here are two I like to do.

- **Neck Stretch.** Tilt your head back with your mouth open, then purse your lips, relax, and repeat for a minute or two. When you purse your lips, you should feel the stretch in your neck muscles, which can help firm the area under the chin.

- **Lion's Breath.** This is a classic yoga exercise. Traditionally you do the Lion's Breath while sitting back on your feet with your hands splayed out in front of you, but the key part for us is the face: Open your mouth as wide as you can, stick your tongue out as far as you can, and look as far up as you can. Hold for a few seconds, then relax. Repeat a few times.

Strong Muscles, Firm Joints, Graceful Movement, and Upright Posture

How you move is the result of an intricate dance of muscles and joints, strength and flexibility, and even mood. Posture, too, indicates strength and flexibility. Many older people develop a hunched back due to years of slumping as well as unhealthy bones, but those who stand and sit upright with energy and strength always look younger. Slumping, shuffling, and hunching can all be habits that accumulate over years, but they usually also indicate physical weakness, low energy, and often a depressed mood. As I've said before, regular exercise is the number one contributor to beautiful movement as well as good posture, and we also know it improves mood and can be an effective therapy for depression.

When I evaluate someone for these traits, I look for muscles I can see, well developed and not hidden by fat. I look for graceful joints without nodules and movement that is smooth and easy, not awkward or stilted. Posture when standing should be tall and lifted from the crown of the head, and while sitting, should be upright, not slouching against the back of the chair.

One study evaluated risk of death in older adults (ages 51 to 80) who could not sit down on the floor in a cross-legged position, then stand back up without support.[7] Six years after the study, more people unable to perform this task had died than those who were able to do it. If you aren't fit and don't exercise, this is pretty difficult to do. Give it a try! It's really just a measure of fitness, but it's worth practicing, in case you fall someday and need to get yourself back up.

THE PSYCHOLOGY OF GLOW

Surprisingly, beauty that seems purely physical is sometimes mostly psychological. Humans have an innate ability to judge the emotional status of others. This was probably a part of our early survival as social beings and integral to the formation of relationships. I believe that is one reason why, when we feel good, happy, cheerful, positive, or engaged, we look more attractive to other people. Mental health shows on the outside, and is just as important to cultivate as physical health. You can be well fed, well rested, well hydrated, and physically fit, but if you are unhappy, depressed, or suffer from anxiety, you won't look healthy (although poor physical health does make depression and anxiety more likely).

On the other hand, even if you don't always eat the best diet or get enough sleep, even if you forget to drink plenty of water or have a ways to go before you are physically fit, if you are happy, content, calm, interested in life, and are passionate about something (or someone), your whole being can radiate beauty and glow. You may also be more easily motivated and better at sticking to healthy habits, so even if you aren't quite where you want to be physically, nurturing your mental health can help you to get there.

TIME TO GLOW

There is no magic pill for beauty, or for health. When something on the outside is indicating a problem on the inside, we know it is never as simple as "take this supplement" or "eat that food." Let's say your hair is thin and dull. You can't just decide to take some B vitamins and get the results you want. Your hair isn't unhealthy because of a lack of B vitamins (or not just because of a lack of B vitamins). It's unhealthy because the cells in your body aren't turning over and restoring themselves quickly enough. Because you aren't absorbing the vitamins, or synthesizing the protein. Because your systems aren't synchronized or they don't have the energy to do what they need to do.

Your hair is reflecting that your circulation may be sluggish. Your hormone production may be off. You may be under a ton of stress. Your immune system may be overreacting. All of these things could be connected and they are all influenced by every aspect of your lifestyle. That's why you can't just throw a pill at a problem or fix your skin with a laser any more than you can get physically fit with plastic surgery or become a happy person because you took some medication. (Please don't stop taking an antidepressant if you need it.) I'm also not saying you shouldn't take supplements or use lasers or even get plastic surgery. These may all be fine things to do for you—but none of them are panaceas. This is why it's so important to look at health from so many different angles. This is the essence of lifestyle medicine.

All the techniques discussed in this book support inner health and, therefore, contribute to beauty and glow. Other chapters cover dietary choices, exercise, sleep, habit adjustment, supplements, and more. Here, I want to talk about just four additional factors that can light up your glow from within, and that are not covered in other chapters in this book.

- **HYDRATION:** Nothing in your body will work as well as it should without sufficient hydration. It is critical to drink enough water every day. Divide your body weight in pounds in half, and aim to drink that many ounces of water per day. For example, if you weigh 150 pounds, you should try to drink 75 ounces of water. It may seem like a lot if you aren't used to drinking that much, but once you start, you'll be surprised at how much better you feel and look.

- **THE TRIPLE OIL TREATMENT:** You need enough healthful fat in your diet, especially EPA and DHA, to have supple, resilient skin, shiny hair, strong nails, and good organ function. Be sure to eat deep cold-water fatty fish, like salmon, mackerel, ahi tuna, sardines, and anchovies, at least a couple of times a week. You can also take a fish oil or algae supplement with EPA and DHA. Extra-virgin olive oil, avocado oil, and grapeseed oil are also great additions to your diet, in moderation. Externally, I recommend coconut oil, for moisturizing your face, elbows, knees, feet, nails, and cuticles. (Ladies, coconut oil can also be used topically to help with vaginal dryness, which is a common problem when estrogen levels begin to drop during perimenopause.)

VIBRANT PRO TIP: The combination of 1) EPA/DHA supplements, 2) extra-virgin olive oil and other healthful oils in the diet, and 3) the external use of coconut oil is your vibrant Triple Oil Treatment.

- **BEAUTY BREATHING:** Deep breathing not only helps to oxygenate your blood, which is good for all parts of you, but when your breathing technique lengthens the exhalation to be longer than the inhalation, the effect is to calm your mind, ease anxiety, and reduce the effects of stress. Try this Beauty Breathing exercise, which not only lowers your stress hormone levels but also helps to oxygenate your blood and will take the worry right out of your face. Set a timer for five minutes. Then:
  - Inhale slowly and as fully as possible to a slow count of four (or about four seconds).
  - Hold your breath for a slow count of five (or about five seconds).
  - Exhale slowly and as fully as possible for a slow count of eight (or about eight seconds).
  - Hold your breath after the exhale for a slow count of two (or about two seconds).
  - Repeat until your five minutes are up.

- **PASSION:** Cultivating a sense of purpose and interest in life will bring you psychological energy and give your life more meaning. Being passionate about something leads to contentment and happiness . . . which leads to beauty.

BEAUTY WINS

Every small step you take toward vibrant health on the inside will eventually show up on the outside, so try one or more of these three beauty wins and get ready to glow!

DRINK MORE WATER. Drink half your body weight number in ounces of water every day. If that's too much, start with half that amount and work your way up.

○ *I tried it! Here's how it felt:* _____

_____

BEAUTY BREATHING. Once a day, take five minutes to stop what you are doing, close your eyes, and practice the Beauty Breathing exercise in this chapter, to calm your mind, bring peace and contentment to your face, reduce your level of stress hormones, and oxygenate your blood.

○ *I tried it! Here's how it felt:* _____

_____

TRIPLE OIL TREATMENT. Take an EPA/DHA supplement daily, have a daily salad with a tablespoon of extra-virgin olive oil and a squeeze of lemon juice, and put coconut oil on your skin wherever you notice dryness. Your skin may absorb the coconut oil best if you do it in the evening before bed since skin repair and renewal happens more rapidly at night (supposedly peaking around 2 am).

○ *I tried it! Here's how it felt:* _____

_____

PART II

Deeper

Let's go deeper. In this section, we will explore the Vibrant Triad. It is your touchstone for a vibrant lifestyle. To achieve the energy and glow that makes you vibrant requires a mindful three-pronged approach, so we're going to go in depth about how to eat for vibrancy, how to move for vibrancy, and how to connect for vibrancy. These three primary life-style factors are the most influential in establishing vibrant health from the inside out. So, together, let's drill down and get these three pieces right. When you master all three sides of the Vibrant Triad, you will begin to experience dramatic changes. It's time to fully believe in your-self and do this!

Food

Vibrant

Movement   *Connection*

CHAPTER 4

The Communicator: How to Use Food to Feel Better

When I was a very young doctor—I don't think I was even 30 years old yet—I ran an integrative medicine clinic in the Midwest. I treated adults, helping them to feel better, and because I was trained in functional medicine (among other things), I typically ran a lot of lab tests to try to get to the bottom of disquieting symptoms. There was a local woman, a nurse, whose father was a well-loved and respected general surgeon in the community. The woman had a son with autism, and she kept calling my office to try to get my staff to let her come in so I could see him.

I didn't know anything about autism back then. My brother had Down syndrome, so I was acquainted with developmental issues in children, and I'd seen ADD, ADHD, and Tourette syndrome, but autism was out of my wheelhouse. I couldn't imagine there was anything I could do for this woman. And yet, she persisted. She insisted. Finally, I agreed to see her for a consultation—but not her son. I was not a pediatrician, so I planned to let her down gently, telling her that there was nothing I could do, but at least she would be satisfied that we had met face-to-face and had a talk about her situation.

When we met, the first thing I asked was what she thought I could do for her. She told me that I was the only healthcare provider she knew of who would run food sensitivity tests, and that is what she wanted from me. Fair enough, I thought, but even if I did run a food sensitivity test on her son, I wasn't sure if I could guide his case, not being a pediatrician. Furthermore, I couldn't believe her father, that trusted local surgeon who was quite traditional in his approach to medicine, would support such a thing. And yet, she told me he was the one who directed her to me. She told me: "He said he thinks you're crazy, but he also thinks you're smart."

Then I got a bit more information. This woman told me that her son was only five years old, but that he was already suicidal, had ADHD, and was severely underweight, on top of his autism diagnosis. I thought about one of my very first patients, a man who was schizophrenic and told me his "head was talking to his stomach." Food sensitivity testing had revealed a severe dairy intolerance in him, and when he went completely off dairy, his symptoms subsided dramatically and he was eventually able to go off his medication. That had been the first time I'd ever really thought about how food can affect the brain, not just the gut. Today you would never know he had once been diagnosed with schizophrenia. (I'll talk more about his case in the chapter about the brain.)

Although I knew schizophrenia was completely different than autism, and a child is much different than an adult, the mother's report about her child's mental health issues alarmed me. I was scared and intimidated, frankly, but I made an agreement with the boy's mother to be her partner in working out this problem—as long as she understood I was not a pediatrician and not an expert on this issue.

I did a lot of reading before the appointment. I often dealt with food sensitivity in my patients, and I knew what reactions to food could do. There are the regular things, like inflammation and autoimmunity, but I began to think about what all the adult cases I'd seen had in common— depression, anxiety, no motivation, foggy dull thinking, inability to focus—all those things that are tough to get adults to recognize because they get good at compensating or making excuses. But in kids, these symptoms are more obvious because they don't compensate, and I thought, *Am I staring the same animal in the face here? Is food really so linked to the nervous system?*

That really opened my mind to the neurological impact of food. Maybe there wasn't really all that much difference between a schizophrenic adult and an extremely intelligent but tortured, suicidal five-year-old, from a dietary perspective. In any case, I thought, what could a food sensitivity test hurt?

It turned out the boy was severely reactive to both dairy and gluten, and also had some lead toxicity. It took us a year and a half to repair the damage, but by the age of seven, that little boy was thriving in private school.

FOOD IS FIRST

Here is a simple truth that can help you prioritize your way through the rest of this book:

> FIX YOUR FOOD, AND THE REST
> WILL BE SO MUCH EASIER.

In this chapter, that is where we will start. Food is at the top of the Vibrant Triad because it is the communicator: talking to the body with every meal and every snack, talking to the organs and hormones and microbiome, and creating you literally by giving your body what it needs to build bones, muscles, organs, and skin. Food keeps you alive, and you become the food that you eat. Choose wisely, and your body will become strong and wise. Choose poorly, and your body will eventually break down, causing stress, energy depletion, and cellular-level dysfunction.

At the most basic level, food is energy and you cannot create energy without food. We've discussed how your mitochondria use the components of the food you eat to create ATP inside your cells. Externally, food also affects your appearance, often within a single day. You can't glow without glow-inducing food. Since you can't be vibrant without energy and glow, you can't be vibrant without getting the food piece right. What you put in your mouth may be the single most powerful influence you have over your health.

You hear a lot these days about our broken food system. I agree that we have a problem. The food most available to most people is overly processed, genetically modified, hybridized beyond recognition, and adulterated with chemical residue from pesticides and herbicides as well as chemical preservatives and artificial colors and flavors. Yes, our soil is depleted and the food we grow today tends to be less nutrient dense than food a hundred years ago in a less polluted world. Yes, processed foods are shadows of their former selves and a far cry from the fresh whole foods I recommend you eat. Yes, there are fast-food restaurants everywhere, in practically every country on the planet. It's hard to travel so far that you won't run into a Starbucks, a McDonald's, or a KFC.

Temptation may lurk around every bend in the road and call to you from every billboard and every advertisement, but remember that you still have plenty of choices. Organic whole foods are *also available*, and have become more affordable than ever before. Even Walmart carries organic food now, and it's also much more affordable than it once was at stores like Aldi and Trader Joe's. We hear a lot about food deserts— those areas where you supposedly can't get healthful food—but I think the problem is more a knowledge desert than a food desert. Good food doesn't have to be expensive.

Here in the middle of the country, where I live, farmers markets abound, and while we have our fancy artisanal vinegars and olive oils and cheeses and our adaptogenic mushrooms and handpicked wild strawberries that rival anything on the coasts, we also have good basic vegetables on the cheap. You can get a big bag of tomatoes or peppers or kale or fresh baby greens for a couple of dollars. You can get boxes of zucchini or winter squash or sweet potatoes for a few dollars more. Garlic, onions, collard greens, romaine lettuce, even meat from small family farms and fish from small family fisheries are all available and cheaper than what you'll find at the grocery store. Buy in bulk, freeze what you don't use right away, and you can actually save money. Real food is everywhere. You can even grow it in your backyard or in pots on your deck or patio.

If you find yourself tempted to spend money on drive-through food and dollar-store frozen meals or discount-store boxes of snack cakes, add up those costs and put that same money toward healthful ingredients to prepare at home. If money is a concern, scrutinize your budget carefully: Is it true that you can't afford to buy good-quality foods, or is it rather that you don't know where to look, or haven't learned how to prepare whole foods? It's a learning process but it's also primal knowledge that is widely available for anyone who wants it. Your health and your family's health are at stake. Food habits are hard to break, but no habit is impossible to break if you really want to change. Your health, your choice.

Once you've found real food, you have a few more things to consider: Will you deep-fat fry or lightly sauté? Will you drown your salad in Ranch dressing or dress it with a drizzle of olive oil and a squeeze of lemon? How will you fill up that plate? You can choose whether to eat more vegetables, less sugar, more lean protein, less saturated fat. You can choose wild-caught fish and grass-fed or pastured meat. You can choose food grown near to where you live. You can choose your portion size, and whether or not to take second helpings. Your choices, despite your proximity to a food system that could be doing much better than it's doing now, are still practically infinite. It's all up to you. But what matters is that you know the impact of your choices on how you feel right now and how your health will fare in the future.

Every food choice you make directly impacts your health in multiple ways. Food contains messages for your cells, via the amount of carbohydrates, fats, and proteins it contains as well as the delivery vehicles you choose for those macronutrients—a strawberry cupcake versus a cup of strawberries, butter versus olive oil, bacon versus salmon, etc. It also contains the micronutrients and phytochemicals that send signals to your cells and support your biochemical processes. Food affects how many fat cells you make and how much fat you burn. It controls how high your blood sugar goes. It helps to determine which microbes thrive inside your gut. It influences how well your endocrine system can balance your hormones. It influences your inflammation levels, how much water you retain, and how likely it is that you will develop a chronic disease, from heart disease to autoimmunity, diabetes to cancer. Food is the primary way you can transform what the mirror says, what the scale says, and what your doctor says. Every bite you take is a missive to your body, saying what you want your health to be. So choose well!

I'm here to help you with those choices. In this chapter, I'm going to show you how the foods you eat send messages to your body, and how you can send better messages, for better results. Whether you are trying to lose weight, feel better, or support your goals (like running a 5K or having a sharper mind), food is your number one power play. So let's get this right. How should you eat if you really want to optimize your health, not just prevent disease? How should you eat if you want to be vibrant?

THE MYSTERIOUS MICROBIOME

You can't see it, but it lives within you, influencing everything about you. You are populated with microbes that have their own DNA, and they live symbiotically with you, for the most part. Microbiome management has become another big trend in the health world because the more we learn about the bacteria, fungi, viruses, and other microscopic creatures that live in us and on us, the more we recognize how much we rely on them. They can control our moods according to how much serotonin they produce.[1] They have evolved along with our immune systems and are in constant communication, helping immune function with their own molecular signaling in exchange for the immune system accepting their presence.[2] They can even determine what foods we crave![3] The next time you're dying for a chocolate chip cookie, you can blame your inner microbes. It's like we've got tiny little alien overlords ruling us from within. Thank goodness most of them are friendly, since our survival means their survival.

However, the gut microbiome is not without its troublemakers, and you either empower or disempower those mischievous microbes with every meal. Food has a rapid and dramatic effect on your microbiome.[4] Despite its significant influence, your dietary decisions put you in charge of who is doing what inside your gut. Scientists have observed patterns in people with different diets. While vegetarians have similar microbiomes to each other,[5] vegetarian microbiomes are much different than those in people who eat a lot of meat. Some bacteria, such as Lactobacillus and Bifidobacterium, are friendly, helping to keep you healthy. They thrive on fiber and resistant starch (those parts of fruits and vegetables you don't digest—they digest it for you). Others aren't so friendly, like the sugar-devouring Candida fungi and the saturated-fat-loving Bacteroides bacteria, both of which are inflammatory and can cause serious health problems when they overgrow.

The next time you reach for a snack, give a thought to your microbiome. Do you want those microbes telling you to eat steak and cake, or do you want to send them some vegetables to munch on and let them know who is really in charge?

DISEASE DIETS VERSUS WELLNESS DIETS

It goes without saying there are thousands of diets out there, and trends come and go. Many of these diets are extreme, drastically increasing or reducing some macronutrient or food group, and they often promise extreme results. A part of you may know that when something sounds too good to be true, it probably is, but what I'd like you to understand about many of these extreme diets is that, originally, they did work . . . for people with extreme health conditions.

Consider two very famous doctors: Dr. Robert Atkins and Dr. Dean Ornish. Both Dr. Atkins, who recommended a very low-carb diet, and Dr. Ornish, who recommends a very low-fat diet, have had success treating people with advanced heart disease. They used opposite approaches, but they both improved the health of cardiac patients with their interventions. It's my opinion that both diets worked because:

1. **Both intervention diets were an improvement** over the standard American diet their patients were likely eating.

2. **Some people don't do well on carbs.** Inflammation from too many carbohydrates, or a genetic or environmental sensitivity to carbohydrates, can cause arterial dysfunction, so drastically reducing carbohydrates can help the body to reduce inflammation. It can also help to increase HDL cholesterol, which is beneficial for heart health, and reduce triglycerides,[6] which can be a risk factor for heart disease, when elevated. There are some intriguing studies that support the link between a low-carb diet and a reduction of cardiac risk factors.[7]

3. **For others, fat is the problem.** Inflammation from too much saturated fat, or a genetic or environmental sensitivity to fat, can cause atherosclerosis (hardened arteries), so drastically reducing fat could help the arteries to clear. There is also a lot of good research linking low-fat diets to improved heart health in cardiac patients.[8]

Both of these diets were disease intervention diets. They were not originally designed for people without heart disease. And *both* of these diets have also been used to intervene with certain cancers, dementia, autoimmune diseases like multiple sclerosis and rheumatoid arthritis, and more. You can find studies that support the use of low-fat or low-carb diets for all of these conditions as well as research that doesn't show any benefit. (I suspect this is largely due to different people needing different kinds of diets and is an indicator of the need for personalized medicine—but I'll talk more about that later.)

The ketogenic diet is another good example of a successful disease diet. In children with epilepsy, the ketogenic diet has in some cases almost completely stopped severe seizure disorders that were not responsive to medication.[9] Newer research shows that the ketogenic diet can also help control epilepsy in adults.[10] Ketogenic diets have also been shown to help improve symptoms in people with neurological disorders like multiple sclerosis, Parkinson's disease, and Alzheimer's disease. There is also some evidence that it can be helpful in slowing the growth of some cancers.[11] As expected, however, since nothing is simple, there is also some evidence that ketogenic and other high-fat, low-carb diets can increase the risk of some cancers. As an article from the Fred Hutchinson Cancer Research Center put it, "It's complicated."[12]

In my work with the Cancer Treatment Centers of America, I've seen a vegan diet used successfully as a therapeutic intervention for certain types of cancer. The research for this is most robust for prostate cancer[13] and breast cancer. (One large study showed that women on a low-fat plant-based diet, which was not necessarily strictly vegan but contained no more than 20 percent of total calories from fat, were no less likely to develop breast cancer, but were much less likely to die from it.[14]) Again, these were used as disease diets—for many people, a very low-fat vegan diet would be just as extreme as a very high-fat ketogenic diet.

It *is* complicated because for every study that says an extreme diet helps some disease, you can almost always find another study that says the opposite—either that such a diet doesn't work, or that an opposite diet also works, or works better. Even in the case of obesity, studies show that when you pit a low-carb diet against a low-fat diet, over the long term, the results are about the same. They both help with obesity by intervening in some extreme way.

Unfortunately, when a diet shows great promise at successfully treating a disease, somebody always gets the bright idea that there could be profit potential, and goes on to translate that disease diet into a wellness diet—for better or for worse. This is why millions of people have been convinced to go keto, or on the opposite side of the spectrum, eat an extremely low-fat vegan diet. This is why so many people are confused about what to eat, what to do, what to think about food. Every theory is supported somewhere, and debunked somewhere else, so eventually many people give up and go back to eating the Standard American Diet—the one we know actually causes chronic disease!

Enough about disease diets. My question is: What is a *wellness diet*? What is a diet that can prevent chronic disease from happening in the first place? That's what has always interested me. Sure, disease diets can be useful and might make a meaningful difference for many people, but if you are not drastically ill (and most people aren't), I don't believe a disease diet is appropriate for you. I want you to be drastically *vibrant*, so let's talk about what we can do to achieve *that* goal.

I believe that eventually, as genomic, food-sensitivity, and microbiome testing become more sophisticated and more accessible, every person will have a clear picture of their disease risk and can customize a diet designed to prevent the diseases to which they may be prone. That may happen sooner than later, but for now, I do not recommend that you go on a disease diet. I recommend you go on a wellness diet, and by diet I don't mean "diet." I mean a chosen way of eating that can optimize your health, help you reach a healthy weight, increase your energy, and provide your body with everything it needs to thrive. Chances are, eating that way will also go far in preventing chronic diseases in your future. But let's look at what you can do right now.

THE BEST WELLNESS DIET

There is one diet that has been shown, over and over, to be the most beneficial for wellness across the board.[15] It is the Mediterranean diet: a diet based on whole fresh foods and rich in vegetables, fruits, seafood, nuts, seeds, with some legumes, whole grains, olive oil, and small amounts of meat and eggs.

When I advise people about what to eat, I embrace most of the tenets of the Mediterranean diet, but I tweak this diet just a little, in ways I believe are even more conducive to building health. I call this a modified Mediterranean diet, or the Vibrant Diet.

1. The Vibrant Diet skews toward both lower carb and lower saturated fat.

2. The Vibrant Diet eliminates foods containing gluten, dairy products, and sugar.

3. The Vibrant Diet allows for one processed item: a daily high-quality protein shake.

Let's talk about why I've made these alterations to a classic diet that has been shown to be the most beneficial diet known to us so far.

Why Lower Carb and Lower Saturated Fat?

As discussed above, disease diets often drastically reduce carbohydrates or fats. You need carbohydrates and fats for energy. They should be balanced with protein, and they should come from high-quality nutrient-dense sources of food, so you have plenty of information and resources to deliver to your body.

But let's face it: We live in a culture of excess, and it's hard to break out of that all-or-nothing mentality. I do not believe you should ever go no-carb or no-fat. Not only can that cause you to miss out on valuable nutrients, but it's simply not sustainable for most people. You know that old saying that the best diet is the one you'll actually follow? That's about sustainability, and extreme diets, whether disease diets or their mainstream equivalents, usually aren't sustainable. Sustainability is easiest when a diet is balanced because you won't feel like you're missing anything, and eliminating a macronutrient, or even limiting it too much, can upset the balance. The consequence of low-fat diets is often overconsumption of carbohydrates, and the consequence of low-carb diets is often the overconsumption of fat.

When I say "lower-carb, lower-fat," what I really mean is balanced carbs and balanced fat, but in this culture of eating too many carbs and too much fat, I feel I have to say "lower" to achieve that true balance. Balance applies even with healthful carbs like those in quinoa or sweet potatoes or apples; and healthful fats, like those in avocadoes, olive oil, and walnuts, can lead to trouble if you eat too much of them. Those foods are all great for you, but just because something is good doesn't mean more is better. The most common health problem in the Western world right now is excess weight. The best way to get that under control is to lower your carb intake while still having some healthful carbs, and lower your fat intake (especially saturated fat) while still having some healthful fats (especially monounsaturated fat and omega-3 fatty acids). This makes weight control so much easier, while still delivering enough micronutrients (like vitamins and minerals) and microbiome-feeding fiber for all-around glowing vibrancy.

DIETARY SUPPLEMENTS FOR A DE-MINERALIZED DIET

The depletion of much of the soil in agricultural America as well as hybridization to make crops more pest- and weather-resistant has resulted in food with lower nutrient density than it once had,[16] and minerals in particular have been stripped from our food. Keep eating your veggies, but also think about adding back some of what has been lost in our food supply.

- **Calcium:** If you aren't already taking calcium supplements, consider it now. You need it to build strong bones and teeth and also to help deliver messages from your brain to the rest of your body. I recommend taking 1,500 mg per day, for your bones, teeth, and brain.

- **Selenium:** A mineral found in the soil, we only need a little but it's necessary for metabolic function. A supplement (take about 55 mcg per day) or, even better, a daily Brazil nut (which contains more than 55 mcg) will give you what you need.

- **Iron:** Not everyone is iron-deficient, but if you are prone to anemia, have heavy periods, or don't eat any animal products, you may be deficient. I recommend having your iron level checked before supplementing, but if you're low, a supplement can restore healthy hemoglobin and myoglobin levels in your blood. You need these to carry oxygen from your lungs to your muscles and throughout your body where you need it.

- **Zinc:** This mineral is essential for a healthy immune system, including for wound healing. I recommend taking 15 to 30 mg per day.

Why No Gluten, Dairy, or Sugar?

If you follow the health news and have been looped into the diet world for a while, you've surely heard about how "gluten is bad" or "dairy is bad" or "sugar is bad." But if you are new to this world, or are a mainstream medical practitioner, you may have the opinion that there is nothing wrong with gluten, dairy, or even sugar, for a "healthy" person. Yes and no. Much depends on the form and how much you eat, although I would argue that even for healthy people, there is no reason to include any of these three potentially hazardous products. Let's talk about each of the three in turn.

Gluten Issues

You may be thinking, rightly, that earlier in this chapter, I gave you the whole speech about disease diets, and that is also what I was talking about at the beginning of this chapter, when I told you about my adult patient who had schizophrenia and my pediatric patient who had autism and suicidal thoughts. You are absolutely correct. But . . . when it comes to food sensitivity, it can become a bit of a chicken-and-egg situation. Did the disease trigger food sensitivities, or did food sensitivities trigger the disease?

If food alone is powerful enough to cause psychosis and suicidal thoughts, and the removal of a food completely resolves the problem, then, to me, that is less a disease than a food reaction, and that is relevant for anyone who has food sensitivities. Gluten is an incredibly common food sensitivity.

Gluten is a protein in some cereal grains like wheat, barley, rye, and spelt. We know that people with the autoimmune condition celiac disease can't eat it. In this disease, gluten causes the body to attack its own small intestine, and this can cause a cascade of serious health problems. People with celiac disease are not the only ones who will feel better avoiding gluten. There is a newly discovered condition called Non-Celiac Gluten Sensitivity (NCGS) that mainstream medicine disregarded at first, but the evidence is mounting that this condition is real, and a real threat to health. I think gluten sensitivity exists on a spectrum, with celiac disease on one end, and no reactivity on the other. Many people are likely somewhere in the middle.

We don't have actual statistics at this point, since this is a newly recognized issue, but we do know that about 30 percent of people have at least one of two DNA variations (polymorphisms) for celiac disease (HLA-DQ2 and HLA-DQ8).[17] Only 3 percent of these people will actually develop celiac disease. Something triggers these genes to "turn on." There is a theory that those who don't develop celiac disease may be at least somewhat gluten-sensitive, meaning that eating gluten may be doing damage to them, even if it's subclinical (non-diagnosable) damage. We also know that some people without either of these variations do experience real symptoms after eating gluten. We still have much to learn about this, but what we do know is that, for many people, probably far more than we know, gluten is causing harm. There are millions of people around the world who experience chronic stomach pain, gas, bloating, constipation, diarrhea, or brain fog, depression, anxiety, or joint pain, muscle pain, or other vague symptoms that doctors can't explain. Could gluten be a contributing culprit? I think so.

The man who really put the nail in gluten's coffin is Dr. Alessio Fasano, an internationally recognized expert on celiac disease as well as all things gluten. His book, *Gluten Freedom*, brought new understanding to both the public and scientists about what gluten is and what it can do to people. Dr. Fasano says that the human species was never meant to eat gluten and only started to eat gluten when they began to domesticate crops. Before that, none of the foods humans ate contained gluten, and according to Dr. Fasano, gluten cannot be digested and is toxic for everyone, even though not everyone exposed to gluten will get sick.[18]

Some people can handle the toxic assault without symptoms, or without life-altering symptoms. Those who can't develop celiac disease and a range of other serious gluten-related health issues.[19] More people will develop milder, but still troublesome and ultimately damaging, symptoms. Dr. Fasano's research on what he calls the spectrum of gluten-related disorders is fascinating and implicates gluten in a wide range of health issues beyond celiac disease, including other autoimmune diseases, joint pain, chronic fatigue, fibromyalgia, even schizophrenia.[20]

According to Dr. Fasano, some people experience the release of excessive zonulin when exposed to gluten. Zonulin is a protein that regulates the permeability of the intestinal lining, often called the gut barrier. Too much zonulin can open the "weave" of this lining enough that food proteins leak into the bloodstream. Leaky gut can lead to many different health conditions, especially autoimmune diseases. These include celiac disease but also conditions like type 1 diabetes, Crohn's disease, rheumatoid arthritis, multiple sclerosis, lupus, psoriasis, and more, as well as certain neurodegenerative diseases and cancers.[21] Unfortunately, these conditions can inhibit the absorption of vitamins and minerals, including vitamin D and zinc, which support the healthy functioning of this "gate" function, so as these nutrients are depleted, the problem can grow worse.

Although research shows that people with celiac disease are the most likely to have this excessive zonulin response, Dr. Fasano stresses that gluten causes leaky gut in everyone. He only stops short when asked if everyone should stop eating gluten. He says that some people's bodies manage to process out the toxin without any bothersome symptoms (whether or not there is internal damage), so he isn't yet prepared to say that gluten should be off the menu for all.[22] But I'm prepared to say it! At least until you get to the bottom of any of the symptoms that are holding you back from feeling vibrant, gluten should not be a part of your food plan.

Gluten sensitivity seems to be more common in women, and so I ask each of you reading this book to consider: Is your immune system fighting gluten right now? Are you having trouble digesting the toast you had for breakfast, the sandwich you had for lunch, or the pasta you had for dinner? I'd like you to start paying attention to how you feel after eating a meal containing gluten, and how you feel after eating a meal that doesn't contain gluten. I suspect many of the people who "don't feel anything" after eating gluten just aren't paying close enough attention. Get in the habit of noticing. Although symptoms can show up the next day or even later, it's still a good idea to have this on your radar. The research may not yet show the consequences of gluten exposure in those without diagnosed celiac disease, but in my experience, those consequences are likely to exist, often at a low level or in a way that you would not necessarily link to gluten.

What does this mean for you? If you have persistent digestive symptoms and don't feel well, it's worth getting tested for celiac disease, just in case. If you're pretty sure you don't have celiac disease, you could spend the time and money to get tested for gluten sensitivity, or to see if you have the genetic variations for celiac disease. For some people, getting test results that confirm a gluten sensitivity or susceptibility helps them with their resolve to quit. Or, you could just stop eating gluten. (If you do plan to get tested for celiac disease, don't stop eating gluten until after the test, as this can result in a false negative.) Even if you aren't gluten-sensitive (although you probably are), there are other compelling reasons to give up gluten:

- Many empty-calorie junk foods contain gluten. If you decide not to eat gluten, you could help yourself to eliminate many bad food habits.

- There is no nutritional value in gluten-containing products that you can't get in other, more healthful foods.

- Most people eat too many carbohydrates, so cutting down on gluten can help cut down on carbohydrates. (Avoid packaged, processed "gluten-free" junk food, which is just as bad for you.)

- If you are trying to lose weight, giving up gluten can be a helpful strategy, not because gluten-free foods are always less caloric, but because you will be eliminating some of the most high-calorie, low-nutrient foods from your diet. If you replace one big sandwich, plate of pasta, or pizza with one big salad every day, you are already winning.

- Modern wheat, the main source of gluten in the U.S. diet, is typically heavily sprayed with pesticide and has also been drastically manipulated through hybridization, so it barely resembles its ancient cousins. It is harder to digest, starchier, sweeter, more caloric, less nutrient-dense, and can cause water retention in weight-sensitive people. It is also typically refined, which removes the beneficial fiber. It is no longer (and perhaps never was) what I would call a natural food.

Who knows what troublesome health issues many of us confront might be gluten-related?

You will never know if you don't take it out of your diet for a while (or permanently), so consider giving this a try. (This will be an option for one of the "Diet Wins" at the end of this chapter.) Ultimately, it's your decision, of course, but giving up gluten might just be the key to vibrancy that you've been looking for. You'll never know until you try.

Go here for more information on testing for food intolerances, allergies, leaky gut, and autoimmune conditions like celiac disease, as well as basic lab tests I recommend for everyone.

Dairy Issues

Many people who have gluten sensitivity also have dairy sensitivity. This is quite common in children with autism but also common in people with celiac disease. But many people without any disease or condition also find out they are sensitive to dairy products. For some, dairy is the primary problem.

There are multiple ways that dairy can be problematic. Some people have an intolerance to lactose, one of the sugars in milk. They get stomach issues from dairy but may be able to have lactose-free milk. Others react to casein, which is one of the primary proteins in milk. It is especially concentrated in cheese, so casein-sensitive people may have stronger reactions to cheese than to small amounts of regular milk. Dairy also contains compounds that behave, during digestion, similarly to opioids in the body. These compounds are also more concentrated in cheese. This is probably why so many people say they are "addicted" to cheese.

Are you sensitive to dairy? As with gluten, you might be, but you might not know it. There is a genetic test that can tell you whether or not you are predisposed to be lactose intolerant, but that has nothing to do with casein sensitivity. These are two completely separate problems. Lactose is a milk sugar that can cause bloating and stomach upset in some people, but lactose-free milk doesn't bother them. Casein sensitivity is harder to unravel. Casein is a protein in dairy products (just as gluten is a protein in grain products), and all dairy contains protein, whether it comes from cows, goat, sheep, or camels (no, really, that's a thing). Casein sensitivity can cause digestive problems, but it might also cause skin rashes, joint pain, fatigue, or even neurological symptoms. Many of the symptoms of casein sensitivity are exactly the same as the symptoms of gluten sensitivity, or celiac disease.

Dairy products also contain saturated fat and are inflammatory in many people. High dairy consumption is also a risk factor for certain kinds of cancer, such as prostate cancer—tell your favorite men, as you take away their cheese! Dairy champions argue that it contains protein and calcium, but so do many other foods, without the problems inherent to dairy. If you must continue to eat dairy, treat it like alcohol or a sugary snack, as a once-in-a-while, special occasion treat. There is some research that shows nonfat dairy has microbiome benefits,[23] especially yogurt.[24] There is also some evidence that nonfat milk and yogurt can reduce the risk of type 2 diabetes (but only while also reducing cheese intake).[25] But again, there are plenty of other good ways to strengthen your microbiome and reduce your risk of diabetes. Cow's milk is for nourishing calves, not adult humans. You'll be healthier if you leave it to them.

Sugar Addiction

Refined cane sugar isn't likely an allergen—there isn't much to react to—but it is most definitely inflammatory in just about everyone. It is an unnaturally sweet, highly refined, highly caloric, nutrient-void substance (I wouldn't call it a food) with no merit other than it tastes good. Too good! Refined sugar overstimulates our brain's pleasure centers and causes an addiction-like reaction not unlike cocaine does. Sugar is also an appetite stimulant, so if you are trying to lose weight, sugar should probably be the first thing you cut from your diet, especially if you notice that it tends to trigger overeating.

Giving up sugar can feel very difficult at first, but if you can white-knuckle it through a couple of days, you'll find your urge to splurge lifts like magic and sugar will lose its hold on you. Some people report withdrawal symptoms when they quit sugar, but these should be gone at the seven-day mark. I save sweet treats for special occasions only, and that is my recommendation for everyone. You just don't need sugar, and it also dulls your palate. When you stop for even two days, you'll begin to notice how sweet and special naturally sweet foods like fruit actually taste. Cinnamon and the supplement chromium can help to stabilize your blood sugar while you're working on quitting, making the process feel a little bit easier.

A Slam Dunk for Weight Loss

VIBRANT PRO TIP: If you stop eating gluten, dairy products, and sugar, you're going to have a much easier time losing excess weight.

If you are tempted by fad diets, back away from the diet pills, the fake foods, and the extreme eating (or starving)! Dangling the idea of easy weight loss in front of people is a trick as old as the hills, but it doesn't usually work and it almost never works permanently. There are many reasons to go on a special diet (such as for disease intervention or for ethical reasons), but if you are doing something extreme for weight loss, it is counterintuitive to what really works. A healthy, balanced body and moderate habits will naturally calibrate you to the right weight.

But I know you want a solution. You want to feel like you are doing something to help yourself lose weight, so here's a no-brainer: Just stop eating gluten, dairy, and sugar. Not only will this reduce your inflammation significantly, but when you avoid this troublesome triplet, there isn't much left to overeat. Draw a hard line between you and gluten, dairy, and sugar, and that might be all you have to do to get to your happy weight. Not only will you cut way down on processed food and extraneous calories, but you will likely notice that you retain less water. There is no downside, other than some temporary inconvenience as you adjust. It's better for your bones, your microbiome, your blood sugar, your metabolism, and it can help ward off autoimmunity and other chronic conditions you might not know you are beginning to develop. If you do have a chronic condition, quitting gluten, dairy, and sugar could stop it in its tracks.

It's simply a win, across the board. If you also cut way back on any packaged, processed food (most of these contain gluten, dairy, and/or sugar anyway), you'll find it's pretty hard to overeat. Without bread, pasta, cheese, ice cream, or sugar, you would have to get pretty creative, and I doubt you're going to binge on broccoli. If for no other reason than weight loss, I recommend giving up gluten, dairy, and sugar. Trust me. You're only missing a fleeting "hit," but you aren't missing anything truly good.

Why a Protein Shake?

Candidly, even though it's not a whole food and has nothing to do with a Mediterranean diet, this is my secret weapon for nutrient density and convenience when I don't have time to sit down to a full, healthful meal. I drink a high-quality, nutrient-rich protein shake every day. It contains a wide range of micronutrients I could never get from food alone, based on the food quality we have available to us today. A protein shake will also maximize your macro- and micronutrients for a low calorie cost. It cuts down on the number of supplements I have to take, and I enjoy the taste.

But not just any protein shake will do. Look for brands based on pea protein and/or rice protein, not whey protein. Whey protein is made from dairy, so I avoid it for that reason, but also because the whey used in many popular protein shakes tends to be lower-quality waste whey. Some bodybuilders swear by whey protein, but if you're going for a strong, slim physique and not a bulked-up one, go with pea or rice protein. (Although, for the record, my husband disagrees and prefers whey protein!)

Also, look for formulas that are organic, unsweetened (stevia is okay), non-GMO, gluten-free and dairy-free, with a balanced macronutrient profile, at least 15 grams of protein, a complete amino acid profile, about 5 grams of fiber or higher, and with a wide range of micronutrients.

Some also contain probiotics and vegetable and fruit concentrates. (I am currently working on a Vibrant protein shake that meets all my requirements—keep an eye on vibrantdoc.com for an announcement of availability!) Incorporate one into your daily routine, whether for breakfast, lunch, or snacks. I often recommend half of a protein shake for a morning snack, and the remaining half for an afternoon snack.

VIBRANT FOODS

Changing your eating habits isn't just about going to the grocery store. It's an overhaul. How many times have you gone out and bought healthful foods, but then when it came time for dinner, you chose your old favorites? You kept meaning to use all those veggies, but eventually, they went bad in your crisper. Sound familiar?

To make a change and commit to that change means you have to reorganize. You are going to be shopping differently and stocking your pantry, refrigerator, and freezer differently. While you're at it, rethink that cabinet full of supplements. Toss out everything (food, drinks, supplements) that is expired, bad, or not in line with your goals (if you can't bear to throw away edible food, see if a friend will take it off your hands). You're going to start with a clean slate. If it is processed, in a package with more than five ingredients or any additives you don't recognize, or it contains gluten, dairy (animal milk in any form), or sugar, toss it. It's not vibrant. Take the trash to the curb so you aren't tempted to take any of it back.

After you've purged, give your kitchen a good, thorough cleaning. You are making room for vibrant food! Clean, beautiful food deserves a clean, beautiful kitchen. Clean out all the shelves and drawers in the refrigerator and freezer. Wipe down the pantry shelves. You are getting inspired to be a vibrant cook! You are prioritizing your vibrancy! And you are putting food into perspective. It's not a crutch. It's not a pacifier. It's not an antidepressant. It's not for entertainment. It's to nourish you and help your body do all the magnificent things it is capable of doing. (But that doesn't mean you're not going to enjoy every bite.)

For those of you who live with (and cook for) others, I do want to say that I understand how difficult dietary changes can be when you are the only one in the family trying to get healthier. That is why I always recommend getting the whole family on board. Get them excited about living a vibrant life. Tell them how good you are all going to feel and how much more energy you will all have.

If you are the one who shops and cooks, this is even easier because you can make what you're going to make and the rest of the family won't have much of a choice, but assure them you will still be making tasty food. Only the junk is off the menu. Kids may need more fat and calories than you do since they are still growing, but they definitely don't need gluten, dairy, or sugar. There are lots of kid-friendly foods without them.

If you have a hard time convincing your family (or just your partner), you may have to stand up for your own self-care, even if everyone else in your household is a hot mess or a negative influencer. Sometimes it's hard to take a stand, but think of it as a matter of life or death . . . or at least a matter of becoming the vibrant person you were always meant to be. Your family is going to like that person. A lot. You can do this. Doctor's orders!

This can be easier when the rules are very clear. When I advise people how to eat, I like to give them a list of foods, and set them free to eat those foods in whatever way they like, but a list really helps to keep you in the right zone. If you eat from the food list in this chapter most of the time, you'll be making significant progress toward building health and giving your body everything it needs to heal and thrive. If the only foods in your house are from this list, it gets much easier. The two-week meal plan at the end of this chapter offers ideas for breakfasts, lunches, dinners, and snacks, but it is only for inspiration, to show you how a vibrant diet can work. Or, just use it to spark your own culinary creativity. You'll also find forty Vibrant Recipes, starting in chapter eleven. You don't have to follow the meal plan or use the recipes. You can make whatever you want out of these vibrant foods, or experiment remaking your favorite recipes using these foods instead of less healthful ingredients. But for those who like more direction, you can use the meal plan to practice eating vibrantly, until you get the hang of it.

Once you get used to eating vibrantly, the change will be noticeable, not just to you but to everyone around you. You're going to start feeling fantastic. The initial effort it takes to change your habits will pay off and you will begin to see it as a doorway into a different way of eating, feeling, and living. I bet it won't take long for you to feel more energy, and if you need to lose a few pounds, that will probably start happening very soon. But be patient. Consistency is key, and if you eat vibrant foods in moderate portions, over time your body will recalibrate back to its normal weight.

HOW TO DESTROY A SUPERFOOD

There are certain foods people call "superfoods" because they are particularly rich in health-promoting nutrients. These include things like blueberries, kale, nuts and seeds, salmon, edible mushrooms, leafy greens, seaweed, avocado, broccoli, yogurt, green tea, garlic, and dark chocolate. You'll find that the Vibrant Food List includes many of these superfoods, but a word of caution: When the industrial food system gets ahold of superfoods, it often processes them in ways that neutralize their superpowers and turn them into junk food. It's practically criminal!

For instance, almonds are a fantastic food (in moderation, due to their calorie density), but when you roast them in highly processed cheap industrial seed oils known for being inflammatory and cover them with salt and other artificial flavorings, you can no longer call them a superfood. And just look at what they've done with kale! You can make perfectly delicious and healthful kale chips at home (I've got a simple, clean recipe for you on page 300), but if you buy a bag of kale chips in the store, they are likely to be loaded with inflammatory fats, salt, preservatives, and artificial flavorings, not to mention plasticizers from the packaging. You can hardly call them a superfood.

When blueberries are coated with oil and sugar and dried and packaged, they lose their superfood status, too. They become more like candy than the beautiful low-sugar, high-antioxidant berry they once were. Probiotic-rich yogurt also becomes a dessert when loaded with sugar, artificial colors, and flavorings. The trick with superfoods is to eat them in their most natural form. Fresh veggies, fresh berries, raw nuts and seeds, plain plant-based yogurt. If you prepare them at home with the least invasive cooking methods, like steaming, baking, or a light sauté with a bit of olive oil, you'll be honoring these superfoods instead of destroying them.

Your Vibrant Food List

This food list is divided into animal proteins, plant proteins, non-starchy vegetables, starchy vegetables, fruits, fats, grains, plant-based "dairy," nuts/seeds, herbs/spices, beverages, and miscellaneous. Under each section, some of the foods are noted as Core Foods. These are the foods to eat most of the time. You'll also see Use Sparingly lists. These are foods that have nutritional merit, but they also tend to be easy to overdo, so I recommend you limit them. I'll give more specific advice along with some of the foods in the lists, as needed. I'll also let you know what I consider to be a portion, so you can begin to get used to what a normal amount of food really looks like. (Many people honestly don't know and typically overestimate.)

For a printable
version of this list,
go here.

ANIMAL PROTEIN
FISH 6 OUNCES PER SERVING, ALL OTHER MEAT
4 OUNCES PER SERVING, A SERVING OF EGGS IS 2

CORE FOODS (in order of preference)

- Wild-caught cold-water fatty fish (no white fish, no bottom feeders—ONLY the following):
  - Alaskan wild salmon
  - Ahi tuna
  - Atlantic herring
  - Atlantic mackerel
  - Sardines
  - Trout

- Game meats, all types: venison, elk, buffalo/bison, pheasant, etc., 4 ounces per serving
- Lamb, 4 ounces per serving
- Lean grass-fed beef, 4 ounces per serving
- Organic-only poultry (chicken, turkey, duck, etc.), 4 ounces per serving
- Organic eggs

Use Sparingly (in order of preference)
- Scallops, 4 ounces per serving
- Shrimp, 4 ounces per serving, should be wild-caught only from the Pacific, not the Atlantic or Gulf

> **NOTE:** *Avoid shrimp from India, Indonesia, Bangladesh, Vietnam, Thailand, and Mexico as well as all shrimp that is farmed, grown in ponds, or caught with bottom trawling.*[26]

- All other shellfish, 4 ounces per serving: crab, lobster, clams, oysters, langostino, etc.

PLANT PROTEINS
½ CUP OR 4 OUNCES PER SERVING

Use Sparingly (if you are a vegetarian, these can be core foods)
- Beans, peas, lentils, edamame (canned, rinsed, and drained, or prepared from dried)
- Hummus
- Non-GMO organic tofu
- Non-GMO organic tempeh

NON-STARCHY VEGGIES (FRESH OR FROZEN)
SERVING SIZES UNLIMITED

Core Foods
- All, preferably organic (e.g., all leafy greens, broccoli, cauliflower, Brussels sprouts, asparagus, onions, garlic, mushrooms, etc.) and brightly colored vegetables (tomatoes, peppers, carrots, summer squashes, zucchini, etc.)

STARCHY VEGGIES (FRESH)
SERVING SIZE 1 MEDIUM OR ½ CUP COOKED

USE SPARINGLY
- All except white/yellow/red potatoes, preferably organic (such as sweet potatoes, yams, purple/blue potatoes, winter squashes like acorn and butternut, pumpkin, fresh peas, fresh corn, parsnips, rutabagas, turnips)

FRUITS
SERVING SIZE 1 MEDIUM PIECE OR 1 CUP RAW

NOTE: *No more than 1 cup or piece of fruit per day, preferably in the morning or before exercise.*

CORE FOODS
- All berries, fresh or frozen, unsweetened, no additives

USE SPARINGLY
- All other fresh or frozen, unsweetened, no additives

OILS/FATS
SERVING SIZE 1 TABLESPOON

CORE FOODS
- Extra-virgin olive oil, to eat on salads
- Olive oil for cooking
- Avocado oil
- Grapeseed oil

USE SPARINGLY
- Coconut oil, only small amounts for cooking (no coconut milk) (Children can have more.)
- Cold-pressed raw nut or seed oils, for flavor, all, such as walnut oil, almond oil, sesame oil, hazelnut oil, etc.

GRAINS: GLUTEN-FREE ONLY!
SERVING SIZE ½ CUP COOKED

USE SPARINGLY
- Gluten-free ancient grains only: quinoa, amaranth, millet, buckwheat, and certified gluten-free oats
- Organic brown rice

DAIRY
SERVING SIZES 1 CUP MILK, 6 OUNCES OR ½ CUP OF YOGURT, 2 OUNCES OR ¼ CUP CHEESE:

USE SPARINGLY
- Goat's milk, or yogurt or cheese made from goat's milk
- Sheep's milk, or yogurt or cheese made from sheep's milk
- Non-dairy milks, yogurts, and cheeses made from organic nuts, seeds, or gluten-free grains; must be unsweetened (such those made from almonds, coconuts, oats, hemp, cashew, hazelnut, etc.)

NUTS/SEEDS, RAW ONLY, NEVER ROASTED, SALTED, OR FLAVORED
2 TABLESPOONS TOTAL PER SERVING IN ANY RECIPE

CORE FOODS
- Walnuts, almonds, pistachios, Brazil nuts, sesame seeds, pumpkin seeds, flaxseeds, and chia seeds

USE SPARINGLY
- All other nuts, such as cashews, pecans, hazelnuts, macadamia nuts

HERBS AND SPICES, PURE ONLY, NO PURCHASED STORE MIXES

CORE FOODS
- All, fresh or dried, use liberally—these have many health benefits, unlimited serving size

- Natural unprocessed salt, such as natural sea salt, Himalayan salt, black salt, gray salt, etc., no more than 1 teaspoon per serving in any recipe
- Pepper, all types (black, white, red), unlimited serving size

SWEETENERS, NATURAL ONLY
SERVING SIZE MAX 1 TABLESPOON

Use Sparingly
- Real maple syrup
- Raw honey
- Agave nectar
- Pure date syrup
- Coconut sugar
- Molasses
- Brown rice syrup

BEVERAGES

Core Foods
- Spring water, unlimited
- Green tea, no more than 4 cups of tea total per day
- White tea, no more than 4 cups of tea total per day

Use Sparingly (if at all)
- Organic black coffee, no more than 16 ounces per day
- Organic black tea, no more than 16 ounces per day
- Wine, no more than 4 ounces per day
- Beer, no more than 12 ounces per day
- Unsweetened alcoholic drinks, no more than 2 ounces of alcohol per day, must be gluten-free

Go here for tips on how to eat vibrantly when you're not at home.

YOUR VIBRANT MEAL PLAN

For those of you who love a plan, below is an example of how you could use the Vibrant Recipes in chapter eleven to create a simple, healthful, vibrant meal plan. This is just an example. You could eat any of the recipes you like as often as you like, or make your own recipes from the food list, but I hope this will inspire you to see how delicious, vibrant, health-building, and energy-enhancing your meals can be.

I also want to give you a few words of encouragement here. Some people see a meal plan and think they have to be perfect, but nobody can stick to a food list or a meal plan all the time. Sometimes you're traveling, or extra stressed, or you just fall off the wagon when you're really hungry. That's okay. I do it, too.

What I most want you to remember when this happens is to listen to your body. If you do, you will notice that while overeating or eating things that aren't vibrant foods may feel good for a frantic few seconds of indulgence, it ultimately isn't satisfying. Maybe you'll tinker around with some of those packaged, processed, gluten-free foods or you'll eat something really sugary or fatty or you'll drink too much wine or whatever it is. When you are paying attention to how your body reacts to the messages you are sending it through the foods you eat, you're going to begin to notice that the reaction isn't a good one. You might notice an energy dip or a rise in irritability. You might get puffy or bloated for a while or just feel generally less good than usual. That is your body saying: "Let's not do this too often." You might decide to do it anyway, but just know that you will not feel as good as soon, nor will you lose weight as quickly, and with too many missteps, your weight could stall, or even start going back up.

So, listen up. Your body is talking, and it is wise. Just keep your eye on the prize. Getting healthy is a long game in some ways, but in other ways, every bite you take is effecting changes in your body within minutes, either for better or for worse. You are influencing your weight, your energy, and your health right down to the cellular level. Food is the communicator, so communicate well and that's how you'll feel.

Here's one way to do it:

SAMPLE 2-WEEK VIBRANT MEAL PLAN

	BREAKFAST	LUNCH	SNACK	DINNER
DAY 1	Berry Beautiful Parfaits (page 274)	Ground Turkey Taco Salad Bowls (page 285)	Sliced Blood Oranges with Shaved Dark Chocolate (page 297)	Roasted Salmon with Blueberry Compote (page 309)
DAY 2	Tropic Green Smoothie (page 276)	Creamy Roasted Cauliflower Soup (page 286)	Refreshing Sliced Cucumber with Hand-Smashed Guacamole (page 304)	Roasted Butternut Squash and Kale Hash (page 316)
DAY 3	Mermaid Bowl with Blue Butterfly Pea Powder (page 275)	Smoked Salmon Niçoise Salad with Dijon Tarragon Dressing (page 292)	Date and Pecan Power Truffles (page 303)	Mackerel with Zucchini Wrapped in Parchment (page 308)
DAY 4	Quinoa Breakfast Bowl with Sautéed Apples (page 278)	Gingery Sesame Tuna Poke Bowls (page 289)	Frozen Berry Beauty "Nice Cream" (page 299)	Slow Cooker Bison Stew (page 312)
DAY 5	Chicken Sausage Breakfast Skillet (page 279)	Roasted Beets over Leafy Greens (page 288)	Ruby-Throated Dragon Mocktail (page 306)	Mediterranean Ahi Steaks with Roasted Red Pepper Compote (page 311)
DAY 6	Chocolate Cherry Bomb Smoothie (page 277)	Greek Roasted Salmon Power Bowl (page 291)	Clean Turmeric and Paprika Roasted Kale Chips (page 300)	All-Day Elk Bolognese with Zucchini Noodles (page 315)
DAY 7	Summer Patty Pan Egg Cups (page 280)	Simple Massaged Kale Caesar Salad with Protein-Packed Anchovy Dressing (page 290)	Simple Family Fun Chocolate Stackers (page 301)	Cast Iron Venison Steaks (page 313)
DAY 8	Smoked Salmon and Veggie Breakfast Platter with Chive-Yogurt Sauce (page 282)	Detox Salad with Kale, Pomegranate Seeds, and Forbidden Rice (page 287)	Easy Apples with Cinnamon Raisin Almond Butter (page 302)	Summer Turmeric Chicken over Sautéed Purple Kale and Mushrooms (page 310)

SAMPLE 2-WEEK VIBRANT MEAL PLAN (CONTINUED)

	BREAKFAST	LUNCH	SNACK	DINNER
DAY 9	Turmeric Tofu Scramble (page 283)	Easy 30-Minute Roasted Chicken and Kale Soup with Bone Broth (page 293)	Frozen Banana "Nice Cream" with Madagascar Vanilla (page 298)	Tempeh Taco Lettuce Cups (page 317)
DAY 10	Mediterranean Crustless Quiche (page 281)	Ground Turkey Taco Salad Bowls (page 285)	Sliced Blood Oranges with Shaved Dark Chocolate (page 297)	Slow Cooker Bison Stew (page 312)
DAY 11	Chocolate Cherry Bomb Smoothie (page 277)	Gingery Sesame Tuna Poke Bowls (page 289)	Refreshing Sliced Cucumber with Hand-Smashed Guacamole (page 304)	All-Day Elk Bolognese with Zucchini Noodles (page 315)
DAY 12	Berry Beautiful Parfaits (page 274)	Roasted Athenian Chicken Cobb Salad (page 294)	Date and Pecan Power Truffles (page 303)	Roasted Salmon with Blueberry Compote (page 309)
DAY 13	Quinoa Breakfast Bowl with Sautéed Apples (page 278)	Creamy Roasted Cauliflower Soup (page 286)	Rosemary Release Mocktail (page 305)	Summer Turmeric Chicken over Sautéed Purple Kale and Mushrooms (page 310)
DAY 14	Chicken Sausage Breakfast Skillet (page 279)	Greek Roasted Salmon Power Bowl (page 291)	Clean Turmeric and Paprika Roasted Kale Chips (page 300)	Dijon-Encrusted Lamb Loin Chops with Cauliflower Smash (page 314)

FOOD WINS

I would love it if you jumped right in with the food list and started eating 100 percent vibrantly, but for many people, sudden changes don't stick as well as gradual ones. If you think that might be you, just start with one or two of these food wins, below. If you're more of the all-or-nothing type, go for all three at once. Work them into your day until they become habits. In chapter ten, when we go through 30 days of tips and habit formation work, we'll ease you into other vibrant habits covered in this chapter. Meanwhile, these three wins are a great start.

GO GREEN. Have three servings (cups) of green vegetables every day—anything off the above non-starchy vegetable list. A big salad can take care of all three servings, or you could have a small salad and some steamed veggies with your dinner. Mix it up if you like variety, or find one way to do it that works for you every day. As long as you get in three servings, you'll boost your nutrient intake in meaningful ways, and increase your fiber intake, too, which is great for your microbiome.

○ *I tried it! Here's how it felt:* _____

_____

_____

DRINK A PROTEIN SHAKE EVERY DAY. Find a good one, as I describe above, and let this become a habit. This is a big one to help with weight loss.

○ *I tried it! Here's how it felt:* _____

_____

_____

CHOOSE EITHER GLUTEN, DAIRY, OR SUGAR, AND GIVE IT UP FOR ONE WEEK. Any of these three might make a big difference for you, but it's pretty difficult to cut them all out at once, so pick one and start there. Eliminating gluten means eliminating everything made with wheat (like bread, bagels, muffins, cookies, crackers, cereal including oatmeal, unless it is certified gluten-free, pita bread, flour tortillas, and most baked goods), barley (including beer, unless it's gluten-free), rye (rye bread, pumpernickel bread), and certain ancient grains like spelt and kamut, farro, and freekeh. In my opinion, giving up gluten will have the greatest impact—join me in the gluten-free life!

But maybe you would rather start with something a bit easier. Eliminating dairy means giving up everything made with the milk of an animal (cow, goat, sheep), including cheese, cream, yogurt, ice cream, and anything with milk in the ingredients list. There is an ever-expanding list of non-dairy choices, so going non-dairy is easier than ever before. Try milk, cheese, yogurt, cream, even ice cream made from the "milk" of almonds, coconuts, cashews, oats, rice, hemp, flax, or peas.

Giving up sugar means avoiding all the obvious things (cake, cookies, muffins, candy, desserts) but also reading ingredients labels carefully because many savory foods contain sugar, such as salad dressing, ketchup, soup, and bread. Some people find this easy. For others, it's extremely difficult. Whichever one you choose, challenge yourself to go just one week, and pay close attention to how it affects you. This can result in valuable information from your body.

○ *I tried it! Here's how it felt:* _____

_____

_____

CHAPTER 5

The Activator: How to Move More to Live Longer

In my field of functional medicine, anti-aging medicine, and nutrition, I hear a lot of people quote Hippocrates, the Father of Modern Medicine: "Let food be thy medicine, and medicine be thy food." I have seen this quote at the front of more books than I can count on two hands (even though there is no actual proof Hippocrates ever said this). There is another Hippocrates quote (real or not, I'm not 100 percent sure) that I don't hear very often, and which I first encountered in an academic article in a scientific journal: "Walking is man's best medicine."

Walking may be the most natural human exercise[1] and it is just the beginning of what you can accomplish if you make exercise a part of your life.

AFTER FOOD, EXERCISE IS THE NEXT ELEMENT OF THE VIBRANT TRIAD AND CRITICAL FOR VIBRANCY.

I call exercise my elixir and my fountain of youth, and it's not an exaggeration. Exercise triggers a cascade of positive biochemical effects that influence every part of you, generating energy where you need it, building strength, improving brain power, enhancing flexibility, and increasing endurance. It improves your longevity for the future, it helps you lose weight incrementally, and it significantly lowers your risk of developing a chronic disease.[2] It's also changing you *as you do it*, so there's no need to wait for positive benefits. Incredible health-building changes are happening in real time. Exercise is instant gratification as well as an important investment in your future health. Without it, you cannot maximize your energy or maintain the circulation necessary for glow, which means, without it, you cannot be truly vibrant. Bottom line: Exercise activates your body to work better, defend you better, perform better, and live longer.

Science supports me on this. Over the past sixty years, study after study has demonstrated that even when making allowances for people who are in good health but don't exercise, and even despite body weight, those who exercise the least die sooner than those who exercise the most. Exercise seems to be dose-dependent. Those who exercise a little benefit a little, and those who exercise more benefit more. (There is a limit—the "sweet spot" starts at a burn of around 1,000 calories [Kcals] per week, and goes up to a burn of 3,500 per week, which means burning between 150 to 500 calories every day from exercise. Beyond that, exercise can become stressful.[3])

CALORIES IN, CALORIES OUT?

As soon as calories enter the conversation, some people's brains switch off. The very idea of calories can be stressful for someone who has struggled with dieting for years. However, calories are just energy. I'm not a calorie counter myself, but I do think some initial calculations can be useful as a general guideline. For instance, it's very useful to know your basal metabolic rate, or BMR, so you have a general idea of how to balance what you eat with how much exercise or movement you get in order to maintain your weight, or change your weight—because, of course, calories aren't just about the energy you take in from food. They are also about the energy you burn off from exercise. (That is, after all, what food is for . . . fuel for your life.)

Your BMR is the amount of energy you use just to exist, without actually doing anything active. If you eat the number of calories you need just to exist, then anything else you do above that (exercise and other active endeavors) will have to come from somewhere other than your food, which means you'll dip into your fat stores.

The new smart scales that scan your body through sensors you step on and send the information to your smartphone can tell you your weight, body fat percentage, muscle percentage, and also estimate your BMR. These are great for assessing whether you may have too much body fat or too little lean muscle, even if you are at a normal weight, in addition to helping you determine about how many calories you should be eating. Smartwatches can tell you how many calories you burn from exercise. All this information is useful in figuring out how much to eat and how much to exercise to meet your weight loss goal, or to maintain your weight.

Let's say you want to lose weight. If you have a BMR of 1,400 calories and you eat 1,400 calories a day but also exercise for 30 minutes a day, you'll need to burn fat to fuel that exercise because you used up all your food calories just existing. If you want to maintain your weight, then you can add the calories you burn from exercise onto your BMR. If you burn 300 calories from exercise, then you could eat 1,700 calories that day and not gain weight, or you could eat 1,400 calories and lose weight.

Of course, this is also an oversimplification of how metabolism works. Not everybody burns calories at the same rate from exercise, and not everybody gets the same calories from food. Everyone's metabolism is a little bit different. Still, knowing your BMR and calculating your burn can give you a good general idea of how to lose or maintain weight. That's worth doing a little math, right?

CALCULATE YOUR BMR

If you don't have a smart scale (although I do recommend them, and they have become quite affordable), you can calculate your BMR like this:

First, convert your weight to kilograms and your height to centimeters. Then:

For women: **[10 x your weight in kg] + [6.25 x your height in cm] – [5 x your age in years] – 161 = BMR**

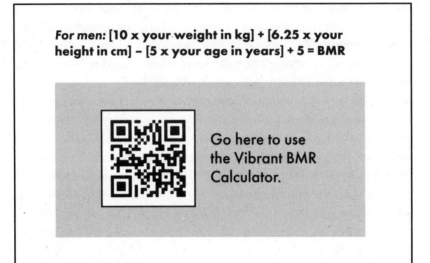

For men: [10 x your weight in kg] + [6.25 x your height in cm] – [5 x your age in years] + 5 = BMR

Go here to use the Vibrant BMR Calculator.

WHAT EXERCISE IS (AND ISN'T) FOR

As you can see, exercise is a powerful way to manipulate your weight. It allows you to eat more without gaining weight because you are burning off the fuel you eat (which, again, is the whole point of food). On top of that, it makes you feel good, sleep better, and get stronger, as I've mentioned. Why, then, isn't everybody doing it?

Why are so many gym memberships unused? Why aren't the sidewalks in every neighborhood teeming with people out for their daily walk?[4] Why do people spend so much time just sitting in front of computers and televisions and smartphones, when their very lives are at stake? I spend the winters in Arizona, and I was noticing recently how many people in my own community don't move well. We live in a state full of sunshine and beautiful weather, perfect for exercising in the winter, but I rarely see people outside walking in my community.

When I do see people walking, I often notice that they can't walk correctly, in ways that reveal their lack of physical fitness. I can tell just by watching them move that they don't exercise. Even if you are thirty pounds overweight, you should be able to move with ease and hold up your own torso without your back collapsing or your knees bowing inwards. You shouldn't waddle or limp, like so many people do because they are stiff, in pain, or weak. You shouldn't get winded walking up a flight of stairs or carrying a bag of groceries. You should be able to move with confidence and good posture and without pain.

The human body is meant to walk and bend, squat and jump, lift heavy things and carry them, and run away if necessary, even as it ages. If you are the slow one, you'll be the one who gets eaten by the bear! Yet, from what I can tell, many people can't do all those things, even in their twenties and thirties. They don't live active lives and have lost the ability to move as humans should, not because they are overweight but because they don't exercise.

I believe there are three straightforward reasons for the epidemic of sedentary living.

1. **SITTING IS EASIER THAN STANDING.** Standing is easier than walking. Walking is easier than running, and our culture prizes comfort and ease. We have designed modern life around having to move as little as possible, so especially at first, exercise *feels hard*. It makes you sweaty. You have to shower more and do more laundry. It takes time, and perhaps it doesn't feel as productive as answering your emails or doing other work at your desk.

2. **HUMANS LIKE INSTANT GRATIFICATION.** We want to do what feels good now, rather than what will feel good later. Candidly, I think people don't really believe they are actually going to die someday. Denial is a happy place, and death seems a long way off, doesn't it? Unless someone gets a wake-up call in the form of a scary diagnosis or the death of a loved one, they often don't feel any urgency to change.

3. **PEOPLE DON'T UNDERSTAND THE STAKES.** They don't always have the information that conveys how urgent exercise is for health and longevity.

I also think there is another somewhat disturbing reason. I think people are getting the wrong message about exercise. In our culture, we teach women basically one thing about exercise: It's for losing fat so you can look thin. Period. And we teach men basically one thing about exercise: It's for building muscles so you can look strong. Period. You can find plenty of research about the health benefits of exercise, but the primary push, the unspoken message we get from models and movies and constant media exposure, is that it's all about weight loss or muscle gain, to achieve some perfect ideal body.

Even if you don't think you believe this, the conditioning is insidious. Women are brainwashed with images of young, slim models with perfect, unblemished figures (often airbrushed), and men are brainwashed with images of young, burly models with bursting muscles (often due to steroids). Many women are terrified to be overweight. Many men are, too, but they are also terrified to be weak or scrawny.

These are dangerous messages, and they do the wonderful benefits of exercise a disservice. Whether it's doctors, advertisements, websites, magazines, or just "the industry" in general, the game is to exploit people's psychological vulnerabilities for profit. They are selling you something, and they depend on your fears of fatness and weakness to do it. Maybe that thing they're selling is something you genuinely want or need, but when money is involved and profit is the motive, there are always people willing to prey on your fear and bend science into a convenient shape.

The truth is that if you want to build health, feel better, and live more vibrantly, you need to get back to basics. Before you worry about any trendy health or fitness innovations, you have to build a solid foundation: Eat real, whole food, and get up and move. Quite simply, this is your one-two punch to get back to reality and back on the path to health.

It's hard. I know it is. The influences are *everywhere*. That is why we have to stay focused on the goal. But when exercise doesn't seem to accomplish those goals the way people hope it will, too often, they give up: "It's too hard." "It takes too much time." "I hate getting so sweaty every day." "It doesn't work."

I can assure you that exercise *does work*, for so much more than losing fat and gaining muscle. Those benefits are really just the tip of the proverbial iceberg.

KNOW YOUR BMI

Your BMI, or body mass index, is what doctors currently use to determine whether you are at a healthful weight or not. While it isn't accurate for every person, especially for someone who has quite a lot of weight from muscle, for most people it is a fair assessment and the range of normal is broad. Normal BMI is between 19 and 25. Obesity starts at around 31.

If you don't already know your BMI or want to keep track as you work the Vibrant Triad, go here to access the Vibrant BMI Calculator.

FINDING YOUR "WHY"

If you don't fully understand all that exercise can do for you, you may feel like you don't really need to do it, or you don't have a good reason to do it. If you've been told for most of your life that exercise is just for losing weight, and then you read that losing weight is "mostly about diet," or worse, "if you are trying to lose weight, don't exercise" (that advice really is out there), then why would you bother to break a sweat?

Our priorities have been manipulated and we are paying the price, with a nation that is fatter and less fit than ever before. Regular exercise may be *the best predictor* of health as well as longevity,[5] but people don't seem to think about that. They tend not to be future-oriented. They only think about how it will make them look, and they want to see the changes on the scale and in the mirror *now*.

The beauty of exercise is that it benefits you both now and in the future. Whenever I'm exercising, especially on those days when I don't really feel like it or exercising feels harder than usual, I remind myself that every minute I am on the treadmill or with every weight I lift, I am sending my body positive messages in real time. If I feel like quitting, I remind myself that I would be interrupting a beneficial conversation I'm having with my body, and I would stop the positive changes happening *right now*. These are changes you can't see on the scale or in the mirror, but they are real and affect how you feel immediately. When you exercise, you are shifting your blood sugar and hormone balance minute by minute, via chemical messengers that exercise sends throughout your system.

Of course, exercise also has longer-term benefits. Hundreds of them. Specifically, here's what happens while you are exercising, whether it's power walking, lifting weights, doing a downward dog pose, or swimming a lap in the pool. When you know how much it is improving your system, you can use that as motivation for why you need and even *want* to exercise regularly:

- **IMMEDIATE BENEFITS:** As you are exercising, your muscles take up glucose so if you are having a post-meal blood sugar spike, exercise can correct it fast. Regular exercise will help your blood sugar to become steadier over time, and it can actually intervene in blood sugar dysregulation immediately.

  You also burn fat as you are exercising, so you can imagine your fat cells shrinking with every step, stroke, lift, or pedal. When you exercise, your skeletal muscles release compounds that communicate with the rest of your system, changing the nature of fat cells to be more beneficial to health and increasing resistance to obesity and diabetes.[6]

  Your blood vessels dilate and your heart beats faster, which increases your circulation so blood gets shuttled around more efficiently and you get a nice glow while also building your cardiovascular fitness. This helps to deliver oxygen via the blood to your muscles, so they have more energy to power you.

  Meanwhile, blood is also traveling more rapidly to your brain, so exercise will make you more alert and aware as you are doing it, and for hours afterwards. In response to exercise, your brain produces brain-derived neurotrophic factor (BDNF), which is a substance that increases plasticity in your brain, increasing your ability to learn new things in the moment and immediately after exercise as well as triggering the release of serotonin, endorphins, and dopamine, which puts you in a better mood and can even induce feelings of euphoria.

  Your pituitary gland produces growth hormone in response to exercise, so your body burns fat for fuel, rather than muscle tissue. Your cells, perceiving the need for energy, start generating more energy, too, and that energy boost continues even after you're done exercising.

- **BENEFITS OVER THE NEXT 24 HOURS:** After a good exercise session, you will likely notice an improved mood all the way into the next day. You are likely to sleep better, with higher-quality sleep and less waking. You may have some muscle soreness if you really pushed it, but that's a good thing because it will remind you that your muscles are now rebuilding and getting stronger than they were before. You are also likely to notice more energy over the next twenty-four hours. In fact, most of the immediate benefits mentioned above are extended over the next twenty-four hours.

- **LONG-TERM BENEFITS:** If you exercise consistently (ideally a minimum of moderate to vigorous cardio 150 minutes a week— enough to get your heart rate up and actually sweat—divided up in any way that works for you) over a period of weeks or months, you will begin to notice major changes accumulating.

    You'll notice your brain works better, with clearer and quicker thinking, as it is getting a consistent dose of BDNF as well as increased blood flow. You'll tend to be in a better mood more often, and mood-related symptoms of premenstrual syndrome (PMS), if you have those symptoms, may diminish noticeably. You will likely notice more self-discipline with other habits, as you are training your brain to know that you are able to keep up with your goals.

    Your blood sugar will tend to be more stable, and you will likely lose excess weight more easily, and maintain a normal weight without much effort. Your health overall will improve as well, with more energy for running all the systems of your body and for living your life the way you want to live it. In short, you will enjoy an improved quality of life as well as health.

- **LONGEVITY BENEFITS:** People who exercise regularly live longer, on average. We know that for sure. We know that exercise can reverse many of the effects of aging,[7] improve mobility, decrease the chances of falling and injury, and decrease the chances that you will develop a chronic disease like certain cancers, heart disease, type 2 diabetes, osteoporosis, and dementia, all of which can reduce your quality of life. We know there is an "inverse, independent, and graded association between physical activity, health, and cardiovascular and overall mortality in apparently healthy individuals and in patients with documented cardiovascular disease."[8] People with active jobs sustain half the rate of coronary heart disease as people with sedentary jobs, regardless of age, gender, smoking, high cholesterol, and high blood pressure.[9] Bottom line: People who exercise are healthier all around and live longer.[10]

There is no arguing that exercise does amazing things for every part of you. What have you got to lose—other than excess weight, pain, and fatigue?

NO EXERCISE EXCUSES!

Do you think you have an excuse not to exercise? Let's see if we can get around your barriers.

- **Excuse:** I don't have time.
- **No Excuses:** Exercise doesn't have to take a long time. If you have a couple of hours, sure, you can suit up, drive to the gym, workout, take a shower, put on fresh clothes, and drive home, but if you don't have two hours to spare for exercise, you can still benefit from taking a quick 15-minute walk in the morning, maybe another at lunch, and maybe another after dinner. A 30-minute sweat session will make you feel much better than no exercise. And if you exercise at home, by walking or running around your neighborhood or doing cardio on a home treadmill, elliptical trainer, or exercise bike, or by following exercise videos, along with some simple weight training with inexpensive dumbbells and even less expensive workout bands, you can eliminate the commuting time and cut your workout time in half.

  BONUS POINTS: *Use your optional social media time, Netflix bingeing time, or your cocktail hour to exercise instead!*

- **Excuse:** I don't like gyms.
- **No Excuses:** I don't either. And gyms count on that. I've read that 63 percent of people with gym memberships never use them, and 82 percent of gym members go less than once a week, while 22 percent stop going after six months, and 31 percent say they never would have signed up to join a gym had they known that they

wouldn't use it.[11] If you join a gym and don't go, you are that gym's dream customer. They get your money for nothing!

Some people love going to the gym, and that's great, but if you don't, then I suggest not wasting your money, and sparing yourself the gym guilt. There are hundreds of ways to get active without going to a gym. Go on a hike, walk your dog (fast!), play an active game with your kids, meet your friend for a brisk walk instead of coffee, go on a bike ride, hit a tennis ball . . . the possibilities are endless. Even if you do nothing more than a brisk walk or an easy jog (or alternating between the two) for an hour on most days, you will enjoy major health improvements.

- **Excuse:** I don't know what to do.
- **No Excuses:** Start with something you like to do. Or, find exercise videos online. Many are free. Or, try a yoga class or join a walking group or try water aerobics.

- **Excuse:** Exercise makes me too hungry and I overeat. I'd rather lose weight by dieting.
- **No Excuses:** Exercise makes you hungry because you need fuel to move your body, but that is the perfect opportunity to practice giving your body what it needs. You can't exercise well on junk food or by stuffing yourself, but if you feed your body with healthful whole foods, like some fruit before you work out for energy and a protein-rich snack like plant-based yogurt or a hard-boiled egg after you work out to give your muscles something to use to get stronger, you won't be compromising your weight loss at all. You'll be helping speed it up. Hunger is not something to fear. It's something to leverage for your own benefit.

- **Excuse:** I don't like exercise.
- **No Excuses:** Then don't call it exercise. Call it play. Call it fun. Call it moving. Or do it anyway because you know it's good for you. You're a grown-up and you know perfectly well that sometimes you have to do things you don't like all that much because it's worth the result. Decide to give more structured exercise a try for two weeks because maybe you will like it if you try it. Who you are now is different than who you were the last time you tried to exercise. Your wisdom, your motivations, your intentions have all evolved. You may find that what you didn't like before has suddenly become a lot more enjoyable as you start feeling better and recognizing how much exercise helps you. In the same way you can grow to appreciate healthful foods you didn't used to like, you can grow to appreciate exercise. There are millions of converts.

START WHERE YOU ARE

I can tell people about the health benefits of exercise until I'm blue in the face, but I know there is a profound psychological element to exercise. If it sounds like too much or it represents a drastic lifestyle change, some people shy away. I've realized over time that it's important to meet people where they are when it comes to exercise. In other words, it's okay to let yourself off the hook just a little. My recommendation is and has always been this:

> EXERCISE, IN ANY AMOUNT, AT ANY LEVEL, IN ANY WAY, IS ALWAYS BETTER THAN NO EXERCISE AT ALL.

Living a physically inactive, sedentary life is self-sabotage. It increases your risk of heart disease, high blood pressure, stroke, type 2 diabetes, certain cancers including colon cancer, breast cancer, and uterine cancer, osteoporosis, obesity, frailty, depression, and anxiety.[12] Any way you can get moving will chip away at that risk and activate healthier functions. That being said, once you are hooked, I quickly follow up with this revised advice:

> MORE EXERCISE IS ALMOST ALWAYS BETTER THAN LESS.

Exercise can be a tough sell if you aren't in the habit, but once you are, it's important to push yourself just a little to keep achieving those benefits, building more energy, increasing glow, getting stronger, improving circulation and cardiovascular fitness, and enjoying the significant boost in mood. Begin where you are. Do a little. Feel how it feels. Work it into your routine, in whatever way you can. Stay activated, and notice how good it feels. Then *keep going.*

The Downside of the Body Positivity Movement

What I'm going to say next is controversial, but I also believe it is important. Yes, I'm getting on my soapbox again, so get ready! I will preface this speech with the assertion that nobody should *ever* have to feel shame or be the victim of any kind of abuse or prejudice due to their weight or shape (not to mention their color, gender, race, etc.). Obesity is a metabolic problem, not a moral failing. I believe 100 percent in "respect at any size." I also believe in "health for any body type."

But "health at any size" simply isn't true, I'm sorry to say. If you are a little overweight, that's one thing, but if you are very overweight (a BMI of over 27 and up—see page 122 or use any online BMI calculator) and you do not exercise, you *are at risk for serious health problems.* There is no argument.

That doesn't mean your weight is anybody else's business. Anybody who says "I'm only saying this to you for your own good" and isn't a doctor has no business telling you what you should or shouldn't be doing. That is shaming, plain and simple. They don't know your life. But I am a healthcare professional and I feel as if, by reading this book, you are asking for my medical opinion, so here it is.

We know *for sure* that overweight and obesity are metabolic disorders that put you at a much greater risk for type 2 diabetes, atherosclerosis, heart disease, stroke, and many forms of cancer, including colon cancer, liver cancer, endometrial (uterine) cancer, esophageal cancer, stomach cancer, kidney cancer, pancreatic cancer, thyroid cancer, rectal cancer (especially in men), breast cancer (especially in postmenopausal women), and ovarian cancer.[13] Other than smoking cessation, losing enough weight so that you are no longer obese is probably the single most powerful cancer intervention and prevention we have. We know *for sure* that overweight and obesity puts you at greater risk for developing an autoimmune disease,[14] as well as high blood pressure, high LDL cholesterol (the kind associated with heart disease risk, so you want it low), low HDL cholesterol (the kind that is protective against heart disease, so you want it high), high triglycerides (another heart disease risk), inflammation, osteoarthritis, fatty liver disease, gallbladder disease, depression, anxiety, sleep apnea, and chronic pain.[15]

But *you can do something about it.* You have the power to mitigate those risks and avoid a future of disease and disability. You really do.

So no, it's not your fault. It's not about shaming you into behavioral changes. We also know for a fact that this doesn't work, and actually has the opposite effect. Sometimes people change because of a health scare, but more often it is inspiration rather than shame that fuels real change. It's not right to shame someone because of their weight, any more than it would be right to shame someone who got cancer or had a heart attack.

But . . . if you have been convinced that your weight is not really a health problem, then I hope you will rethink this. Obesity is not a quality, like hair color or personality. It's a disease, and you will feel so much better if you cure it. But, unlike some diseases, you already have full access to the cure.

$$\text{Obesity} = \begin{cases} \textit{Cancer} \\ \textit{Heart Disease} \\ \textit{Diabetes} \\ \textit{Autoimmunity} \\ \textit{Premature Death} \end{cases}$$

This is not a political discussion or a social issue. It is a public health crisis, and a public health crisis should never be politicized. It's too important. We are talking about lives. You should be able to live a life you love while feeling strong and capable in your body. This is your right! If you care about your health, if you care about *yourself* (and I certainly hope you do, and absolutely believe that you should), and if you want to feel good, age well, and enjoy your life without physical barriers, then it's time to let go of that extra weight, deal with what that means for you psychologically, start eating vibrant foods, and *get moving.*

> NOBODY ELSE CAN DO IT FOR YOU,
> BUT NOBODY CAN STOP YOU FROM
> DOING IT FOR YOURSELF.

Even a little exercise is better than none, so it's okay to start small. What matters is that you start making good food choices in moderate portions and start moving more. Those people who say that "eat less and exercise more" is a lie are lying! This is *the formula*. With patience and commitment, you can chip away at that extra weight, and if you are consistent about it, one day you will wake up and it will be gone. That will be a good day for you, not because of how you look, but because of what it means for your life.

THE FOUR PRIMARY TYPES OF EXERCISE

I hope you've found some really great reasons in this chapter to start exercising. If for no other reason than you will feel better almost immediately, exercise is an undeniable win. Exercise can be *your* elixir, *your* fountain of youth, and *your* psychotherapist. Together, let's keep working the Vibrant Triad and figure out what kind of exercise will work best for you.

 Look here for a quiz you can take to determine what kind of exercise might best suit you.

Any movement is exercise, but to really get a full-spectrum workout, it's a good idea to alternate between four different types. They all have different benefits and strengthen different parts of you. If you only do one thing (such as walking), it's better than doing nothing, but it's not nearly as good as switching it up. Your body adjusts to what it is used to doing, so if you only do one kind of exercise, after a couple of months, you won't get as much benefit from it as you will if you keep changing what you are doing. Here are the four types of exercise I recommend, with examples of each. Think of them as your four activators in your quest to move more and live longer.

- **ACTIVATOR #1—CARDIO:** Fast walking, jogging, running, biking, stair climbing, elliptical training, rowing, and dancing—if it moves fast and gets our heart rate up, that's cardio, which is short for cardiovascular training. This kind of exercise strengthens your heart and lungs, increases circulation, and is the best kind of exercise for boosting your mood. It also releases BDNF, so it is great for keeping your brain young and sharp (more about that in chapter seven). Cardio also burns a lot of calories, and the burn continues for up to a few hours after you are finished exercising.

- **ACTIVATOR #2—RESISTANCE TRAINING:** Lifting weights, using weight machines or Pilates reformers, resistance bands, and lifting your own body weight (such as through push-ups, sit-ups, and certain yoga poses like plank and handstand) are all examples of resistance training. You might also do some resistance training while cleaning or doing yard work, or if you have to lift heavy things as part of your job.

  The primary benefit of resistant training is strengthening muscles. The stress of the weight creates micro-tears or tiny injuries in the muscle fibers. This signals your muscles (specifically, the mitochondria within your muscles) that you need to get stronger, so this generates more mitochondria and the muscle heals to be stronger than it was before. The "side effects" are more energy (because of more mitochondria) and also a higher metabolism because muscle requires more energy than other types of tissue. The more muscle you have, the more calories you burn even when you are doing nothing but sitting and breathing.

- **ACTIVATOR #3—FLEXIBILITY TRAINING:** Healthy muscles are both strong and supple, and connective tissue and joints need to move to stay flexible, so flexibility training, though often neglected, is extremely important for easy, graceful movement. Warming down after working out by gently stretching your muscles can also help reduce post-workout pain. Other types of exercise are mostly devoted to flexibility, especially yoga and some ballet-style workouts. Flexibility training can make you more graceful and less clumsy.

VIBRANT PRO TIP: If you tend to be hypermobile, meaning you are very flexible and loose-jointed or "double-jointed," be careful stretching too far. Strength training can help stabilize your joints to prevent injury and may be a better focus than flexibility training, since you already have natural flexibility.

- **ACTIVATOR #4—HIIT IT!:** HIIT stands for high-intensity interval training. HIIT workouts are short—10 to 30 minutes—but very intense. The basic way to do a HIIT workout is to alternate periods of high intensity with periods of moderate intensity or low intensity. There are many different methods, from Tabata workouts* to intuitive versions. A simple example is to walk at a moderate pace for 5 minutes; run as fast as you possibly can for 1 or 2 minutes; walk for 5 minutes again, alternating until you have done about 20 minutes. If you look online, you can find a lot of different versions, including treadmill, stationary bike, elliptical trainer, stair climber, and calisthenic versions.

WEARABLE TECH

If you love technology (or just your Apple watch), this is your time! Thanks to the trend called biohacking, which is all about finding ways to optimize health and often uses health tracking devices, there are hundreds of new products: watches that measure your steps and calories, rings that track your sleep stages and wakefulness, headbands that help you meditate, and bracelets that monitor your oxygen levels when you sleep, and more products coming out all the time. And it's not just wearable tech—now we have smart scales, workout machines that track your heart rate, and even machines like Peloton bikes and smart mirrors to help motivate and inspire you to exercise more, and more efficiently. It's pretty exciting!

---

* If you are interested in Tabata, you can watch a video of Dr. Tabata, the inventor, explaining it. "Tabata Training Message from Professor Izumi Tabata." YouTube video, 1:54. Posted by Ritsumeikan Channel, July 14, 2015. https://www.youtube.com/watch?v=R6diyOp1TAo.

To be honest, I don't use wearable tech very often, but I also have a lot of experience with fitness so I feel like I don't necessarily need it to motivate me. However, I do appreciate how much it can motivate people, and if it works for you, by all means, use it to the extent you want and can afford. Health technology is one more way that you can gain knowledge and get feedback about your body so you can feel even more empowered to take control of your own health and make good lifestyle decisions. A good place to start is with a smartwatch. Newer ones can measure many aspects of your fitness. Some even have an ECG, which can catch atrial fibrillation (racing or irregular heartbeats). These watches can track what exercises you do, how many steps you took, how far you went, how many calories you consumed, how many calories you burned, and more, all synched to your smartphone and dropped into helpful graphs. You can set goals, do challenges, and monitor your progress, and the watch can tell you when you've been sitting for too long and when to take a minute for deep breathing. And, as I mentioned before, they are likely to be able to do even more in the coming years, like measure blood sugar, and maybe even give you other information about your blood and other body functions.

Fitbit and Apple have long been the major players in the wearable tech game, but many other companies are now making competitive products, so shop around and decide what you like. They also come in a range of styles, from sporty to high-fashion. If the numbers motivate you or you have biohacking tendencies, give wearable tech a try. I expect this exciting market will only continue to innovate, expand, and become increasingly available and affordable.

However . . . one caveat. Once upon a time, a scale, a watch, a pedometer, a heart rate monitor were all either analog or digital but not connected to the internet. Now that all of these technologies are synched with apps and store your information "in the cloud," that information is (or might be) out there, from your weight to your blood pressure to your disease status. This creates a question of privacy because this health data is not 100 percent secure. It could potentially be accessed by other people without your knowledge. It brings up questions of confidentiality and even questions about who actually owns your private information. I would much prefer that only you owned your personal health data, and you may choose not to use these devices in a way that compromises that confidentiality. On the other hand, for many people, that risk is worth the benefits they get from health technology and the convenience of easy access to data and activity tracking. It's your choice, and just something to be aware of.

. . .

Now that you have a good idea about how to approach exercise in a way you'll enjoy, I want to leave you with one final thought:

> # NO EXERCISE WILL WORK FOR YOU
> # IF YOU DON'T DO IT.

It's better to find an activator you love, even it seems less strenuous to you or less like real exercise, than to try to do something you won't be able to keep doing for life. We are meant to move our bodies, but it doesn't really matter how, as long as we do it vigorously and consistently, and even if you start with something easy, the energy, strength, and motivation you will gain will help you to want more. It's your time to glow.

EXERCISE WINS

You may already have a plan, but if you are still thinking about how to ease in, pick one, two, or all three of these exercise wins to get you started. Integrate these into your routine at your own pace, until exercise has become your new favorite habit (or if not your favorite, at least something you can see sustaining for the next ten years or more).

STAND UP FOR YOURSELF. Sitting is the new smoking, as they say, so if you sit for most of your day, easing out of that state is a first step toward a more active life. For three days, keep track of how much time you spend sitting during the day. Include work, computer time, relaxing time, driving time, and evening screen time (whether it's your tablet, your phone, or the television). Once you have an average, see if you can cut that number in half. There are many ways to do this. Walk around when you're on the phone, do other seated tasks standing when possible, see if you can get a standing desk wherever you do most of your work (these are getting less expensive and many are adjustable to multiple heights), or work frequent breaks into your day to get up, do some stretching, and walk around. Could you walk to work, or park farther away? Could you ride your bike? (Riding a bike does not count as sitting time!) Can you walk on your lunch hour, or after work before dinner? Can you do exercises while watching TV instead of sitting on the couch? Every minute of sitting you remove from your day is a minute that moves you toward your health goals, rather than away from them.

○ *I tried it! Here's how it felt:* _____

_____

_____

MIX IT UP. Shake up your routine by trying something new. If you don't currently exercise, try some form of exercise, even if it's just walking. If you normally walk or do cardio, try strength training or yoga. If you normally do weight training and floor exercises, work in some cardio. Or try something you've never done before, like tennis or racquetball, yoga or tai chi, weight machines or resistance bands. Exercise is more interesting if you change it up and give yourself new experiences.

○ *I tried it! Here's how it felt:* _____

_____

_____

PUSH YOURSELF. Exercise can be stressful and you don't want to overdo it, but you definitely don't want to underdo it, either. On the days when you feel energetic, you will benefit a lot by increasing your endurance and strength if you push yourself just a bit out of your comfort zone. Don't injure yourself or go so hard that you feel ill, but just go a little past what you think you can do. Push through the "I can't" feelings. You *can.* The next time you exercise, see if you can go a little bit faster, a little bit farther, or a little bit heavier than what you normally do. Pushing yourself is how you get stronger.

○ *I tried it! Here's how it felt:* _____

_____

_____

CHAPTER 6

The Connector: How Human Connection Supports Physical and Mental Health

The third side of the Vibrant Triad is about something you don't often see discussed in health books, yet it is just as influential to health as what you eat and how much you exercise. You cannot feel vibrant if you don't have meaningful relationships, or if the relationships you have are unhappy or troubled. According to the Holmes-Rahe Life Stress Inventory,[1] which is a widely used stress assessment scale to determine the risk of experiencing a stress-induced health breakdown (since we know for sure that stress impacts health), the top five most stressful life events are about relationships. They are:

1. Death of a spouse or child
2. Divorce
3. Marital separation

4. Imprisonment (I consider this to be a form of social isolation)

5. Death of a close family member

While some of the remaining items are about work and money, overall, most of the 43-item list of top stressors is about relationships, either directly or indirectly. Other relationship stressors on the list include marriage, marital reconciliation, sexual difficulties, major changes in the health or behavior of a family member, troubles with the boss, and major changes in church and social activities.

Go here to take the Vibrant Stress Assessment Test.

Humans are social creatures, so while troubled relationships are our most potent stressors, supportive, loving relationships are perhaps our most powerful stress relievers. When you feel understood, loved, and supported by the people around you—your partner, your family, your friends, your community—you are much less likely to suffer health problems. The science is clear and the results are straightforward. For decades, many studies have illustrated that those with positive relationships live the longest[2] and those without strong social ties are more likely to develop depression and cognitive decline in old age.[3] People who live in isolation without meaningful contact with others are much more likely to develop diseases, including heart disease and cancer.[4] One study showed that those with fewer positive relationships were twice as likely to die prematurely, which is equal to the risk of being obese, never exercising, or smoking fifteen cigarettes a day.[5] There is no doubt that we need each other to be vibrant.

ROMANCE, LOVE, AND MARRIAGE

There are many ways to have relationships and they are all beneficial, but what most people crave is a romantic partnership with one primary person (whether or not they get married), or at least fulfilling, supportive companionship. Most people want to find "their person" sooner or later, even if they are enjoying being single in the moment. It is our human destiny to be in relationships (and I recognize that relationships can have many different forms), and people will do just about anything to create them, even when other people aren't available. That's why we are so bonded to our pets, and even to things like houses and cars. We make relationships out of everything because we all want to love and be loved.

Love is complicated. Especially now, when traditional gender roles are often no longer relevant and nobody is exactly sure what their place is, figuring out how to interact with a romantic partner, especially when living together, can be confusing. Who makes the money? Who is the protector? Who does most of the housework? Who manages the tasks of daily living? Who takes care of the kids? These issues can cause resentments, and feelings of disempowerment.

Love is also social. Are you still "supposed to" get married? Have children? Do your parents expect it? What will the neighbors think? More and more relationships are nontraditional, and that can sometimes still result in stressful social pressure.

Love is psychological. We all have programming from childhood about what love looks like, and many people continue to repeat mistakes from the past because that is all they know.

Love is also definitely biochemical. That initial rush of passion and infatuation is really more about attraction than actual love, though people often mistake that euphoric and irresistible feeling of longing and desire as love. It's hard to be logical about your relationship in those first few months of romance, but what's really going on is hormonal (as are many of our emotions). Hormones are the connection between physical and mental health because they influence how we feel about things. They play a role in every part of the Vibrant Triad, influencing food cravings, motivation, energy, and passion. They have more power than you might realize.

I'm going to put on my doctor hat for a moment and explain what love does to your endocrine system. It's a dance of rising and falling levels of hormones,[6] including:

- **CORTISOL:** The notorious stress hormone, cortisol, rises with initial attraction. This is a stress response but one that energizes and excites you, creating a feeling of tension and sexual desire. It is more like an acute response than a chronic response, and when the relationship settles in, cortisol levels should return to normal.

- **DOPAMINE:** Increases in dopamine can cause that euphoric, weak-in-the-knees, I-can't-be-apart-from-this-person feeling. It is an intense desire for physical and emotional bonding. This can last for a few months or up to a year.

- **SEROTONIN:** Falling serotonin can cause feelings of obsession and rash behavior, like when you're tempted to drive by your beloved's home over and over or secretly track their every move on the internet because you just can't get enough of them. This may be a primal response to help us overcome any barriers to reproduction. This is also temporary and should be back to normal after a few months or up to a year.

- **OXYTOCIN:** Oxytocin is the bonding hormone released by physical contact that helps mothers bond to their babies, makes hugs feel so good, and helps you stay connected to your beloved even after your serotonin level goes back up to normal. This is the hormone largely responsible for the long-term relationship glue, and it is released during intimate contact, which is one biochemical reason why couples who stop having sex often feel like they have lost their connection.

Layer societal expectations, from romantic anticipation ("he's 'the one'!") to familial obligation ("my family expects me to marry her"), on top of that hormonal cocktail, then add a dash of dysfunctional programming (such as choosing partners based on destructive patterns established during past relationships, or assuming a partner will fix all your problems for you) and you've got a complex set of physical, emotional, and psychological expectations going on in your head that aren't always going to be fulfilled. With every new layer, relationships get more complicated. One example is that raising children is, by many accounts, the biggest source of stress in romantic/marital relationships.[7]

Yet, despite the challenges and the emotional roller coaster, eventually most people pair up and settle down into a rhythm, and there are health benefits to doing this. There have been a lot of studies on marriage in particular (although I assume the results would mostly apply to any sort of domestic partnership). People who are married are less likely to be depressed than single people, and when it comes to living longer, married people also have an advantage. Scientists have been researching the effect of relationships on health and longevity for decades, and the results have been pretty consistent that people who are married live longer than people who are not married, including those who have never been married, are divorced, or are widowed.[8]

Most studies show that men are the most susceptible to this (and all) marriage benefits. Married men tend to be happier, less stressed, less depressed, healthier, and more long-lived than married women, which is something worth further study, in my opinion. Conversely, people in unhappy marriages are much more likely to be depressed than single people, including those who have been divorced or widowed, but this effect is more pronounced in women. In one study that looked at both men and women who were single, married happily, married unhappily, divorced, and widowed, women in unhappy marriages had the highest depression rates at nearly 50 percent,[9] higher than any other category. When marriages are happy, however, both partners benefit. So, how do you turn an okay relationship into a vibrant relationship?

If you aren't particularly happy in your relationship, there are ways to fix it. You don't have to go on with your life feeling like your relationship is mediocre or "good enough." There are action steps you can take to prepare yourself to be a better partner, and there are action steps you and your partner can both take to create the relationship you always dreamed of having. Remember, there are three sides to the Vibrant Triad. The daily choice to nurture your human connections is just as important as making healthy food choices and moving your body more. You can eat the purest organic whole foods and exercise every day, and still suffer mentally and physically if you don't also value and foster your relationships, and feel valued and supported within those relationships. Later in this chapter, I'll share some secrets from my relationship coach, with whom my husband and I have been working since we first met.

But not every relationship is a good relationship, and a bad relationship is worse than no relationship at all. Let's talk about that first, because not every relationship is worth fixing.

WHAT I LEARNED FROM AN ABUSIVE RELATIONSHIP

I'm going to get personal here and write about something I've never really talked about publicly before. When I was a young doctor in private practice, I was in an abusive marriage. For a long time, I didn't want to admit that to myself. I didn't think I fit the profile of an abuse victim. I was a successful entrepreneur who worked hard to build a private practice in a Midwestern suburb. I was ambitious, driven, well educated, and had a strong personality. I never experienced or witnessed any abuse in my background. I'm not from a broken home (my parents divorced when I was in my twenties). I had a great relationship with my parents, and they had an egalitarian partnership that was a good marriage role model for me.

And yet, somehow, I ended up in a marriage with a man who physically and emotionally battered me. There were many times when I was threatened, insulted, manipulated, and literally strangled until I lost consciousness. I hid it from everyone because I was ashamed. I didn't want to admit that I had gotten myself into this situation. I didn't want to fail. I thought I could fix it. I made so many excuses for why I didn't leave, but thank God I finally did because, truthfully, I survived within an inch of my life.

During that time, I was under incredible stress, and the health impact was devastating. I had chronic migraine headaches, I barely ate anything, and my hormones were essentially flatlined, as if my endocrine system had given up and turned itself off. As a functional medicine doctor, I had access to the tests I gave my patients, so I knew that my thyroid hormone, estrogen, testosterone, and progesterone were all very low, but my cortisol was extremely high. I had all the symptoms of post-traumatic stress disorder (PTSD), except I was still in the middle of the trauma. Some small part of me (the doctor part) knew that if I didn't take care of myself physically, I was headed for a major health crisis, so I became very strict with myself about the things I could control. When I could manage to eat, it was always gluten-free, dairy-free, and organic. I did yoga every day, and also spent a lot of time meditating and praying. For a time, I didn't know how to get out of my situation, but at least I was doing what I could, and I suspect I never would have been able to fully heal from that trauma if I hadn't been taking those important self-care steps.

The day I told my husband that I was moving out—that I would not see anyone else, nor would I seek divorce, but that I could not live with him anymore—he took out his gun and shot at me three times, at point-blank range. Somehow, he missed, or I would not be here to write this book. That was when I knew I had to get all the way out.

He wasn't arrested for that incident because he didn't hurt me and claimed it was an accident, but we both knew better. I was lucky. I survived, but after I left, he stalked me relentlessly, and stole most of my money and my profitable practice. My work had been everything to me. I had spent years learning and training and investing in my education and my business, and he destroyed it all. He took everything from me but my life, and I had to start all over again.

For many years, I didn't tell anyone about this. I didn't want to involve my ex-husband's family, or put myself at risk by angering him further. But he has since passed away, and I feel a freedom I didn't feel before to share this with you, my readers, because I know that many people are in a similar situation. What I want you to know, if you are a victim of abuse, is that there is a life on the other side of where you are now. (There is also help for you right now. You can call the National Domestic Violence Hotline and talk to someone for free, to get help and support. Call: 1–800–799–7233.) You can come out of this and start over.

Leaving is hard in many ways. For some women, it's not so much the relationship but the finances. I understand the thought that you can take another beating but you can't take homelessness. What about your job? Your bank account? Your kids? There are many reasons to convince yourself to stay, but there are resources out there and people to help you if you leave. Who will stand up for you if you don't stand up for yourself? It was one of the hardest things I did. During that marriage, there were three major episodes of violence, after which I went back to him. It wasn't until the gun incident that I was finally able to break free, but it wasn't until he began aggressively stalking me and threatening to kill me that he was charged and had to leave me alone.

When the police finally took action (because of the stalking and death threats), they told me that, other than the fact that I didn't have any children (thank goodness, in this case), I perfectly fit the profile of someone who would ultimately be murdered by their abuser. I was surprised to learn that someone like me would fit a profile like that, but I guess abused women (and men) don't always "look the part."

It's hard to leave. I get it. But what if I hadn't done it? What if you don't do it?

For a long time after my divorce, I did nothing but take care of myself and try to heal. I decided I could start over with a clean slate. In many ways, I was very happy to be single because I was finally free. I could do whatever I wanted. I could work hard all day and all night, or I could come home and lie on the couch and do absolutely nothing. I didn't have to contend with anyone else, compromise with anyone else, or try to be anyone else. I spent a long time getting reacquainted with myself and thinking about what had happened to me. I found my way back to my own power and my own voice. I was determined never to get into a situation like that again. At first, I thought I would never remarry. I didn't want to get fooled again. And if I were to get into a relationship, I decided I would be very, very careful.

And then I met Mr. Amazing.

I met my husband as I was coming out of an elevator to give a presentation to the board of the Cancer Treatment Centers of America. He was holding a stack of papers and folders, and as I stepped out of the elevator, he took one look at me and dropped them all over the floor. (He loves to tell this story. It's so cute. He also likes to say how I didn't recognize the large formal portrait on the wall of the founder of CTCA—the portrait of him. It's true I didn't know who he was at first.) CTCA was interviewing me as a possible candidate to join their staff because they wanted to bring on a functional medicine doctor. My presentation went well, and I went home, feeling good about the interview. Little did I know that the charming gentleman who had dropped his papers on the floor was already smitten with me. And so, we began, cautiously, to date.

At the time, he, too, was dealing with a contentious divorce, so both of us were nervous about starting up with someone new. We both had emotional scars and were wary. Neither of us was willing to make another big mistake. That's why, when he asked if I would talk to his relationship coach, Dr. Jay Ferraro, I wasn't offended. I was more than happy to have a professional involved in helping us determine whether we were right for each other.

As our relationship deepened, we continued to work with Dr. Jay, and it was the best decision we ever made. He helped us at each step of the way, to stay true to who we were, define what we wanted, avoid the destructive patterns in our pasts, and decide what we were willing and able to do for and in our relationship. He helped us build a rock-solid foundation that gave us both the confidence and support to realize that marriage would work for us.

We recently celebrated our sixth anniversary (after a long and careful courtship), although my husband insists it was actually our tenth anniversary, since, as he puts it, "I married you the moment I met you." (He's so adorable.) We still work regularly with Dr. Jay, to help us navigate the inevitable rough patches, to give us perspective, and to keep us honest and real with ourselves as well as with each other. We both work very hard to nurture our relationship and put it first. Although there is an age gap between us, we have the same values, we want the same things from life, we care about the same issues, and we make each other laugh. He is the love of my life, and he has made all my dreams come true.

My husband made me believe in love again. As a romantic aside, I'll tell you a quick story. All my life, I used to dream that a big, dark-blue airplane was flying overhead. It would slow down as it passed me, and I would look up at it and wonder what it was. I had this dream many times over the years. A short time after my husband and I started dating, he told me we would charter a private plane for a very special surprise date. When I saw it, I recognized it. It looked exactly like the plane I had dreamed about my whole life.

Meanwhile, my husband was trying to get things right in his own life, so one of his friends asked him to write down a description of the perfect woman for him. He spent a lot of time writing this list and it was very detailed. His friend took the list and used it to set him up with various people, but it was never right. After we'd been dating for a while, he showed me the list. It was an exact description of me, almost like he had painted me with words.

This is all just to say that we both feel it was fate. We have a spiritual connection that is beyond anything I could have imagined in my past relationships. Sometimes he says that a part of him always knew he was waiting for me to be born, and to grow up, so we could meet. My life is so different now from when I was in that abusive relationship. If any of my history resonates for you, I want to say that you don't know what's waiting for you out there, but unless you get away from your abuser, you'll never get a chance to find out.

If it wasn't for that abusive relationship, I never would have worked so hard to make my current marriage work, and I might not have waited long enough to find the right person. I was also able to do it because of that time I took on my own, taking care of myself and learning to have compassion for myself. I built up health reserves that I was able to use when my emotional reserves were exhausted, and as soon as I was free, I built my emotional reserves back up before letting myself commit to anyone else other than myself.

What I learned from this experience is this:

1. Where you are now does not dictate where you will always be.

2. You do not deserve to be treated badly by anyone.

3. Healthy relationships do not involve physical or emotional violence, shaming, insults, or being made to feel like you are a bad or inferior person.

4. You can't change other people, but you can change yourself.

5. Self-care and self-development now will help you survive. Don't wait to start taking care of yourself.

6. If you are careful with your heart but willing to keep pursuing your dream life, you can find the relationship that will make your life better, not worse.

YOUR RELATIONSHIP WITH YOURSELF

Do you have that friend who can't be without a romance in her life? Or, maybe it's you. Romance is a lovely thing, exciting and full of promise, but when you are in a romance, it's easy to lose sight of yourself, at least in those initial swept-away stages. It's an addictive feeling, and can come with the side effect of you not doing any self-examination. I think that's why some people can't be without it. If you are focused on somebody else, you don't have to focus on yourself. Sometimes people, women in particular, think it's selfish to focus on themselves, and we put everybody else first, or we're afraid of what we might find out about ourselves if we look too closely. Yet, you can't be in a truly healthy relationship until you know who you are.

Our relationship coach, Dr. Jay, talks about this. After a divorce, he decided to spend a year working on himself. He calls it his "year in a cave," and it helped him realize many things about himself that he hadn't been willing to face before. I was also very hesitant to begin another relationship after my first marriage ended. I wanted to be sure I had spent enough time with myself to realize who I was again. Candidly, I was also enjoying myself too much to get into another serious relationship! I felt fulfilled, not having to do anything for anybody else. My work was demanding, but I loved it and it was the only thing I had to do: make money to live on, and do what I wanted. It was great. I liked having my own house and doing my own personal development on my own schedule. I loved feeling empowered. It was a time in my life that I remember with great fondness. I never expected to be in that position, but once I was, I took full advantage of it. As mentioned, I didn't happen to have kids, and I wasn't dating very much. I focused on sleeping and relaxing. I had to wrestle the twin beasts of my trauma and my financial devastation, and I had a huge mountain of healing to go through, but I gave myself the time and space to do it.

I didn't like dating at all. This was a time in my life when I had no desire to hear anybody else talking about themselves and their ex-wives and their blended families and their work problems. No, thank you. I think I probably would have stayed single forever if I had not met my husband. There is enormous value and fulfillment in owning your own space and not having to compromise.

Ladies (and gentlemen), being single for a while is a gift. Trust me when I tell you it is much, much better to be single than to be in an unhappy relationship. Even if partnering with someone is your ultimate goal, those times in your life when you are single offer a great opportunity to work on your relationship with yourself. If you just got out of a relationship, take some time just for you, to really dive into who you are and what went wrong. Be honest and figure out what you don't want. Don't waste time jumping back into the exhausting world of dating apps and blind dates until you have figured out what patterns to avoid and what warning signs to look for. Doing all that work to dig yourself out of a trauma will take all your energy. This is your chance to decide what matters to you, and figure out what your purpose is in this life.

Besides, it's the 21st century. You don't need a partner. You are your own person, not somebody's property. You don't need anybody to "complete you." You can have your own life, your own home, your own career, your own identity. When you really know who you are, why you are here, and what you want in this life, you will be in the best possible position to find someone else equally evolved, equally self-aware, and equally capable of the kind of deep, lasting, loving partnership we all crave. Or, they will find you. Often, when you are ready, the right person appears.

So put yourself first. Become whole. Dysfunctional relationships are relationships where two people need each other in order to be whole. Healthy relationships are about two whole people who choose to walk side by side into the future. Become the person capable of that, and you will be a person capable of a truly vibrant relationship.

HOW TO LOVE FOR LIFE

Here is the sobering truth about marriage (according to Dr. Jay):

- Up to 53 percent of first marriages end in divorce.
- Over 60 percent of second marriages fail.
- And 73 percent of third marriages also fail, suggesting we're not getting it even after multiple failures.
- One in three divorces are attributed to emotional infidelity (largely due to social media).
- Finally, 57 percent of men and 54 percent of women admit to having an affair while being in a committed relationship such as a monogamous marriage.

According to the renowned relationship expert Dr. John Gottman, there are four primary signs that a relationship is going in the wrong direction. This is something that has been out there for a while so you may have heard of it. Dr. Gottman calls this quartet the Four Horsemen of the Apocalypse—not the ones from the Bible that foretell the end of the world, but the ones that foretell impending marital doom. They are:

1. **CRITICISM.** When couples constantly criticize each other, they are focusing on the negative and not the things they love and respect about each other. Criticism focuses on someone else without taking any responsibility on yourself, and it damages the relationship. It's typically a "You" statement. *Example:* "You're overly sensitive," or "You don't care about my feelings." There is never a need for it. You can always express what you want to express without criticism.

Start your sentences with "I" instead, such as: "I'm sorry I hurt your feelings," or "I feel hurt by what you said."

2. **CONTEMPT.** This is criticism combined with a personal attack that makes the other person feel worthlessness or shame. *Example:* "Did you do anything worthwhile today? You are a hopeless case," or "Why do I even bother talking to you? You are incapable of listening and it disgusts me." Instead, stick to the facts, not your anger, such as: "Do you want to talk about what's holding you back from doing everything you wanted to do today?" or "I feel unheard. Can we talk about how we can both communicate better?"

3. **DEFENSIVENESS.** This is when you feel attacked so you respond by attacking. *Example:* "The only reason I forgot to pay the electric bill was that you didn't remind me." Instead, "I'm sorry I forgot to pay that bill. Let's come up with a system so I can remember next time."

4. **STONEWALLING.** This is shutting down completely and cutting off communication. When an argument escalates, it can be tempting to do this, but it's better to explain that you need to take a time-out so you don't feel so overwhelmed and can get control of your emotions again.

Dr. Gottman has said he can tell within minutes if a couple is headed for divorce based on whether they do these four things. I bet at least one of them sounds familiar, yes? These are common bad habits, especially after people have been in a relationship for a while, but they destroy relationships. When people behave in this fashion, they often don't understand how damaging it is, and they don't know how else to relate to each other anymore. If you can begin to recognize the "Four Horsemen" before they take over the conversation and instead switch into a different mode where you don't escalate or attack but honestly ask for a collaborative solution to problems, you will be investing positive energy into your relationship.

THE SEX BOX

I can't write a relationship chapter without talking about sex. As my team was reading early drafts of this manuscript, several of them said,

"Shouldn't you have a sex box?" So that's exactly what I'm calling this box. The Sex Box.

It's an apt description, not just because these lines have a square around them but because couples who have been together for a while often do put sex in a kind of box. It's that thing you used to love doing, but you eventually started doing less. It's that thing that sounds good in theory but in practice may seem too exhausting.

Sex keeps intimacy intact, and it's healthy physically, both for hormonal balance and to keep tissues young and vital. It fosters the bond between two people and it's absolutely an act of physical and mental health. If your sex life is healthy, hooray! Keep it up (so to speak)! Fit it in whenever you can. If it's been awhile, know that the more you do it, the easier (and more fun) it gets. But what if there are barriers to (ahem) entry? Let's talk about that.

Hormonal fluctuations may have you or your partner or both of you feeling a lack of desire, but stress is often the culprit. How do you get interested in having sex? You're already trying to be good at your job and keep the house clean and pay the bills and take care of your kids, not to mention eat better and exercise more and cook dinner and make your own homemade organic ketchup because you just found out ketchup is full of sugar and preservatives? Oftentimes, sex ends up as one of the last items on your to-do list, and I know most of us never get to the bottom of that list by the end of the day. You may even find yourself thinking, *Why do there have to be three sides to the Vibrant Triad? It's too much!*

If it feels like too much, it is too much. If your body is telling you that you are overextended and stressed out, believe it. Self-care is necessary for a healthy libido. The reason women so often feel like they don't have enough energy for sex is because they don't have enough energy, period. This is the elephant in the bedroom that most health books don't talk about. Perfection is the enemy of progress, but if your body isn't feeling good, sex won't ever feel like an option, so to get you to the third side of the Vibrant Triad, we have to get you feeling good.

Do one thing at a time, and when you feel overwhelmed, remember that the Vibrant Triad does not have 50 sides. It has just three: Eat well, to give your body nutrition to fuel the production of energy and glow. Exercise, for energy, strength, flexibility, and circulation. And prioritize time for physical and emotional bonding. Human connection makes all the effort you put into your physical health feel more worthwhile. If hormones are part of the problem, you might mention lack of desire to your doctor, and get some testing done. Women as well as men can have low levels of testosterone, and supplementing this can help boost energy and desire. Estrogen dominance can cause irritability and mood swings, which can interfere with that romantic mood, and a natural progesterone supplement or cream could help. When estrogen levels drop, desire may also drop, along with natural lubrication. There are many pros and cons to hormone replacement therapy, so I advise discussing your individual situation with your doctor, but a diet rich in whole organic plant foods, evening primrose and black cohosh supplements, and a little coconut oil can help to lubricate the interaction (so to speak).

VIBRANT PRO TIP: Don't take hormone supplements without guidance from your doctor. Integrative and functional medicine practitioners will be most open to guiding you toward natural solutions to your hormonal imbalance, while also considering whether more conventional pharmaceutical treatments might be the best fit for you.

Finally, remember stress management. Some deep breathing, yoga, plenty of sleep, lots of water, and some basic human contact can go far in restoring your emotional and physical bond. Start with a long hug and see how it feels. You can find your way back to each other, even after a sexual dry spell, if you are both willing. When sex is good, it shouldn't feel like one more thing on your to-do list. It should feel like a mini vacation, during which you can forget about your to-do list for a while and reconnect with what's really important.

Love is not something you get to have for free, like a present. It's something you work to create with another person, like a collaborative project. I've talked about some of this already in this chapter, but here are some words from Dr. Jay himself, when I asked him what he would say to my readers about how to make relationships work better:

> *People tend to be confused about love. When I ask them what they want, I find out that their priorities do not align with their expectations. They want a Ferrari for the cost of a Ford. What people expect from their relationships today is at an all-time high because they live in a culture of entitlement: I need, I want, I deserve, I should have. Yet, they want it all without making any sacrifices.*

What's wrong is the other person's fault. "They aren't giving me what I need."

What most people don't realize is that, except in cases where one partner is abusive or incapable of giving, love is not about finding the right person. Helping people find the perfect match is a billion-dollar industry, but love isn't about how someone looks or smells or tastes, about how many likes or followers someone has, or about which digital platform you found each other on. Love is about you. Soul mates are not found. They are created, but you don't create them by changing anyone else. You don't find a soul mate by focusing on what your partner should be, or how they should act, or how they should treat you. You don't create them by feeling anger or resentment or contempt toward them to punish them for not fulfilling your fantasy of a perfect partner.

No, love requires more of you. It requires the decision to stop blaming your partner for what isn't right in your relationship and in your life, and take responsibility for your own situation. True love begins with holistic self-development. If you really want to love somebody, you have to establish your relationship with yourself first. You have to deal with your own stuff. It takes courage to know yourself, in order to have the courage to let yourself be known by someone else. If you want to be loved but you don't want to take the trouble and time and do the work to become someone capable of loving another person, I suggest you get a dog. They are much easier to love than people.

But if you really want love with another human being, if you really want a soul mate, then you can create your soul mate by becoming someone capable of loving the person you have chosen, and becoming the right partner for the person you have found. To do that, you have to come to terms with some important questions. We all have lofty intentions, but there is an important difference between intention and commitment. Do you just intend to have a good relationship, or are you actually committed to having a good relationship, even when you don't feel like making the effort?

Ask yourself:

1. *What are you available for?*
2. *What do you really want?*
3. *Why is what you want important to you?*
4. *Does your availability match what you say you want?*

Most people want a level of love, intimacy, and eroticism that they are not actually available for. Most people think love should make them happy all the time, and that this is the other person's job. Love is not about the unrealistic notion of constant happiness. Happiness is a temporary state, about as useful as an orgasm. In a relationship, of course you want to be happy, but a healthy relationship is about fulfillment, not happiness. Fulfillment comes from being aligned with your highest self and with each other.

This is difficult for people to do, especially later in life, when they've already been through difficult relationships that didn't work out. It's hard to see that you are reenacting your old patterns. This is where some of that self-development work comes in. You are not the victim of your experience. You are the creator of your experience. Most people are just reactive, stuck in a Pavlovian stimulus response, dealing with obsolete conditioning from past relationships. You have to be willing to look at all of that and bring it into the light. When you know who you are and what you are willing to do, then and only then will you be able to really work on your relationship.

If you're wondering what this might look like in practice, Dr. Jay says there are seven things successful and happy couples generally do.

1. **They have high standards,** both for whom they choose and for themselves, as someone in a relationship.
2. **They put the relationship first,** above all else, regardless of what else is happening in their life. (Hardly anyone does this.)
3. **They have crystal-clear boundaries** around their relationship. They have articulated to each other exactly what they have established that it will mean to love each other.

4. **They say "I love you" every day.** And mean it!

5. **They have rituals of connection,** like always having dinner together or always kissing each other goodbye.

6. **They have regular sex** and are comfortable talking about their sex life.

7. **They have a common vision, common values, and common interests.** They like doing things together.

Look here for a worksheet on how to integrate Dr. Jay's Six Habits of Soul Mate Couples into your relationship and life.

JUST FOR MEN

Hello, gentlemen! This sidebar is just for you. Let's face facts: You probably don't want to go to the doctor or live on salads and yoga. We know. However, staying healthy means you'll feel better about yourself and be a better partner in your relationship. You'll also look better, and I know you care about that, even if you don't talk about it a lot. But it could also mean the difference between a long, vibrant life and a life cut short.

I want to tell you about a dear friend of mine, whose brother was a very athletic, fit runner. When he died of a massive heart attack in his driveway at the age of 57, everybody said he was "the picture of health." I've heard this story many times, and it is almost always about a man. They are always "the picture of health." But when you peel back the layers, you realize there were things someone could have caught if our medical system did a better job at prevention and screening.

It's easy to point fingers—they should have had this procedure or that test; they should have had a faster medical response or it was genetics. All those things may be true, but the focus is always on the end-stage result. My question is: What was going on 30 years ago? No medical system is always going to catch every medical anomaly, but your "health insurance policy" isn't really about your health insurance policy. It's not about your government, your politics, your employer, or your primary care provider. You are your health insurance policy: you, your behaviors, and your lifestyle. It is your responsibility to take care of yourself, to listen to your body, and to respond. If you have a family history of something, get screened. If you feel like something is wrong, get checked. It's not weak to take care of yourself. It is strong and responsible. I also want you to recognize that being physically fit doesn't mean you are exempt from eating right, and eating right doesn't mean you are exempt from fostering supportive relationships. Remember the Vibrant Triad, gentlemen—it belongs to you, too.

I want to drive home the necessity of personal empowerment when it comes to health. You are the master of your body, your mind, and your behaviors. Don't forget why you are making these efforts. Now . . . let's figure out how you can get healthy *your* way.

In my experience, when men have come to me for help, they are usually concerned with one or more of the things on this list, so let's look at these areas of health and see what we can get you to do about them:

- **Strength and fitness.** Most men want to look strong. You know we've seen you flexing your muscles in front of the mirror, right? You want to feel like you can save the day. While your partner is likely to love you no matter how strong you are, there is no arguing that it is healthier and more vibrant to be strong and fit. We all know what that means, gentlemen. You need to exercise, including vigorous exercise (such as HIIT) for cardiovascular fitness, resistance training for muscle strength, and stretching or even yoga for flexibility (yoga can be manly—in fact, men invented it). All the exercise advice and guidelines in chapter five apply just as much to you as to women, so give it a look, or just do what you already know you should be doing: Move more and lift heavy things. You'll feel better, look better, and be in a better mood.

- **Sex and problems with sex** like erectile dysfunction or low desire. As men age, testosterone levels tend to go down (the so-called "male menopause"), which can lead to problems with desire and function. My best advice for combating this gradual ebbing of sexual function is to talk to your doctor about testosterone supplements. Taking a testosterone supplement can make a big difference in your desire (this can also help women). Having sex regularly can also keep things working, for both men and women. The phrase "use it or lose it" is particularly appropriate when it comes sex, so if you've been having a dry spell, maybe it's time to plan an evening of romance. There is also some research that the aptly named herb called horny goat weed can help with erectile dysfunction.[10] Dr. Liu recommends 9 to 15 grams of horny goat weed (called Yin Yang Huo in Traditional Chinese Medicine) for hormonal balance daily, divided into two doses, morning and evening.

- **Prostate health.** According to the American Cancer Society, prostate cancer is the most common cancer in men other than skin cancer, and one in nine men will develop prostate cancer during their lifetime.[11] The most important way to prevent prostate cancer from progressing is to know the early symptoms and obtain early screenings, as your doctor recommends. One accepted and routine screening analysis that you can obtain with your primary provider every year is the PSA (prostate-specific antigen) urine test. It doesn't diagnose cancer, but shows if your level of cancer risk is elevating and you need more aggressive analysis. In addition, there is some evidence that you can reduce your risk through lifestyle changes. Men who are overweight or obese are more likely to get advanced prostate cancer, so getting to a healthful weight is probably the most powerful way you can mitigate your risk. Exercise and a diet rich in fruits and vegetables also may reduce risk, and there is some research suggesting that men who have diets high in dairy products like milk and cheese are at higher risk. The eating style described in chapter four is an excellent diet for reducing risk of all cancers, including prostate cancer, and I highly recommend eliminating dairy from your diet. Taking selenium and zinc supplements may also help; there is some research showing higher selenium levels are associated with lower prostate cancer incidence,[12] and that zinc can inhibit prostate cancer cell growth and invasion.[13]

- **Stress and heart health.** Heart disease is the number one killer of both men and women, but men are often exposed to the stereotypical image of the stressed-out man who clutches his chest and drops dead in the middle of a high-stress moment. Stress does increase your risk of having a heart attack (for both men and women), so stress management is extremely important. Fortunately for men, marriage greatly reduces stress, disease risk, and premature death risk, much more so than for women (as I've previously mentioned). If you aren't married, perhaps it's time to propose?

- **Weight loss.** I know you are worried about your weight. I've seen a definite increase in men asking me about weight loss, both for health and for vanity. As men age, elevated cortisol and depressed testosterone can cause that belly we like to blame on beer. Men who develop a large midsection but lose muscle in their legs are showing the telltale signs of metabolic dysfunction. Chronic stress, a junk-food, high-fat, and/or high-carb diet (right or wrong, the stereotypical "meat and potatoes" meal is still thought of as "masculine"), the wrong kind of exercise, and sleep apnea can all contribute to this downward spiral of dwindling reserves and fading health. I know you want to feel good and look attractive, and weight loss is one powerful way to achieve those goals if that spare tire and paunch have been steadily expanding. The same weight loss principles that apply to women also apply to men—eat more nutrient-dense food, control your portions, and exercise on most days.

You *can* reclaim the energy, drive, and positive outlook you once had. After changing their lifestyles, many men tell me that they feel better and look better and are in better shape in their forties and fifties than they were in their twenties and thirties! Let's get you there, boys! You have the power. It's all about how you choose to nourish yourself, move your body, and connect with people you love. Do it for your partner, your kids, your family, but most of all, do it for yourself.

MY FAVORITE RELATIONSHIP RESOURCES

One of the many ways my husband and I make our marriage a priority is to continually seek ways to get smarter about our relationship and how to make it work better. There are a few books and other resources that have had a profound impact on us. We often give the books as gifts and refer friends to the other resources. We also go on two marriage retreats every year. If you want to get better at relationships, here are the resources we both recommend:

- **Book: *The Five Love Languages*,** by Gary Chapman. This book has been on and off (but mostly on) the *New York Times* best sellers list for years and has sold over 13 million copies. It is a classic that is just as relevant today as when it was first published in 1992. It includes a quiz, which you can also take online, to discover what your love language is, and what your partner's love language is. Taking this quiz early in our relationship was very enlightening to my husband and me because we both got the same test results. Our top two love languages were quality time and physical touch. This wasn't what I expected. I didn't think at first that my husband—an extroverted and high-performing executive—really valued quality time, but I was reassured when I saw his quiz results. I knew that if we could both be true to our love languages, it would work out.

- **Book: *The Seven Principles for Making Marriage Work,*** by John M. Gottman, PhD, and Julie Schwartz Gottman, PhD. We also recommend all the resources from the Gottman Institute, which takes a "research-based approach to relationships." Their website (www.gottman.com) contains many resources.

- **Relationship coaching.** To me, getting relationship coaching or counseling before you have problems is like practicing preventive medicine. If you go to the doctor after you're already very sick, it's much harder to fix the problem than it would have been to prevent it from ever advancing that far. I highly recommend working with a relationship coach as early into a relationship as possible, so you have a better chance at getting it right.

- **Couples or marriage enrichment retreats.** My husband and I have benefited greatly from marriage retreats. One of the highlights was the retreat at the Gottman Institute, which we did about two years into our relationship, and it helped us understand our relationship better *before* we got married. Couples retreats are like taking a (working) vacation that yields major relationship benefits. I highly recommend doing one of these if you get the opportunity. Many churches have them, but there are also secular versions. The Gottman Institute still offers small-group two-day couples retreats, which you can read about on their website.

• • •

No relationship can be created or fixed overnight with "seven easy steps" or pithy phrases from any relationship guru. All relationships are challenging. They do take work, and it's work some people aren't really willing to do. But it is also work that can make your life better. Are you ready to make a commitment to becoming someone capable of true, deep, lasting, meaningful love? Until you know the answer to that, you won't be ready to be a good partner, which means you won't be ready to have a good partner. And that's fine. When you are ready, you'll be ready! When you are willing to do the work on yourself and for yourself, you can get there. The most difficult barriers are the ones in your own head. Pay attention to the messages from your heart, and do what is right for you, always.

RELATIONSHIP WINS

Here are a few ways to start improving your relationships for better human connection. Try one, two, or all three and complete that third side of the Vibrant Triad, for full-spectrum vibrancy.

WORK ON YOURSELF. All the advice in this book about how to become vibrant is also advice about how to work on yourself: your energy, your glow, your lifestyle habits, your stress management, and more. Every good thing you do for yourself will put you in a better position to *be* a soul mate, which is the first step to *having* a soul mate. Commit to yourself, and you'll be committing to better relationships of all kinds, right now and in the future.

○ *I tried it! Here's how it felt:* _____

_____

_____

HOLD YOUR TONGUE. That is, when you want to say something negative. One of the most important things to do is to stop being negative about your partner. Saying negative things is mostly a bad habit, but words matter. They hurt your partner and they influence how you feel about your partner, so practice stopping yourself before you criticize. Either turn it around to something positive, or just don't say anything. It really is possible to disagree, even have an argument, without criticizing. Your life will be better if you can stop this destructive habit.

○ *I tried it! Here's how it felt:* _____

_____

_____

CONNECT WITH A FRIEND. Romantic relationships aren't the only kind of relationships that benefit your mental and physical health. No one person can be everything to anyone, and having a close friend you can confide in (a sibling counts) can make a big difference in how well you can manage stress. Friends who have good health habits can also be a good influence. Reach out to a friend you admire, whom you know has your best interests at heart and has similar goals for health and life, and commit to spending more time together.

○ *I tried it! Here's how it felt:* _____

_____

_____

PART III

Deepest

The Vibrant Triad is your keystone, but we can go even deeper in order to appreciate how the Vibrant Triad can improve three critical systems that govern all aspects of your health and life. You are an astonishing and complex biochemical miracle, and knowing a bit more about what's going on inside of you and how you can make it all work better can be motivating and empowering. In this next section, we're going to explore three primary systems hard at work within you right now—each one of these plays an essential role in how vibrant you feel and how well your body and mind work:

1. Your Nervous System
2. Your Detoxification System
3. Your Immune System

Food

Nervous,
Detoxification,
and Immune
Systems

Movement   *Connection*

NOTE: *The one system I wondered about including here but decided not to include is the endocrine system. Hormones influence every aspect of health, but I ultimately decided this is exactly why I would not include it. Just as stress management is not a part of the Vibrant Triad because it impacts and is impacted by every part of the Vibrant Triad equally, so does the endocrine system affect, and so is it affected by, all the other systems. I'll mention hormones throughout as relevant, but just remember that they influence practically everything about you, so a balanced endocrine system is essential for all these other systems to work.*

The Indicator: Glow

The root of the word vibrant is "vibration," and its original meaning was "light." To me, this perfectly describes what it means to be vibrant—to be full of lightness and the vibration of positive energy.

CHAPTER 3 | PAGE 65

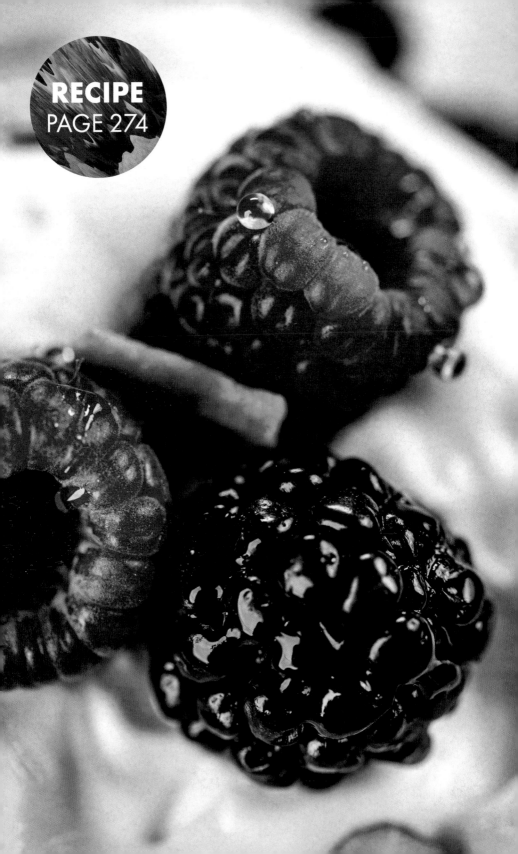

RECIPE
PAGE 274

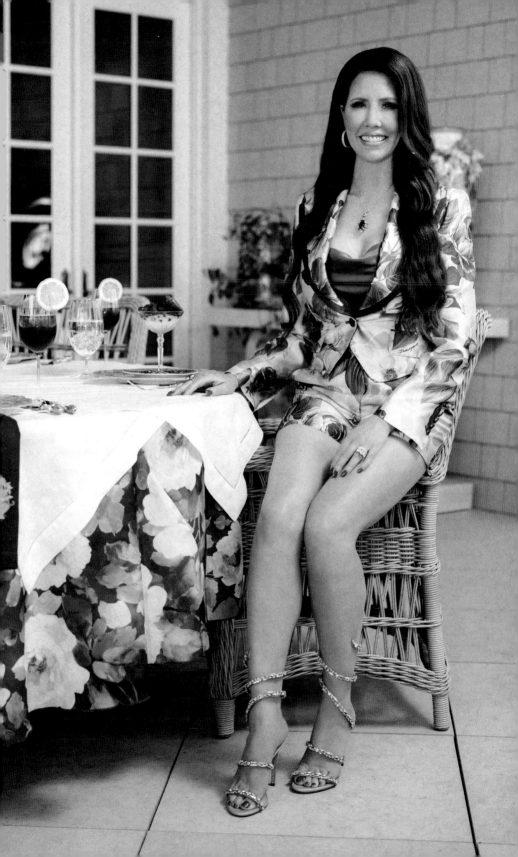

The Mainframe: Brain

Whether your focus is on God or nature or love or your own inner light or something else that feels spiritual to you, give it some of your energy and your energy will grow.

CHAPTER 7 | PAGE 167

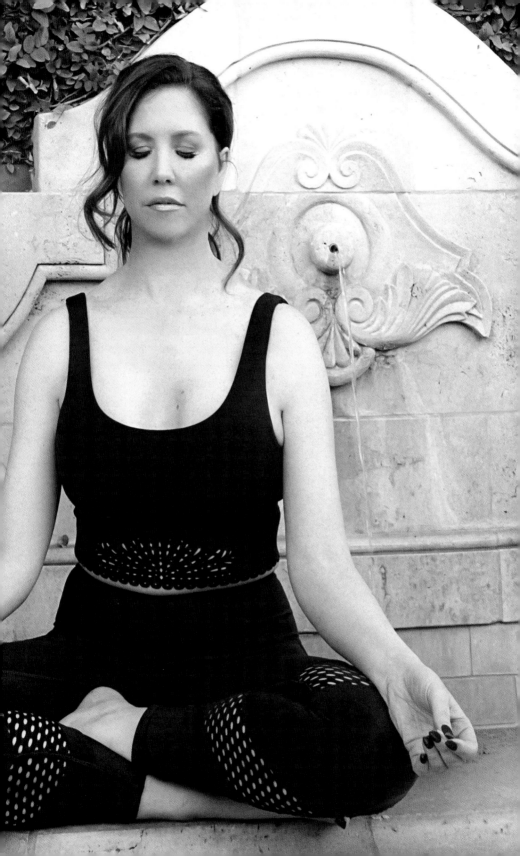

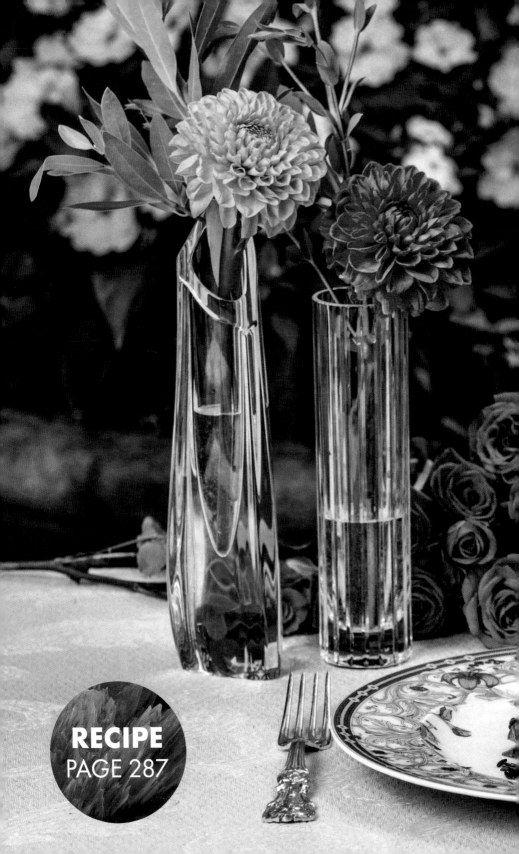

RECIPE
PAGE 287

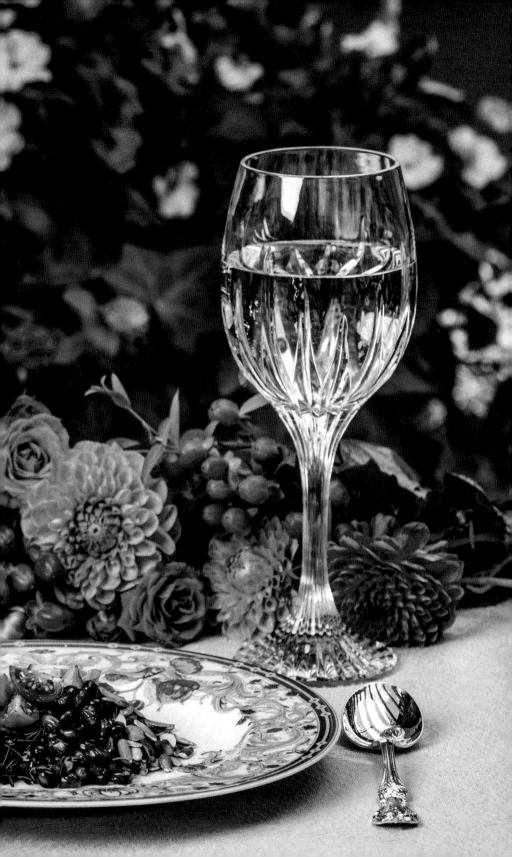

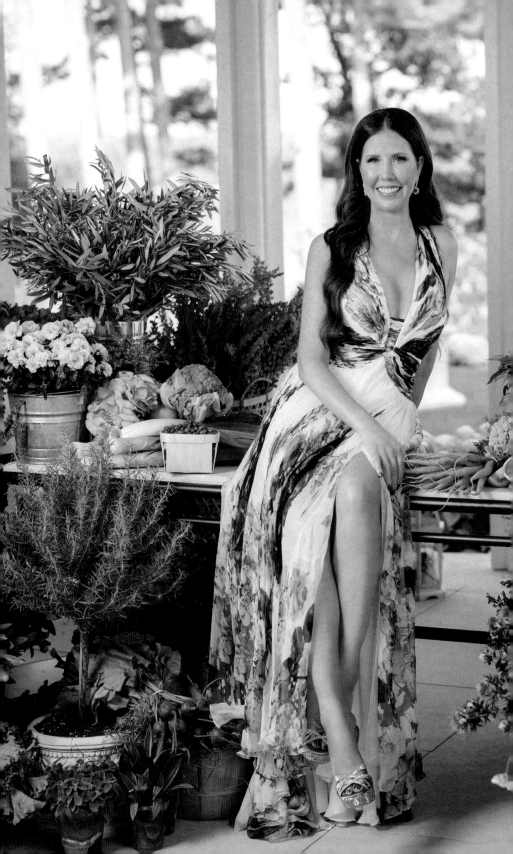

The Communicator: Food

The more vegetables in your diet, the better. Not only do many vegetables contain high levels of antioxidants to reduce oxidative stress in the brain, but they also contain fiber to improve microbiome health.

CHAPTER 4 | PAGE 85

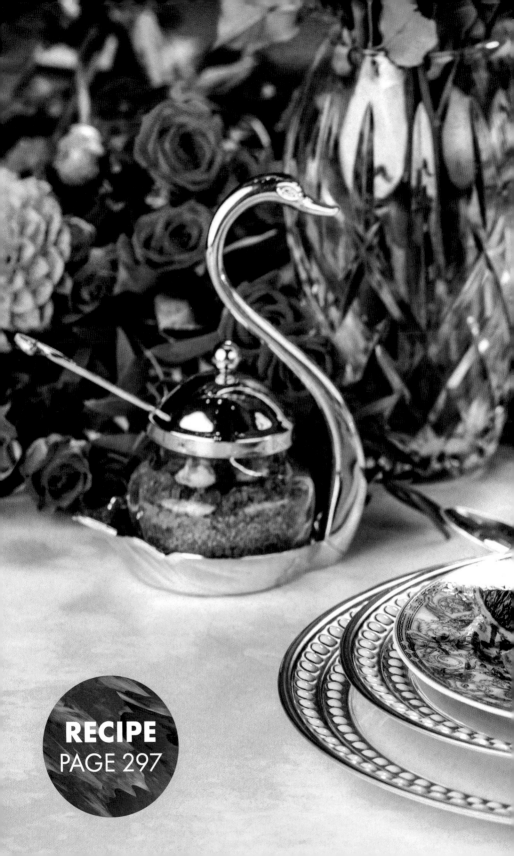

RECIPE
PAGE 297

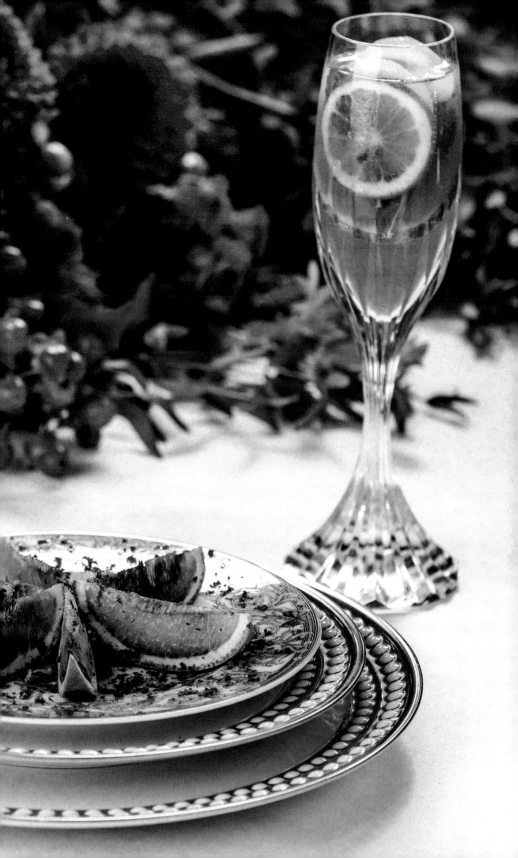

The Rejuvenator: Detoxification

The more vegetables in your diet, the better. Not only do many vegetables contain high levels of antioxidants to reduce oxidative stress in the brain, but they also contain fiber to improve microbiome health.

CHAPTER 8 | PAGE 191

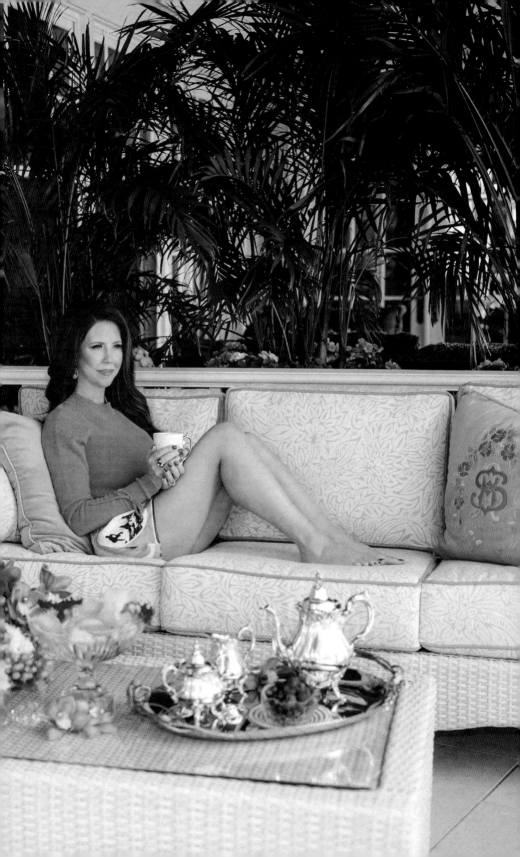

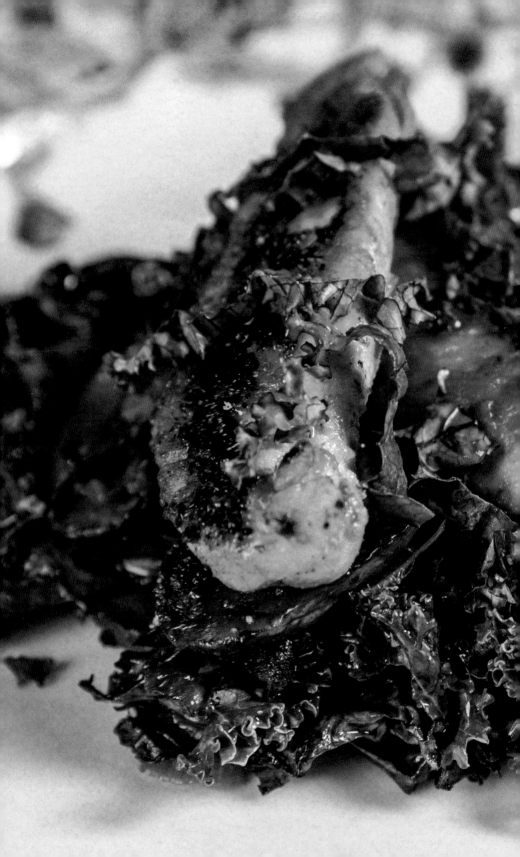

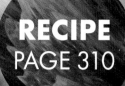

RECIPE
PAGE 310

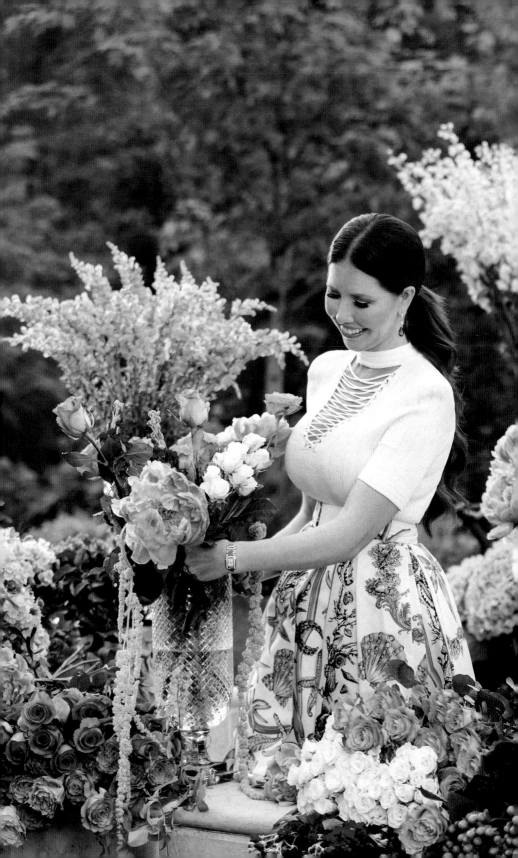

The Fountain: Energy

You know it when you see it—that glow radiating from someone in a way that makes it difficult to stop staring. In the same way your body is sending messages to you about things that are going wrong, it's also sending you messages about things that are going right, in the form of beauty indicators.

CHAPTER 2 | PAGE 41

The Connector: Relationships

There is no doubt that we need each other to be vibrant. When you feel understood, loved, and supported by the people around you—your partners, your family, your friends, your community—you are much less likely to suffer health problems. The science is clear and the results are straightforward.

CHAPTER 6 | PAGE 139

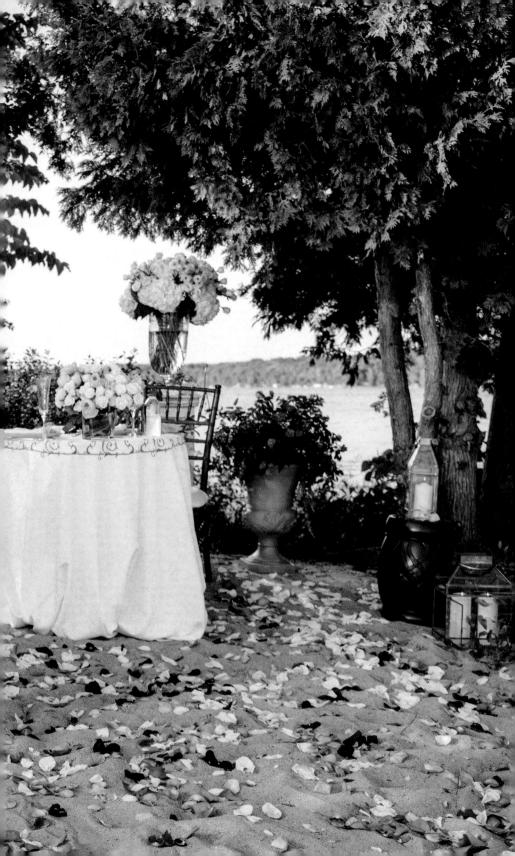

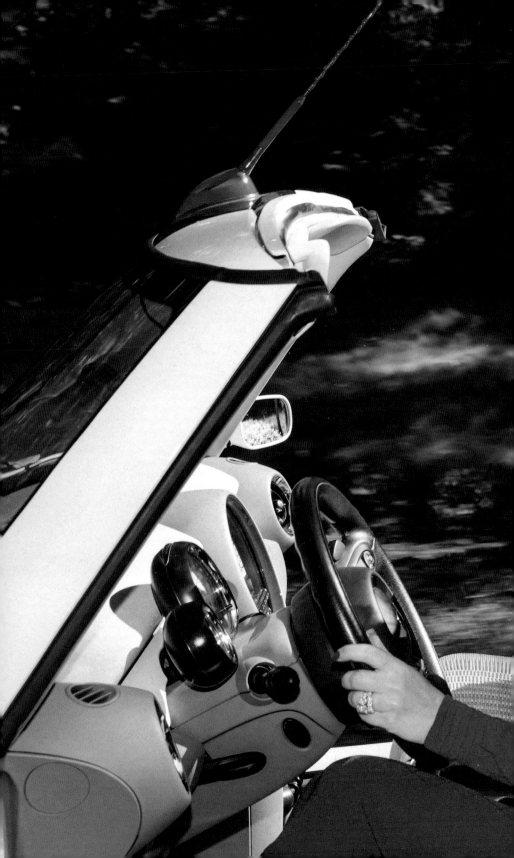

The Activator: Movement

Do you look energized, alive, and bright, or do you look tired and dull? Energy is perhaps the most obvious and most powerful indicator of vibrancy. It is ethereal, intangible, but you can see it.

CHAPTER 5 | PAGE 117

RECIPE
PAGE 315

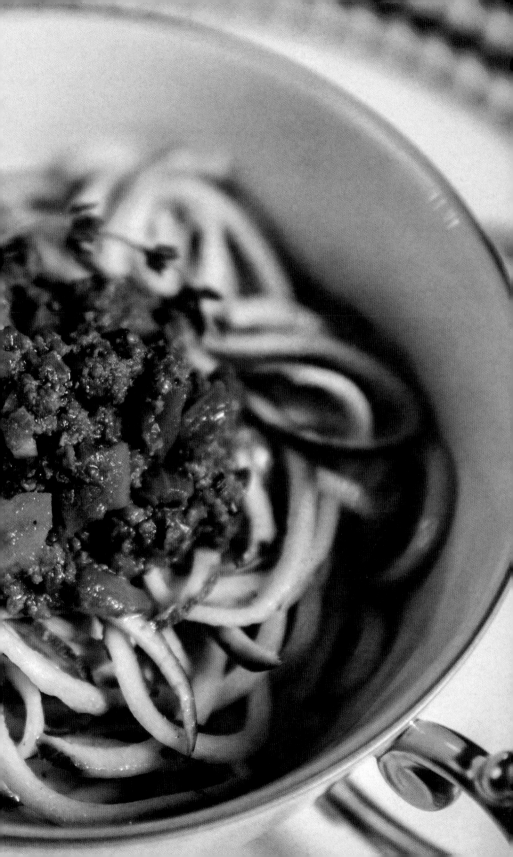

The Sustainer: Immunity

Never, ever give up on yourself, your health, your wellness, and your potential to be vibrant. There is always more you can do to bring vibrancy into your day and energy into your life if you so choose.

CHAPTER 9 | PAGE 215

CHAPTER 7

The Mainframe: How to Fine-Tune Your Brain and Nervous System

Everything you perceive yourself to be is a product of your own thought, so it's no exaggeration to say that your brain and entire nervous system are critical elements in determining who you are and how you experience life. When your brain isn't working as well as it could, you aren't working as well as you could. We all have our moments of forgetfulness, disorganization, and foggy thinking. Most people have periods of sadness or worry. Many a woman in her thirties or forties who walks into a room and can't remember why she went in there fears dementia is imminent. However, it's a myth that we must accept reduced brain function as a natural part of aging. Your brain should work as well today as it did when you were twenty or twenty-five years old, and you have the potential to stay sharp well into your eighties, nineties, or even longer.

Brains are fascinating, complex organs that are influenced by a wide range of lifestyle factors. When it comes to your brain, genetics may play a part but it is certainly not destiny. People often talk about the brain as if it's something separate from the body—perhaps you've heard of the so-called "brain-body connection." There is a separation between the brain and the rest of the body called the blood-brain barrier that (mostly) keeps toxins out of your brain, but your brain is connected to the rest of your body through the spinal cord and the vagus nerve, which connects your digestive system to your brain, so you can hardly call it separate.

Many of the endocrine glands responsible for your hormone balance live in your brain, but others don't and they communicate biochemically with your brain constantly. Because your brain is connected to your gut via the "gut-brain axis" (this is that vagus nerve and the biochemical signaling that runs along it), what you eat directly impacts your brain, and so does the content and health of the microbes in your gastrointestinal tract (your gut microbiome).

Because exercise triggers the release of the protein BDNF—or brain-derived neurotrophic factor—your activity level also directly impacts your brain, and a lack of activity is a notable brain stressor.

Because healing and repair happen during sleep, and both deep sleep and dream sleep (REM sleep) restore different parts of your brain, how you sleep is also a direct influence on brain health.

Because chronic stress shrinks the prefrontal cortex,[1] which is responsible for your memory, and may increase the size of your amygdala,[2] which can make you more emotionally reactive and extra prone to stress,[3] and because it also interferes with the process of neuronal signaling within the brain,[4] how well you manage stress directly influences your brain.

Toxins, especially heavy metals, can also have severe brain effects, even at levels conventional medicine may disregard.[5]

Habits that may seem unrelated to your brain, like using computers and your smartphone frequently, or drinking wine every night, or that little matter of your sugar addiction, can have profound brain impacts.

If your brain is already showing signs of wear and tear—if you are already experiencing anxiety, depression, brain fog, forgetfulness, or you are having trouble concentrating or focusing, and especially if you have a family history of Alzheimer's disease, Parkinson's disease, or other neurological diseases like vascular dementia or multiple sclerosis—then it's time for a brain health intervention.

There are many types of brain dysfunction, from mild to life-threatening. Doctors still don't know for sure why some people suffer from depression, others from anxiety, or why some people develop mental illnesses like bipolar disorder or schizophrenia, or have attention deficit disorder (including many adults), or why some people develop dementia while others are still sharp in their nineties. We are pretty sure there is a genetic component to all of these brain issues, but as with most genetic disorders, something has to happen to turn those genes on. How you live, your exposures, your childhood experiences, your education—all play a role. You could have a genetic susceptibility to depression or schizophrenia or Alzheimer's disease and never get that problem because the genes for it were never activated, based on how you lived your life.

Your brain can compensate for a lot of stress and degradation . . . until it can't. Your best chance at optimal brain function is to take care of your brain with a brain-friendly lifestyle, starting right now. There can be signs of brain dysfunction long before full-blown disease. You might already be experiencing some of the buildup of protein fragments and dead nerve cells that are a sign of dementia. People get mild cognitive impairment before they get Alzheimer's, but there is increasing evidence that you can turn this around, the earlier the better, and never get that dreaded disease. There are warning signs that could signal a mental illness is coming, such as subtle changes in personality and behavior, unusual moods, changes in sleep or appetite, or noticeable changes in attitudes or interests.[6] These could be early warning signs of serious depression or a panic disorder, or even a psychotic disorder like schizophrenia. But early intervention could also head off a more serious condition.

Ideally, you can start taking care of your brain now before you get any negative brain symptoms. Your brain may be your most precious organ because it is the seat of all you know and all you remember. It determines who you are to yourself and to the world by governing your perceptions and personality. Your best chance at avoiding ever having to experience noticeably impaired brain function, and instead getting smarter and sharper, thinking more quickly, and boosting your brain performance in ways that make your life so much better, is to give your brain everything it needs to thrive. In this chapter, we're going to work on some targeted brain TLC to boost your brain performance. Like other aspects of your health, you can come at this problem from multiple angles for maximum impact. Let's start with the Vibrant Triad.

DO BRAIN TRAINING GAMES WORK?

Brain training has become a popular pastime for people who want to preserve their mental function. Programs and apps like Lumosity and BrainHQ claim that, with regular training, you can get smarter and maybe head off brain deterioration with aging. While a few studies have shown mixed results,[7] some before-and-after tests have revealed that, after a period of regular brain training, cognitive function really does improve in healthy adults[8] as well as in those with mild cognitive impairment.[9] If you enjoy these brain games, they can't hurt, and they really might help. The trick, though, is to make them a regular habit, rather than something you do every once in a while. As with anything, consistency + time is what really makes a difference.

EAT FOR A HEALTHY BRAIN

Your brain uses more energy than any other part of your body—it accounts for 20 percent of your total energy expenditure[10]—so fueling it is important. If the brain doesn't have enough fuel, your neurons will be less able to effectively communicate with each other, impairing function, and your brain will be short on the resources it needs to flush out the excess proteins and metabolites and other waste it produces just by doing its brain business.

The Vibrant Diet discussed in chapter four will give your brain all the fuel it needs, in the form of glucose and healthful fats, along with protein for building and nutrients to keep the brain's natural waste removal system functioning. Good nutrition, especially the many antioxidants (compounds that protect your cells from oxidative stress and damage) present in vibrant foods, can also help to reduce oxidative stress and inflammation, which can damage brain tissue, kill neurons, and compromise the blood-brain barrier, letting toxins into your brain that aren't supposed to be there (some people call this condition "leaky brain").

Because your brain and your gut are also connected through the gut-brain axis, your brain knows how your gut is feeling and your gut knows how your brain is feeling. This is why you can get butterflies in your stomach when you're nervous, or feel depressed when you have a digestive disorder. Getting enough fiber and polyphenols from fruits and vegetables to feed the microbes in your microbiome will feed the good gut bacteria, keeping your gut in good condition, which signals the brain that all is well.

You can also target your brain with specific foods that are particularly brain-friendly.

- **FATTY FISH:** Oh, those delicious salmon fillets . . . I love them, and they are so good for so many aspects of your health! The omega-3 fatty acids they contain help create healthy brain cell membranes and have also been shown to improve cognitive function by increasing blood flow to the brain.[11] Mackerel, low-mercury tuna, trout, and sardines are other great sources.

- **EGGS:** The B-vitamins in eggs have been shown to reduce cognitive decline in people with mild cognitive impairment by reducing homocysteine levels[12] (homocysteine is an amino acid that is often high in people who eat a lot of meat, and is associated with brain atrophy and increased oxidative stress as well as heart disease). Egg yolks are a potent source of choline, which also reduces damaging homocysteine by converting it into beneficial methionine, another amino acid associated with improved memory. Choline also helps promote the process of clearing waste from the brain, and may be useful in helping to reduce the risk of Alzheimer's disease.[13]

- **BERRIES AND DARK CHOCOLATE:** Do I have to tell you twice to eat these? Many studies have shown that the high flavonoid content (a type of antioxidant) in berries and dark chocolate that contains at least 70 percent organic cacao can reduce oxidative stress in the brain and is associated with improved learning, memory, and cognitive function. Berries are also a good source of fiber, which feeds the health-promoting microbes in your gastrointestinal tract, leading to a healthier microbiome, which also leads to healthier cognitive function.

- **VEGETABLES:** The more vegetables in your diet, the better. Not only do many vegetables contain high levels of antioxidants to reduce oxidative stress in the brain, but they also contain fiber, to improve microbiome health. There are also some studies that suggest there is at least a mild association with vegetable intake and a lower risk of glioma, a type of brain cancer.[14] Non-starchy vegetables in particular will give you the most nutrition with fiber and without a high carbohydrate content. You can't eat too many non-starchy vegetables. They should be the primary feature of your lunches and dinners.

- **COFFEE:** Brewed coffee has been associated with improved cognitive function, partially due to the antioxidants coffee contains, but also because the caffeine in coffee stimulates the central nervous system. Other studies have identified other components of coffee as neuroprotective, including against the aggregation of the plaques and tangles associated with Alzheimer's disease.[15] I don't recommend more than a couple of cups a day, however, due to caffeine's negative effect on the adrenal glands, ultimately reducing rather than increasing energy.

OXIDATIVE STRESS, ANTIOXIDANTS, AND YOUR BRAIN

To live is to create free radicals. The atoms that make up your body are always losing electrons due to the normal processes of living, metabolizing food, and operating the immune system and all your other functions. Electrons are stable in pairs, but if an electron gets detached from its partner, it becomes a free radical, seeking another electron, stealing one from another atom. This causes a chain reaction of electrons seeking electrons (like some scary biochemical dating site), causing collateral damage to the body, called oxidative stress.

Antioxidants in foods offer up their electrons to stop this destructive process. This happens all over the body, including in the brain, and it's a normal process, but when you are under increased stress or exposed to toxins (such as cigarette smoke or pollution or chemicals in junk food), you may begin to produce more free radicals than your body can handle. Brain tissue is particularly susceptible to damage from oxidative stress, and the damage it causes can compromise healthy central nervous system function. This process could contribute to an increased risk of serious degenerative brain conditions like Alzheimer's disease, Parkinson's disease, and Huntington's disease, especially in those who are genetically susceptible, as well as to anxiety disorders and depression.[16] For this reason, a diet rich in antioxidants is critical for brain health, especially in people who experience chronic stress. Which is most of us.

EXERCISE FOR MAXIMUM BRAIN POWER

Exercise is the best thing you can do for your overall health, and obviously exercise strengthens muscles and builds cardiovascular capacity, but it's also one of the best things you can do for your brain. Remember that exercise triggers the release of BDNF, and that protein has amazing brain rejuvenation powers.

BDNF is like a fountain of youth for your brain. It's been linked to better memory, easier learning, less depression, and reduction of the brain diseases of aging, like Alzheimer's disease and other forms of dementia. Remember how people used to say you can never make more brain cells? Not true. BDNF maintains healthy neurons and creates new ones. It may also lead to easier weight loss and better sleep. To tap that magic and start enjoying all those benefits, all you have to do is move your body.

The exercise that releases the most BDNF and that keeps BDNF in your system the longest is cardio. For maximum BDNF production, step up the pace to at least a moderate effort (easy walking won't do it). Try to get your heart rate up enough that you sweat, and keep it there for at least thirty minutes. If you can work up to a good active hour on most days, you'll be flush with BDNF. You also make BDNF during meditation (which I'll tell you more about later in this chapter), and in the deep sleep stage. Two things that block BDNF production are stress[17] and a high-fat, high-sugar diet.[18]

BACK TO SCHOOL?

It's a no-brainer that learning is beneficial to your brain.[19] People with more education tend to have fewer brain issues and lower rates of dementia, while people with less education seem to develop dementia more often. One study showed this is probably not due to poorer lifestyle habits in less educated people, but has more to do with the brain directly, perhaps due to the expanded brain reserves in more educated people.[20] The more you use your brain, the smarter it gets.

If you've always wanted to go back and get your college degree, knowing it will improve your brain health might be just the extra push you need. But even if you don't have a degree (or the degree you wish you had), you can spend your entire life continuing to learn new things. Never stop learning! Practice learning another language, or learn to play a musical instrument. Stimulate your brain by reading books on complex subjects that interest you. You can never know it all, but you can sure try.

One of the wonderful things about the internet is that it gives you access to advanced learning in just about any field. Try pushing your brain all the time, just a little. Short bursts of stress from learning help your brain to grow stronger and get better at understanding, focusing, and retaining information, as long as you also give your brain time to regenerate with good sleep and stress management practices like meditation and deep breathing (I'll say more on these topics later in the chapter).

CONNECT FOR BETTER BRAIN FUNCTION

As you've already seen, healthy relationships and human connection can greatly reduce the risk of depression. There is also evidence that strong relationships can reduce the likelihood of developing dementia,[21] and can improve symptoms, outcomes, survival rates, and quality of life in people with other nervous system disorders such as Parkinson's[22] and multiple sclerosis.[23] Relationships can even influence the gut-brain connection because people who encourage each other to eat well and make good lifestyle choices may have healthier and more robust gut microbiomes, which can influence the brain through the gut-brain axis, resulting in less risk of neurodegenerative diseases[24] as well as less stress and better resilience.

Beyond the Vibrant Triad, there are some other important ways to maximize your brain power and nervous system health: especially sleep, stress management, and meditation.

BRAIN HEALTH SUPPLEMENTS

There is quite a lot of research showing that certain supplements can improve memory, focus, and concentration, and reduce the risk of or severity of cognitive impairment and dementia. To keep your brain function sharp, these are the superstars:

- **EPA/DHA, but especially DHA:** DHA is the primary omega-3 fatty acid in your brain, and people with neurodegenerative diseases have low levels. If you aren't already taking it, do it for your brain. I recommend taking at least 2,000 mg of EPA/DHA daily from fish or krill oil, for maximum brain health. This can also help with anxiety,[25] lower your triglycerides[26] (elevated levels are a risk factor for heart disease), reduce pain in people with rheumatoid arthritis,[27] and could even be preventive or therapeutic for breast cancer.[28] Be sure to look for high-quality, mercury-free supplements.

- **Ashwagandha:** An important ancient Ayurvedic remedy for stress and anxiety, ashwagandha is considered a "nerve tonic."[29] It is adaptogenic, meaning it intervenes in the stress response and has been shown to improve signs of mild cognitive impairment.[30] Although the mechanisms for its action aren't well understood yet by Western science, research does show it has a neuroprotective effect,[31] and many people anecdotally report its effectiveness in alleviating chronic stress and anxiety. It is also part of the Bredesen protocol developed by Dr. Dale Bredesen in his groundbreaking book, *The End of Alzheimer's*,[32] in which he demonstrates how he has reversed cognitive impairment in many patients through lifestyle interventions. Dr. Liu recommends a dosage of 9 to 15 grams daily. If you take it before bed, it can help you feel calmer so you can sleep better.

- **Bacopa monnieri (also called Brahmi):** Another Dr. Bredesen–recommended neuroprotective Ayurvedic herb, bacopa has been shown to improve learning rate, memory consolidation, and the speed of processing visual information, suggesting it is instrumental in optimizing higher cognitive processes.[33] It has also been shown to intervene into anxiety with regular use.[34]

- **Choline:** Choline helps brain cells produce acetylcholine, which is a neurotransmitter your brain uses to learn and focus as well as execute other nervous system functions.[35] It can also improve feelings of fatigue. You can get choline from egg yolks, but to give your brain an extra boost, I recommend a choline supplement. Start out with 100 mg per day.

- **Melatonin:** Sleep is critical for brain repair, but if you are having trouble sleeping and are already practicing the sleep hygiene suggestions in this chapter (see page 177), you might benefit from supplemental melatonin. Melatonin helps regulate your sleep/ wake cycle[36] (I explain this in more detail below), and your pineal gland makes melatonin to induce sleep in response to darkness. Melatonin supplements can help if you don't make enough.

SLEEP SOUNDLY FOR BEST BRAIN REPAIR

Your brain, like the rest of your body, takes care of itself to some extent. We've known about the lymphatic system for centuries, but we only recently discovered that the brain has its own waste removal system, called the glymphatic system. When you sleep, the glymphatic system shuttles excess proteins and metabolic waste products out of the brain like a cleaning crew.[37] This mostly happens during the deep sleep stage, which is one of the reasons why a sufficiently long and high-quality sleep with an adequate amount of deep sleep is so critical for your brain.

How well you sleep has a lot to do with your circadian rhythm, which is the natural rhythm of your body in response to (among other things) light. When we see the full-spectrum light of the sun, our brains are triggered to begin the process of shifting hormones, such as cortisol, to help us naturally wake up. When we are exposed to darkness, our brains are triggered to begin the process of shifting hormones, primarily melatonin, to help us fall asleep. If you are exposed to light that isn't in synch with day and night, your circadian rhythm can get confused. Before the invention of electric lights, not to mention computers and smartphones, nobody would ever see blue light after sunset. Blue light is for morning. It's present in the full-spectrum light of the sun, and also comes from computer screens and smartphones. Blue light suppresses melatonin release and increases alertness,[38] so being exposed to light, especially blue light, at night can make sleeping difficult. Red light, the kind from firelight, does not seem to have the same stimulating effect as blue light. This may be because early humans only had firelight and moonlight to see by at night, so they adapted in a way that made these lights less stimulating.

You can use this natural process to your benefit by stepping outside into full sun or exposing yourself to blue light in the morning to help wake yourself up[39] or when you feel tired during the day. At night, you can encourage melatonin release, and drowsiness, by turning off all electronics/screens at least two hours before bed. If that's not realistic for you, consider wearing blue-blocking (amber) glasses in the evenings, after sundown. These filter out blue light so your pineal gland doesn't get confused, thinking night is day. This can correct circadian rhythm disruption and improve your sleep quality. You might feel strange wearing them around the house, but trust me, it's a popular trend.

Research also shows that even red light can interfere with sleep by triggering the release of cortisol, which is stimulating—not nearly as much as blue light, but it can still have an effect.[40] While it's fine to wind down with red light, once you do go to sleep, it's important to sleep in the dark, and I mean actual complete darkness. If you tried the suggestions at the end of chapter two, you may already be turning off all electronics, even digital clocks, at bedtime. Invest in blackout curtains or use a sleep mask, and keep the lights off until the sun comes up in the morning, if possible. Your sleep will be much more replenishing.

Sleep Hygiene

As you are seeing, sleep impacts many parts of your brain in complex ways,[41] and each stage of sleep—light sleep, deep sleep, and REM sleep—affects brain repair and restoration. You know that during deep sleep your glymphatic system clears waste from your brain. During REM sleep, your brain consolidates your memories and processes newly learned information. It is also likely important for mood regulation. You may be able to tell that you've had enough deep sleep if you feel refreshed and awake in the morning. You may be able to tell that you've had enough REM sleep if your brain feels sharp and you are in a good mood. Obviously, you want enough of both of these kinds of sleep.

To get it, you may have to improve your sleep hygiene. To have good sleep hygiene means to spend those few hours before you go to sleep in ways that will help you sleep better. Besides limiting your exposure to blue light, there are some other key habits to cultivate for best sleep. When you have a sleep routine that you practice regularly, you are much more likely to sleep more soundly and get more quality deep and REM sleep. Here are some important and proven ways to improve your sleep length and quality:

- **WIND DOWN.** It may sound obvious, but I'm surprised how many people don't make an effort to wind down in the evenings by relaxing, disengaging from work, and making an effort to slow their brains down after a busy day. If you are laboring over your to-do list until moments before getting into bed, you probably won't sleep as well. Instead, right before dinner, try making a list of all the things you have to do the next day, putting it on your desk for tomorrow, then mentally letting it all go. Focus on quiet activities like a warm bath or reading (from a real book, not a screen emitting blue light), easy pleasant conversations (this is not the time for bringing up sensitive issues with family members), and letting your brain and body prepare for sleep. Think low-stimulation.

- **AVOID LARGE, HEAVY MEALS AT NIGHT.** If you eat a large or heavy meal in the evening, especially if it is high in fat and/or sugar, your body will have to spend some of your sleep time digesting and less energy will be available for sleep quality and brain repair. Most people experience more sensitive blood sugar in the evenings, likely because our bodies do not expect to be eating food after dark. A heavy meal at lunch is likely to result in less of a blood sugar rise than a heavy meal at night. If you need something to eat before bed, keep it light and low in calories. Ideally, you should avoid eating anything for at least two or three hours before you go to sleep. If you are always hungry in the evenings, try eating more food earlier in the day. Late-night snacking can also be a habit, rather than something based in genuine hunger. If you skip the after-dinner snacks for a few days, the urge may fade.

- **EXERCISE EARLY.** You are likely to sleep much better on the days you exercise, but exercising too late in the day could inhibit sleep quality because it's stimulating. For most people, exercising in the morning or at least before dinner will have the best impact on sleep. (If evening is the only time you can exercise, it's better than not exercising at all. Just be extra committed to winding down before bed.)

- **CREATE A SLEEP SANCTUARY.** Everything about your bedroom should make you feel relaxed. First of all, like your mother always told you: "Clean your room!" A clean, neat, orderly, beautiful room will put you in a good mode to relax. Keep bedding clean and fresh and decorate your bedroom in a way that makes you happy *but calm*. Your bed should be comfortable. An air purifier or a few green plants can improve your bedroom air quality, and if flowers make you happy, it can be nice to have fresh ones in the bedroom (remove them as soon as they begin to wilt). To some extent, getting a good sleep is a mental game. When your bedroom cues you to feel relaxed and sleepy, you will sleep better. Is it time to refresh your bedroom? It's an investment in your health! Also, just to reiterate, I discourage any electronics in the bedroom—no television, no computer. Not only do they emit blue light, but they can trigger you to think about work or tempt you to turn on an exciting movie. I'd really like it if you would put your cell phone in a different room when you sleep, too, although I realize that's crossing a line for some! If you can't move the screens out of your room, at least drape light fabric over them while you sleep, so your brain doesn't register their presence.

- **GO TO BED SOONER.** Brain-cleaning, body-repairing deep sleep normally happens primarily in the first half of the night,[42] so while you may cycle in and out of it throughout the night, you are most likely to get most of it earlier. If you stay up late, you could be shorting yourself.

DE-STRESS YOUR BRAIN

There is a book I love called *Why Zebras Don't Get Ulcers*[43] written by primatologist Robert Sapolsky, which makes the point that while zebras undergo acute stress when a predator is chasing them, as soon as the lion takes down one of the herd, everybody else immediately goes back to munching on grass. They don't spend their days fretting and worrying that a lion might come along. They are very good at going back to baseline after a stressful event. Humans aren't so good at that. I've already talked a lot about chronic stress in this book, which is exactly what zebras don't have.

We are not created to experience constant stress. And yet we fret, worry, and tear ourselves down with stress even when there aren't any lions in sight, and one of the victims of the damaging effect of chronic stress is definitely the brain. I've mentioned earlier that chronic stress can actually shrink the prefrontal cortex, which is not only responsible for memory but for learning and other higher cognitive functions.[44] Stress can also kill brain cells, suppress the production of BDNF,[45] and have a measurable effect on cognitive function, memory, learning, and the ability to concentrate and focus. In severe cases, such as with trauma or prolonged extreme hardship, stress can result in chronic PTSD, chronic depression, or even cognitive impairment. Over time, some of these changes can even be permanent, so it's important to learn how to manage your stress now. Your brain has no resources to waste.

Stress is an inevitable part of life, but with stress management, you can give your brain a chance to relax and repair. Here are some of my favorite, and the most proven, ways to do that:

- **EXERCISE.** I'll keep saying it: Exercise fixes so many problems! One of them is stress. Exercise has been proven to reverse stress-induced suppression of BDNF,[46] and moderate-intensity exercise has been shown to reduce the effects of oxidative stress.[47] Even five minutes of cardio can stop an anxiety attack.[48]

- **MINDFULNESS.** Mindfulness is a broad term that can encompass many techniques with the same underlying focus: noticing the present moment. In one study of medical students under stress, those who practiced a variety of mindfulness techniques, including focusing on the breath, scanning the body for sensations, eating meditation, walking meditation, and guided imagery, along with daily twenty-minute guided meditation, which they listened to on a recording, experienced statistically significant reductions in tension, anxiety, fatigue, inertia, confusion, and bewilderment. (Trust me—medical school can be quite bewildering.) In the control group not practicing mindfulness, there were statistically significant increases in each of these categories. After the study, 88 percent of the students in the mindfulness group said they felt the techniques were helpful or very helpful, and 71 percent said they felt more mindful in their daily lives, suggesting these techniques have lasting effects.[49]

  To practice mindfulness, all you have to do is what I've been encouraging you to do from the beginning of this book: Tune in to your body and how you feel in response to what you eat, how you move, and what you do. Mindfulness also means focusing your attention on what is going on around you, including the people you are with, the things you see, and the experiences happening to you *right now*, rather than constantly thinking about the past or the future. Your life is happening right now, and mindfulness is how you can be present for it.

- **DEEP BREATHING EXERCISES.** You know that stress triggers the sympathetic nervous system (the so-called "fight or flight" response) to engage, resulting in a cascade of effects based on the release of stress hormones like cortisol and adrenaline pumped out by the adrenal glands. Deep breathing has the opposite effect. A few minutes of deep breathing can calm the body enough to switch back into parasympathetic mode (the "rest and digest" mode). Research has demonstrated that not only does deep breathing change someone's subjective perception of their own stress level and mood, but these changes are measurable in terms of heart rate and cortisol levels in saliva.[50]

The Beauty Breathing exercise in chapter three is one great way to use deep breathing to reverse the stress response. Also, see the mantra meditation in the meditation section below.

Another method is diaphragmatic breathing (sometimes called "belly breathing"), which has been proven to reduce stress in healthy adults.[51] Diaphragmatic breathing is a technique used in yoga and some meditative practices. It is also the way singers are trained to breathe. Your diaphragm is a domed muscle at the base of your rib cage that expands and contracts as you breathe. This happens involuntarily, but you can learn to control the process. At first, it's hard to feel it. Here's an easy way to practice:

1. Lie down on the floor on a yoga mat, or on any firm surface. (It's harder to feel if you lie on something soft like a bed.)

2. Rest one hand on your upper chest, and rest the other hand on your stomach.

3. Feel your breathing and notice where your hands are moving. Most people tend to move their chests as they breathe, which indicates shallower breathing. If the hand on your chest moves as you breathe, you are chest breathing. Notice if that is happening.

4. Now, breathing in through your nose, imagine that you are slowly filling up your belly with air. Try not to move your chest or your shoulders at all. Let the air move the hand over your stomach/upper abdomen only. This may take some time to get the feel of it. Not everyone can do it at first. Just keep trying. Focus all your attention on your lower hand and try to make that move as you breathe.

5. When you are able to do this, it indicates that you are expanding your diaphragm and breathing deeply. Continue to do this for five minutes or so. It should feel very relaxing because you are triggering the parasympathetic nervous system.

6. Practice diaphragmatic breathing once or a twice a day. When you get the hang of it, you should be able to do it while sitting or standing. The sign that you are doing it correctly is that, no matter what position you are in, your chest and shoulders do not move *with the breath*. Only your stomach or abdominal area expands with the inhalation.

- **YOGA.** I try to do some yoga as often as I can. There are different kinds of yoga, but they can all help to reduce stress by increasing mindfulness as you focus on doing different poses. There isn't a huge amount of research on this, but a few studies have shown that yoga does reduce cortisol and measurable signs of inflammation.[52] It's a wonderful therapy for the adrenal glands! People who practice it also report feeling calmer, more positive, and more compassionate toward themselves and others. If you already know how to do yoga, getting back to a regular daily practice can make a big difference in your stress levels. If you aren't sure how to do it, there are yoga classes everywhere, both in person and online. Yoga also happens to be great exercise, increasing strength and flexibility along with its stress-relieving benefits. My favorite calming yoga pose is Child's Pose. Hold this position and completely relax for as long as you can.

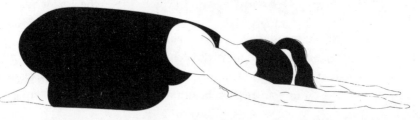

Vibrant Pro Tip: If you have physical limitations that prohibit you from getting into this pose, you can put yoga blocks or pillows under your buttocks and chest to reduce the bend in the knees and hips. Or, try another relaxing pose: Lie down by a wall and prop your legs up straight against the wall (many people just call this "Legs Up the Wall"). This is also very relaxing.

• **MEDITATION.** If you really want to take your stress in hand, meditation is the way to do it. Of all the stress-reducing techniques, meditation is the most studied and the most proven to intervene into the stress response. There are thousands of studies showing that meditation can reduce pain, improve blood pressure, ease anxiety and depression, fix insomnia, and improve the ability to stick to better health habits in general.

Most interesting for this chapter is the way meditation can actually structurally alter the brain in positive ways. While stress can shrink the prefrontal cortex, meditation can increase the size of the hippocampus, which also influences memory and learning, and the thickness of the cerebral cortex. It may also be able to shrink the amygdala, which, as you may remember, increases in size due to chronic stress, increasing stress susceptibility, reactivity, and emotions, especially fear and anxiety.[53] Meditation can restructure the brain in other positive ways. In 2012, researchers examined images of the brains of fifty people who meditated and fifty people who didn't meditate. Those who had practiced regular meditation for many years had more of the folds on the outside of the brain that contribute to the brain's processing ability.[54]

Meditation may not feel like it's doing anything in the moment, and some people find it frustrating to just sit there "doing nothing," but you are definitely not doing nothing when you meditate. Your brain is changing, and your entire body is recovering from stress. Although meditation can have an immediate effect on the stress response, meditating every day over the long term is the real secret to growing a healthy brain, reducing the risk of dementia, and becoming impervious to the damaging effects of chronic stress. Its effects go even further. Meditation has also been shown to help you connect to people better, raise your emotional intelligence,[55] make you more confident, improve your ability to master your own emotions, make you more thoughtful and introspective, help you get better at focusing and paying attention, make you more creative, and make you a happier person overall.[56] It may be the most powerful thing you can do to improve your mental and emotional health.

HOW TO MEDITATE

There are many ways to meditate, and many people will tell you there is a right way and a wrong way, but I don't think there is any wrong way to meditate. Like exercise, the best kind of meditation is the kind that you will actually do. You could pay a lot of money to get trained in transcendental meditation (TM), which is a widely studied form of meditation requiring a teacher, and some people swear by it, but you could also just sit down, close your eyes, and focus on the sound and feel of your breathing.

Some people like to keep it simple, repeating a word or phrase to themselves to focus the mind, and some people like to get creative with detailed visualizations. If you aren't sure where to start and don't already have a favorite style, try either one or both of these simple meditation techniques. The first is a form of mantra meditation, and the second is a guided visualization. It's a way to dip your toe in, try this powerful practice, and enjoy immediate stress reduction benefits.

To practice either one of these meditations, find a quiet place where you won't be distracted. Sit on the floor (or the ground outside) with your legs crossed. If this is difficult, you can sit on a cushion or pillow to raise your hips, which can make it easier to cross your legs. You can also sit on a chair with your feet on the floor. Sit up straight, without support if you can (if not, you can work toward that). Shift a bit until you settle into a comfortable position. If music helps you feel calm, you could play any peaceful meditative instrumental music or nature sounds. Put your palms on your knees, either facedown or faceup, depending on what feels more comfortable for you. If you like, you can touch your thumb and index finger together. This gesture is called a "mudra," and it is meant to channel energy moving out of your body back inside by closing the circuit of the fingers. Close your eyes. You are ready to begin.

Mantra Meditation

To practice a mantra meditation, you focus on breathing and repeating simple words such as OM, which is considered a sacred syllable in

Hinduism and Tibetan Buddhism. It is similar to the Christian "amen." In this meditation, which is one of my husband's favorites, you will repeat two words: "I am" and "calm." Calm has a similar sound to OM when used in this way. You could also use any other words that make you feel relaxed.

1. Bring your attention to your breath. Don't make any effort to change it. Just notice it and feel it moving in and out of you.

2. Inhale slowly for four seconds as you think the words: I AM. Or, say the words out loud after inhaling.

3. Hold your breath for six seconds.

4. Exhale for 12 seconds while thinking the word: CALM. Or, say the word out loud after exhaling.

5. Repeat this breathing for as long as you have decided to meditate. If this is difficult, start with just five minutes and see if you can work your way up to 15 to 20 minutes each morning and evening.

Guided Visualization

1. Bring your attention to your breath. Don't make any effort to change it. Just notice it and feel it moving in and out of you. Stay with your breath for a minute or two.

2. Now, imagine a peaceful, serene place you love to be. It could be a place you know well, perhaps a quiet beach or a forest where you like to hike, or maybe somewhere you went once a long time ago. It can also be a make-believe place, such as a field of flowers next to a sparkling stream, or a tropical grotto, or on a boat at sea, or even a beautiful room you design in your mind.

3. In your mind, look around at this place and notice all the details of what you see, feel, hear, smell. Try to feel it with all your senses.

4. Imagine yourself in the space. What are you doing? How does it feel to be there? Are you relaxing on the beach? Wading through the water? Lying under a tree? Walking through the soft grass? Imagine that you feel complete and utter peace in that place. You feel protected, safe, loved, and happy. Stay there for as long as you want to. Meditation is more about doing it regularly than about how long you do it, so if you only stay there for five minutes this time, that's okay. If you stay there for half an hour, that's okay, too.

5. When you are ready to leave your happy place (for now), feel your breath moving in and out of you again. Let your mind come

back to where you are sitting. Slowly open your eyes. Sit for a moment until you feel ready to move. Think about how you have done something good for yourself. If it was difficult, be compassionate with yourself. You are on a journey, and every time you practice, it will get easier and more enjoyable.

6. Do it again tomorrow.

WHAT TECHNOLOGY DOES TO YOUR BRAIN

When it comes to brain health, technology is a double-edged sword. Technology that helps you exercise more, like fitness trackers, or technology that helps you reduce screen time by showing you how often you've been looking at your phone, or technology designed to monitor your sleep quality, can all be useful in improving your lifestyle habits in ways that benefit your brain health. Anything that gives you feedback about how your lifestyle is impacting you is likely to be a brain booster. Keeping up rewarding relationships over social media, whether with friends and family or with support groups or social groups of like-minded people, can also make you feel happier and more fulfilled, which benefits your brain. One study demonstrated that adults who used computers more often scored higher on cognitive function tests than people who hardly ever used computers.[57] Being online may help keep you engaged and aware of what's going on in the world, especially for older adults. Research does seem to suggest that the younger you are, the worse screen time is for your brain,[58] but the older you are, the better it is for your brain.

However, there is a dark side to technology. Smartphones, tablets, and computers can become addictive, and the source of compulsive behavior that interferes with life and puts you at risk for developing problems with impulse control, loneliness, attention issues, and the loss of the ability to think deeply or be creative. Compulsive behavior surrounding technology can negatively impact face-to-face relationships and is associated with mental health issues like anxiety, depression,[59] and low self-esteem.[60] If you find that you can't stop looking at your phone or you get very uncomfortable when you don't have your phone with you, or you notice that you can't stop checking your email or spend way too much time on a particular website (more than an hour a day, unless it's actually your job), or if you feel compelled to look at your phone when you are talking to an actual person, you may have a problem that is increasing stress on your brain and could even be rewiring your brain in ways that will inhibit your ability to concentrate and focus on things (or people!). In this case, I suggest a digital detox.

To do a digital detox, take a period of time—it could be an hour, or a day, or a weekend, or even longer—during which you turn off your phone and put it away. You can also turn off your computer. During this specified time, you will not look at any screens. Instead, spend time fully engaged in the real world around you. Spend time with real people who are physically with you. Go out into nature and experience the real scenery in front of you, and remember how to look at life in three dimensions again. If you have developed a compulsive habit of looking at your phone, this might feel really hard at first, like giving up sugar or quitting smoking. (Addictions are addictions.) But the longer you go without it, the easier it gets. It can feel like waking up to your life again. (If that's too intense for you, you can also ease into digital detoxes by using our old friend the Rule of Halves. See how in the brain wins, below.)

• • •

If you think about it (a brain pun?), your brain is everything because, without it, you would have no awareness of your own existence. For something so precious, it's surprising how little care most people give their brains. But that's not the vibrant way. Instead, give your brain more love, more care, more nurture, and listen to your body for the signals that your brain needs more support. You should be able to think quickly, clearly, and complexly. Working the Vibrant Triad will get you there, but special attention to your amazing brain in all the ways this chapter suggests can keep you sharper longer so you can maintain focus and enjoy happier, healthier moods. What better way to fully enjoy your vibrant life?

BRAIN WINS

These brain wins can start impacting your intelligence, cognitive function, and mood for the better almost immediately. Pick one or two, or try them all. Let these become part of your life, and watch yourself get smarter, sharper, and happier.

SLEEP BETTER. Choose the sleep hygiene habit (pages 178–179) that you think will make the most difference for you and put it into practice. Maybe it's turning your bedroom into a peaceful sanctuary, or not eating three hours before bedtime, or turning off all screens an hour or two before bed. Notice each morning if you feel more rested when you've done that one thing. If you can tell a difference after a week, you will know this new habit is making a positive change in your sleep quality, and in your brain health.

○ *I tried it! Here's how it felt:* _____

_____

_____

DE-STRESS. Spend 5 to 15 minutes in the morning and/or evening doing either the diaphragmatic breathing exercise on page 181 or the meditation exercise on page 184. See if you can work up to 15 minutes every morning and 15 minutes every night.

○ *I tried it! Here's how it felt:* _____

_____

_____

TRY A RULE OF HALVES DIGITAL DETOX. Figure out how much time you spend looking at your phone every day (many phones can calculate this for you), or keep track by jotting it down.

Start your detox by cutting that time in half. You can still check, but when you've reached your limit for the day, you have to put it away. Try it for a day. If you can do it, try it for a weekend.

○ *I tried it! Here's how it felt:* _____

_____

_____

CHAPTER 8

The Rejuvenator: How to Detoxify, Inside and Out

To be alive in this modern world means to be exposed to toxic metals, plastics, and industrial chemicals, many of which are neurotoxins, endocrine disruptors, obesegens, and diabetogens (these last two are just what they sound like: substances that increase toxic body fat and impair blood sugar control. We are all exposed every day—even newborn babies. Samples of umbilical cord blood from newborns reveal a long list of toxic chemicals, including mercury and lead, sometimes in concentrations even more potent than those in the mother.[1] The world is so toxic that it's amazing we are still walking around! For that, we can thank our body's amazing and brilliant detoxification system.

Your body is always on the job, working to detoxify your system day in and day out. This is why you have a liver, kidneys, a lymphatic system, and why your digestive tract doesn't just have an entrance but also an exit. You are exposed to far more environmental toxins than your parents or grandparents ever were. It was not anticipated by our creator that our bodies would ever have to be this good at detoxification. We have outpaced our body's natural detoxification rhythm with exposure to the by-products of industrialization, from the burning of fossil fuels to the chemical enhancements that increase food yield. Many of these new-to-nature molecules, which weren't around when our detoxification systems developed, are hard to get rid of. For example, polychlorinated biphenyls have half lives in humans (the time it takes to get rid of half the body load) ranging from three to a worrisome 25 years! That means some of the toxic chemicals typically found in farmed fish can take your whole life to eliminate. The best strategy is never to let them into your body in the first place.

Still, your body does a pretty good job, even under these less than ideal conditions. The primary method for detoxification in your body is a two-phase process that happens in the liver, but detoxification also happens to a lesser extent through the lymphatic system, the lungs, and the skin. The body also traps toxins it can't immediately eliminate in fat cells so they are essentially sealed away and harmless (until you burn those fat cells, such as during weight loss.[2] I'll talk more about that later in this chapter).

HOW YOUR LIVER "TAKES OUT THE TRASH"

The liver's primary function is to neutralize and eliminate toxins to keep you alive and functioning. The process happens in two phases: Phase 1 can immediately detoxify some chemicals like caffeine, but mostly it prepares fat-soluble toxins for Phase 2 elimination via cytochrome P450 enzymes. It's a complicated process but for our purposes, what's important is that this phase preps toxins for Phase 2, and in doing so, makes them temporarily even more toxic because they are activated for the next stage. That's why Phase 1 is always followed by Phase 2—activated toxins must be eliminated.

Phase 1 can be hard on your liver, which needs heavy nutritional support, especially when you have a lot to detoxify. Antioxidants support Phase 1, which produces a lot of free radicals. Antioxidants neutralize them (free radicals can cause cell damage). Also supporting Phase 1: B vitamins, zinc, and the amino acid cysteine, which helps to produce glutathione, critical for detoxification.

Phase 2 essentially converts fat-soluble toxins into water-soluble form so they can be eliminated via the kidneys and urinary tract as urine, or through the bile duct and colon as stool (and secondarily through the lymphatic system and through skin as sweat and lungs as breath). Phase 2 nutrient supports are vitamins C, B4, and B12, as well as magnesium and multiple amino acids.

The best way you can support this process is to eat a nutrient-dense diet[3] full of the nourishing substances necessary to support this natural detoxification process. Your other job is to stay out of the way by living in a manner that supports and does not interfere with your natural detoxification process. Unfortunately, our modern lifestyle, with its low-fiber food, insufficient water consumption resulting in chronic dehydration, and sedentary living, tends to slow down the natural elimination processes through the digestive system, the lymphatic system, and by stressing and distracting the liver with other jobs. Every margarita, every dose of ibuprofen or allergy medication, every processed food meal requires the liver to step up and detoxify the alcohol, drugs, and food chemicals you ingested.

Sometimes you can't help giving your liver extra work, like if you need to take antibiotics for an infection or get food poisoning or you are exposed to a lot of pollution you can't avoid. Meanwhile, your body also makes its own waste in the form of the by-products of metabolism, digestion, and the many biochemical reactions that take place inside of you all the time, and all that has to be processed and eliminated, too. Dead cells, dead microbes, excess estrogen produced from fat cells and during early perimenopause—all have to go.

MENOPAUSE AND THE DETOXIFICATION OF HORMONES

As you reach the end of your childbearing years (and the beginning of what could be some of the most interesting years of your life), your hormones will begin to shift, and depending on your health status, those shifts may feel uncomfortable or even interfere with your lifestyle. Some women never have PMS and sail right through menopause without a blink, but most women feel the upheaval in their bodies for up to 10 years. I bring this up in the detoxification chapter because some of the endogenous (internal) waste products your body has to process through the liver are your own hormones.

One of the early signs that menopause is coming is estrogen dominance, which can cause brain fog, sore breasts, headaches, irritability, and rapid weight gain. This is often due to decreasing progesterone, which skews the progesterone/estrogen ratio. Fat cells can act like an endocrine gland and produce their own estrogen, so obesity can further imbalance estrogen, and excess estrogen must be cleared by the detoxification system. Get as toxin-free as you can during this time, to free up your liver. Your body is always trying to balance your hormones, and a toxic load can exacerbate the symptoms of perimenopause because it interferes with your body's ability to manage that balance. As menopause nears, estrogen drops, and hot flashes often kick in. Detoxification is still important, especially if you are on hormone replacement therapy.

A note about hormone therapy: Purposeful hormone manipulation is extremely complex, expensive, and takes expertise. Hormone replacement can cause many side effects having to do with sensitivity, incomplete transformation, and toxicity. A healthy detoxification system is critical if you are adding hormones! But you may not need them. Before you consider hormone therapy, solidify your health foundations. Please, get your diet right, get your exercise right, and clean up your health before you fully engage in another complicator. Working the Vibrant Triad alone could resolve many of the symptoms of menopause. If it doesn't, then you might determine that bioidentical hormone replacement therapy could be beneficial for you, under the guidance of someone who can work with you individually and can monitor your detoxification. Everyone reacts to hormone therapy differently, and to do it correctly requires a lot of testing and a personalized approach. First, I hope you will put your energy into those critical and broadly influential basics, which could render hormone replacement therapy unnecessary.

In addition to the other resources in this chapter, here are a few herbs that Dr. Liu recommends for hormone balance:

- **Tu Si Zi (Chinese dodder seeds):** Dr. Liu recommends this for hormone balance in women, at a daily dose of 9 to 15 grams.

- **Black cohosh:** One of the most popular herbal remedies for menopausal symptoms, this is an ancient Native American remedy for women's hormone problems. Researchers think its effective action has to do with helping to slow the uptake of serotonin, in a way similar to antidepressants.[4] Black cohosh has been shown in some studies (but not all) to significantly reduce hot flashes.[5]

- **Red clover:** Red clover has more bioavailable isoflavones than soy (soy is often suggested as a remedy for menopausal women). It's been shown to reduce hot flashes while not increasing estrogenic activity,[6] so it doesn't appear to increase the risk of any hormone-sensitive cancers.

- **Licorice root:** Here's another supplement that has been shown to significantly reduce hot flashes without estrogenic activity to sensitive tissues.[7] Dr. Liu recommends a daily dose of 3 to 6 grams for hormone balancing.

- **Vitex (Chaste Tree Berry):** This herb can help with all stages of hormonal imbalance. It's been researched for its effects on the symptoms of PMS, endometriosis, and infertility.[8]

Imagine if you never took out your trash. The trash cans in your home would fill up and overflow. Soon, there would be trash on the floor, spilling out the doors and windows. Eventually, you wouldn't be able to live there anymore. You have to take out the trash, and in your body, that means making sure your elimination system is able to work. You need to be having a daily bowel movement, and drinking enough water so that your urine is always a very pale yellow (although if you are taking B vitamins, your urine can turn bright yellow). Those two things alone will make a big difference in how well your body can keep the trash moving out the back door (so to speak).

What about when your body really can't keep up with the toxic load? Let's keep going with our metaphor. Imagine the trash is starting to pile up. It's not dysfunctional yet, but there is definitely a lot of clutter on the tables and other surfaces. What if you find out somebody important is coming over for dinner and they're going to arrive in 20 minutes?

You look around at the mess and panic. No time to clean! So you run around grabbing clutter and stuffing it into drawers and cupboards and closets. (That's what I do!). You think you could probably throw some of it away, but there's no time to sort through it so you stash it all out of sight. You tell yourself you'll deal with it later because, right now, you have to deal with what's in front of you—that person coming to visit.

When your detoxification system becomes overburdened, something similar happens. When your liver has to deal with something important, but has to keep up with its very important job of keeping you clean and not poisoned, it stuffs toxins away into your fat cells,[9] and to a lesser extent your brain, bones, and organs (especially your thyroid), to be dealt with later. The next time your liver has some free time, it can get to those toxins, but during the busy times, your body knows those toxins can't hurt you if they stay isolated and neutralized inside your fat cells.

We all know what it's like to never get around to cleaning out those closets and junk drawers. Out of sight, out of mind. If you never get any free time—if your liver never gets that resting period—it will keep stuffing more and more toxins into your fat cells, even making more fat cells to accommodate the need. You are accumulating toxic fat. This is a survival response—but at a price.

While fat cells make a pretty good toxin storage unit, they can also cause a lot of health problems for you, if you keep gaining more and more toxic fat. They can begin to interfere with hormone production and cause inflammation, both of which can cause weight gain and hinder weight-loss efforts. Your brain and thyroid are sensitive to toxins, which can disrupt their healthy function, and toxic fat can accumulate around the liver and invade liver cells, causing liver disease. If you continue to let the toxins in by eating a poor diet, not exercising, and continuing to hinder your body's efforts with a sedentary lifestyle, not drinking enough water, and adding in regular exposure to alcohol, medications, and environmental pollutants, it will get more and more difficult to get your detoxification system back online. Detoxification takes an enormous amount of energy, so when your body starts tossing the trash into the drawers, it's like giving up and saying, "I can't handle this anymore."

Your body doesn't want to hoard fat, and I'm sure you don't want this either. This is why so many people ask me about cleansing, detoxing, and fasting. I'll tell you what I tell them: You don't need to do a cleanse. Remember that your body is always cleansing. What you need to do is stop inhibiting and start supporting that natural process. In this chapter, I'm going to show you the best ways I know for how to do that, but it really boils down to just two things.

1. Taking out the trash every day (making sure your elimination system is moving).

2. Making less trash.

EASING YOUR BODY'S TOXIC BURDEN

If your detoxification system is working pretty well, that's great. You can continue to support it to make sure it stays functional. For many people, however, detoxification is already getting bogged down. You can tell if your natural detoxification system is overburdened if you:

- **Feel tired all the time.** A toxic burden can interfere with your body's normal energy production.

- **Have skin issues.** Acne, rashes, and skin infections can all be signs that the body is trying to purge excess waste through the skin.

- **Are constipated.** When your digestion slows down or stops, you aren't getting the waste out in a timely manner. To be constipated is to be accumulating waste.

- **Feel moody or irritable, or worse.** Environmental exposures can lead to psychiatric symptoms, from minor mood swings to depression, panic, and anxiety disorders.[10]

- **Have unexplained joint pain or headaches.** This can be a sign of inflammation due to toxicity.

- **React to every food.** Unaddressed food sensitivities may have your digestive system on high alert.

- **Have restless legs syndrome (RLS).** This condition can be a symptom of heavy metal toxicity. (RLS can also be caused by inadequate cellular potassium or low iron.)

- **Feel generally unwell.** Whether you are catching every virus or have the early signs of an autoimmune disease (see the next chapter), this can be a sign that your body is breaking down in response to increased toxic load.

- **Have gained a lot of weight in a short period of time.** It could be your body making more fat cells for toxin storage.

In more severe cases, toxicity can result in more serious neurological conditions. There is evidence that toxic exposure, especially to heavy metals, can be a cause of or contributor to ADHD,[11] autism,[12] bipolar disorder,[13] schizophrenia,[14] severe depression,[15] anxiety disorders,[16] severe headaches,[17] unexplained neurologic conditions such as when people develop Parkinson's-like symptoms[18] as well as actual Parkinson's disease,[19] multiple sclerosis,[20] Alzheimer's disease,[21] and other types of dementia.[22] In addition to triggering these many conditions, toxicity itself can also mimic pathological illness, and it can be very difficult to tell what's wrong. Once you are at this point, you are pretty far down the line and should seek guidance from a medical professional who has experience with detoxification.

Fortunately, most people haven't progressed to the point of serious neurological dysfunction from toxic overload, even if they are showing some symptoms. Remember, that's your body telling you something is wrong and asking you for help. If that is you, it's time to answer those calls with some critical assistance to help your body take out the trash. Here are the most important ways to do that.

THE WORST TIME TO DETOX IS WHEN YOU ARE TOXIC

Ironically, the worst time to "do a detox" that involves severely limiting calories or fasting is when your body is overburdened and your detox system is sluggish. The latest one I've heard about is the celery cleanse, but this has been going on for decades. Do you remember the Master Cleanse? I do, and I hope I never have to start my morning with lemon juice, maple syrup, and cayenne pepper in my glass of water ever again! When you do a juice or water fast or use some extremely low-calorie cleanse recipe or product, your body can begin aggressively releasing toxins, but without fiber and nutrients to support the entire detoxification process, and especially if you are constipated and your liver is already overburdened and inflamed, those toxins will just keep circulating and concentrating, and you won't have the resources to get them all the way out. You'll be dumping the trash cans onto the floor instead of taking them out to the curb!

Constipation and sluggish lymphatic flow are hallmarks of a toxic state, so withdrawing fiber and nutrients can make you even more toxic, and if you are already feeling sick, you'll get worse, as the toxins your body worked so hard to stash safely away are now at liberty, running rampant through your bloodstream. You can also start to break down muscle, which is what happens during starvation. Even if you are obese and eager to lose weight, "cleansing" is not the way to do it smartly. Instead of focusing on detoxifying, it's better to let your body take care of that part, while you focus on dietary and lifestyle changes that will get your digestive system and lymphatic system moving again, and also will support your liver and other organs of detoxification with the nutrients, fiber, fluid, and movement they need. This is not a time to stress and starve. It's a time to mentally relax and flood your body with good, clean nutrition.

Get Regular

Let's not tiptoe around it: Most of the waste leaves your body through your colon and you should be taking out the trash, so to speak, *every day*. In other words, you should be having a good complete bowel movement at least once per day (more is just fine, as long as your stools are soft but solid—they should not be like hard little pebbles). Ideally, you would go after every meal. That's what babies and animals do. Instead, adults often get in the habit of waiting, and that can hinder regularity. I really do think that sometimes people forget that most of the waste goes out through the urine and bowels and it's relatively easy to keep these waste removal pathways moving with some fiber intake and a few targeted supplements, when necessary.

Look here for a visual chart showing what different kinds of stool mean for your digestive health.

My best remedies for constipation are:

- **Eat more fiber.** You should be getting at least 30 grams a day, preferably more like 50 or more. When our detox systems evolved, humans typically consumed more than 100 grams of fiber per day! To get enough, eat as many vegetables as you can, along with fruit and legumes.

- **Drink more water.** To keep your kidneys in good working order, it's important to drink a lot of water—ideally, half your body weight number in ounces per day. Drinking enough water also helps your bowels to move. Dehydration is a common cause of constipation.

- **Move more.** Regular daily cardio does so many great things for you, and one of them is to help ease constipation.
- **Relax.** For many people, stress can cause constipation. In others, it can cause diarrhea. The effect of stress on the digestive tract is likely related to both the release of stress hormones and to the disruption of the gut microbiome (see page 90),[23] both of which affect intestinal movement. Stress management practices such as deep breathing and meditation, along with the aforementioned high-fiber diet to improve microbiome health, can help alleviate this problem.

BEST SUPPLEMENTS TO EASE CONSTIPATION AND SUPPORT YOUR LIVER

Of all the reasons to take supplements, detoxification may be the most important, which is why I list more supplements in this chapter than in any of the others. In this toxic world, your liver and your colon probably need help, and every one of these supplements will accomplish that much more naturally than with drugs or harsh laxatives. Instead, try these:

- **N-Acetyl Cysteine:** This is the supplement form of cysteine, an amino acid your body makes naturally to aid in the production of glutathione, a powerful antioxidant you manufacture internally. The amount of available cysteine determines how much glutathione you make, so it is especially important. Its antioxidant superpowers block cell damage, bolster brain health, and decrease work for the liver and immune system.[24]
- **Magnesium citrate:** I've mentioned this before, but I'll remind you here that this is an excellent remedy for constipation.
- **Dandelion root:** Dandelion root is an ancient folk remedy, both in Eastern and Western countries, for treating the liver, but science has shown it is indeed hepatoprotective (protective of the liver) and also has significant antioxidant and anti-inflammatory properties.[25] It's also been studied as a therapy for type 2 diabetes.[26] Dandelion root tea is an easy way to get the benefits, and its roasty taste is reminiscent of coffee, but without the caffeine. (Chicory has traditionally been used as a coffee substitute, and dandelion and chicory are in the same family.)
- **Triphala:** An important digestive and general health tonic in Ayurvedic medicine, triphala is a combination of three berries with powerful antioxidant action: amla, bibhitaki, and haritaki. It is

> • excellent for constipation and regularity because of its gentle but effective laxative action, but it also has adaptogenic (anti-stress) properties, and polyphenols that feed beneficial gut bacteria, among many other benefits.[27]

Reduce Your Exposure

You can't eliminate every toxic exposure, but minimizing exposure in the places where you spend the most time can make a big difference in how much your liver has to do on a daily basis. Don't stress about what you can't control, but change what you can. You have more control than you might think. Here are some big-impact ways to live cleaner by taking action on:

• **THE AIR YOU BREATHE.** Indoor air pollution can be much worse than the air outdoors. Chemical cleaning products, air fresheners, candles, fireplaces, and stoves can all pollute your indoor air. I remember when I was in college, I used to buy those Yankee Candles and think I was being so Zen, even though they made black smoke! I can't even tell you how much I spent on those expensive candles, thinking I was relieving my stress, when all I was really doing was inhaling particulates.

You can improve your indoor air quality significantly just by removing some obvious sources of indoor air pollution. Let's start with where you sleep: You spend a good one-third or so of your life sleeping, and breathing deeply, in your bedroom. This is a good place to keep an air purifier, to reduce your exposure to indoor air pollution. Look for one with a true HEPA filter, which can reduce dust, pollen, smoke, and pet dander. It doesn't reduce gases like volatile organic compounds (VOCs) and radon, but it can definitely circulate fresher air with greatly reduced particulates.

To tackle those VOCs, open your windows as often as you can, unless you live in an area where air pollution is a problem. Stepping outside and deeply breathing the fresh air during the day will make a difference, even when you are at work. Well-tended, healthy green plants can also absorb these compounds, so if you can manage the maintenance, fill up your home, and your office if you can, with beautiful greenery.

You can also reduce the introduction of these compounds and other air pollutants by making sure stoves and fireplaces are well vented to the outside. Gas stoves in particular may be preferred for those who love to cook, but they are worse for your indoor air. Be sure your exhaust fan is operating at optimum efficiency. All gas appliances burn petroleum. If you smell gas, you are inhaling petroleum! Electric stoves as well as other electric appliances are less polluting than gas. Wood-burning fireplaces and stoves also pollute your indoor air. If you do have these, keep your flue clean and well maintained. Be sure it is open during use, and closed when not in use.

Another good way to reduce indoor air pollution (that you don't always know is there) is to use more natural materials in your home. Synthetic carpets, flooring, paint, and furniture off-gas chemicals into the indoor air. Unless you are already planning to remodel and can choose natural materials like ceramic tiles, hardwood or bamboo, and low- or no-VOC, nontoxic or "natural" paint, integrate these changes a few at a time, as they come up. If each new item you bring into your home is made of natural materials, your indoor air quality will improve slowly but surely.

I also strongly recommend switching over all cleaning and so-called air "freshening" products to natural and organic. There are many natural cleaners available now, but you can also do a lot with just water, vinegar, baking soda, salt, lemon, and rubbing alcohol. For air freshening, try natural essential oils and essential oil diffusers rather than chemical and spray air fresheners.

- **THE WATER YOU DRINK.** Tap water is filtered by cities, but it can still contain many toxic substances, including agricultural and industrial chemicals and heavy metals. The best way to get clean water is either to purchase pure (or purified) natural spring water for drinking, or to filter the water in your home. The most effective filters are reverse osmosis systems, but these can be quite costly. Less expensive carbon filters also filter out many contaminants. Even filtered water pitchers help. The Environmental Working Group (EWG) has an online page (www.ewg.org/tapwater/)

you can use to search your zip code for information about your local water quality and whether it contains contaminants above federal limits.

- **THE FOOD YOU EAT.** My number one recommendation for detoxifying your food is to buy organic food whenever possible. Clean out your refrigerator of all junk food and focus on whole, natural organic food. There is a lot of debate about whether or not organic foods are more nutritious, but that's not why I want you to use them. The most important reason to go organic is to reduce your intake of pesticides, herbicides, cadmium, and preservatives. Organic foods deliver nutrients without over-burdening the liver.

Don't feel nervous if your refrigerator looks somewhat empty. Just try it. I find that a lot of Americans still fill up their freezers and pantries with processed food so they feel like they are "well stocked," but this isn't stocking up on food. It's not food. It's bordering on poison! It's certainly burdening your liver and is deleterious to your health. Instead, think of your pantry as smaller and go as nutrient-dense as you can with organic fruits and vegetables; nuts and seeds; legumes; a few whole, intact, gluten-free ancient grains; and lots of fresh or dried organic herbs and spices. Add low-mercury, wild-caught, deep-water fatty fish; organic eggs; plant-based yogurt; wild game; and organic grass-fed or pastured meat and poultry. Your refrigerator won't be empty, after all. It can be intelligently and strategically stocked with whole, fresh foods to build your health and provide your body with full-spectrum nutrition.

YOUR DETOX DIETARY SECRET WEAPON

The two-step detoxification process that happens in your liver needs nutritional support, and some of the most powerful supporters of both phases of this process are cruciferous vegetables, such as broccoli, cabbage, Brussels sprouts, cauliflower, kale, collard greens, arugula, radishes, turnips, and watercress.[28] These super-powered detox veggies[29] contain inflammation-reducing antioxidants, including vitamins C and E, carotenoids, and polyphenols, but their secret weapon is sulfur-containing compounds called glucosinolates, which, in partnership with an enzyme called myrosinase, offer significant support for both phases of liver detoxification. To activate myrosinase and produce maximum glucosinolates, chop your cruciferous veggies and let them rest for 5 minutes before eating or gently cooking. I recommend one serving per day.

- **THE THINGS YOU TOUCH.** Remember that your skin is a semi-permeable barrier. Everything you put on your skin has the potential to enter your body. Take a look at the chemicals you are directly exposed to every day: cleaners, soap, detergent (and clothes and bedding washed in detergent), shampoo, conditioner, hair styling products, lotions and other skin-care products, antiperspirant/deodorant, makeup, perfume, and so on. If you color your hair or have other chemical procedures done at a salon, that counts, too. (Of course, we all have our detox priorities.) There are natural, nontoxic (or at least less toxic) alternatives to most of these products. Don't forget lawn-care products and outdoor pest control products, which can potentially expose you, as well as your pets and children (not to mention local wildlife), to poisons. If you have old wood climbing toys in the yard, get rid of them immediately. The wood was preserved with highly toxic metals and chemicals which children playing on them can absorb. There are much better alternatives now.

- **THE DRUGS YOU TAKE.** Every single thing you ingest, like ibuprofen, acetaminophen, or aspirin for a headache or menstrual cramps, antacids for heartburn, antihistamines for allergies, or any prescription medicine, has to be processed through your liver and kidneys. Many people are in the habit of popping a pill at the slightest sign of any discomfort, but this is a big burden on your liver. Both over-the-counter and prescription medications can be necessary when symptoms are extreme, but if you don't really need them, don't take them, and you will give your liver a break. Natural remedies may not work as quickly, but they are almost always easier on your body. (Please don't stop taking your prescription medicine without the okay from your doctor.)

Do Some Yoga

You already know yoga is good for your flexibility and, depending on what type you do, your strength and cardiovascular fitness. I love it for its stress-reduction effect, but certain yoga poses, especially twists, can also invigorate and activate your liver and colon, which can relieve constipation and increase detoxification. Yoga can also help to get the lymphatic system moving (as can all exercise and even deep breathing). Try some spinal twisting poses, which have a "wringing out" effect on internal organs. This seated spinal twist is my favorite detoxifying yoga pose:

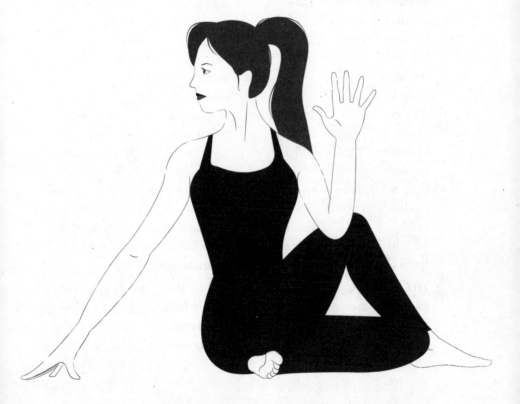

Move Your Lymph

Your lymphatic system is just under your skin and it moves waste out of your body through small vessels and into lymph nodes, which process waste out through the liver. Because it is so close to the skin, it's easy to manipulate, but it doesn't have a pump other than your muscles. Exercise and deep breathing activate it, but you can activate your lymphatic system in even more effective ways.

Lymphatic massage is a gentle form of massage specifically for moving lymph. Not everyone can do it, so look for a massage therapist who has been trained in this technique. It feels fantastic! You can also help out on your own. Dry brushing your skin with a soft brush toward the lymph nodes is very effective. Just brush your skin with gentle pressure, up your arms and legs and around your torso.

When your lymph is flowing freely, you won't feel puffy. You'll feel light, and you will look noticeably thinner. It's amazing what backed-up, toxic lymph can do to add the appearance of excess weight and poor health, so get that lymph moving! Here is a diagram of where your primary lymph nodes are, so you can brush toward them:

HEAVY METAL EXPOSURE AND TREATMENT

Some of the most dangerous, health-destroying, neurotoxic compounds in our environment are heavy metals, especially metalloid arsenic, cadmium, lead, and mercury.[30] Because of their common use, they are widespread and a significant source of toxic pollution. We all have some of these substances inside of us, but when levels get too high, they can lead to DNA damage, cell death, neurological dysfunction, and cancer as well as behavioral disorders and lower IQ in children.

Doctors will treat lead poisoning in children and mercury toxicity at high levels, but conventional medicine doesn't recognize heavy metal toxicity at sub-emergency levels. But subclinical levels can do quite a lot of damage. I have seen many, many people with heavy metal levels too high for vibrant health but too low for conventional medicine treatment. A functional medicine doctor can test you for heavy metals, and I advise having this done if you have been exposed.

Those who work in industrial jobs and are directly exposed to heavy metals probably know it, but there are less obvious exposures, like from air and water pollution (especially if you live in or near an industrial area), food storage products, adulterated supplements, mercury-contaminated fish, and "silver" (mercury) dental fillings.

If you do have heavy metal poisoning or high levels in your blood or brain, you might want to explore chelation therapy. This is a controversial procedure (at least among conventional medicine doctors) in which a chemical such as ethylenediaminetetraacetic acid (EDTA) or dimercaptosuccinic acid (DMSA) that physically binds the metals like a magnet is injected into the bloodstream or taken orally. The chemical grabs the metal and sends it through the liver—and to a lesser degree, the kidneys—for removal. In conventional medicine, EDTA and DMSA are primarily used for treating lead poisoning, but integrative practitioners sometimes use them to remove other heavy metals, when patients show through testing that they have high levels that could be causing health problems. They can also be used to treat atherosclerosis in people with a high risk for cardiovascular disease. For this use, EDTA binds the calcium in arterial plaque that can cause heart disease and carries it out of the body. It also reenergizes the body's enzyme system to open up the small arteries, restoring better circulation. You can learn more about the benefits of this therapy from the American College for Advancement in Medicine (acam.org).

Another method sometimes used by holistic practitioners is the Myers' cocktail, which is an IV infusion of vitamins for intensive support of the body's natural detoxification process. With the addition of coenzyme Q10 and some glutathione, the process can have a mild chelating effect.

Concerning your fillings, more dentists are using composite and ceramic fillings, and some of us (myself included) have had our silver fillings carefully removed by an experienced biological dentist (also called a holistic or ecological dentist). Composite and ceramic fillings are non-toxic and look better because they match the color of the tooth. It amazes me that some dentists are still using silver fillings, since the legal safe limit of mercury in the brain and bloodstream is zero.

If you do decide to have your fillings removed, I recommend going extremely clean with your food and exposures for a few months in preparation, so your detoxification system is ready for the event, and never have more than two or at most three small fillings replaced at a time. The removal process can release mercury gas, but a good biological dentist will know how to minimize this effect, and it may be better to deal with a single exposure event (the removal) with lots of nutritional support than the slow release of mercury gas from fillings over years.

To get tested for heavy metals or to find out more about chelation or other heavy metal detoxification methods, find an experienced and reputable integrative, holistic, or functional medicine practitioner. In the meantime, do your best to minimize your exposure to heavy metals, and keep supporting your liver with daily concentrated optimal nutrition and exercise.

SHOULD YOU TRY INTERMITTENT FASTING?

Many people have an intuitive sense that fasting is a good idea. They can feel it. They are curious, and wonder about those times when they don't feel hungry. They wonder if they should try it. I don't usually recommend intensive long-term fasting unless it is under direct medical supervision by an experienced and reputable physician, but intermittent fasting is something different. In my opinion, it's not really fasting. It's a return to a more normal, human way of eating.

Just the other day, I had a chicken breast and some veggies for lunch. By evening, I wasn't hungry for dinner. I kept checking in with myself to see if I was missing something, but I felt no hunger. Sensing my body wanted to channel energy elsewhere, I drank a lot of water, but by the time I was ready for bed, I still hadn't had dinner and didn't want it. So, I skipped it, and felt great the next morning. Although I didn't call it that, what I was doing was intermittent fasting.

In our culture, people are eating all the time—between meals, in their cars, on trains and airplanes, even while walking down the street. It's like people *can't stop eating*, and they don't really even think about it or plan it. The consequence of this is that the body never gets a rest from constantly digesting food. When you eat all day long, your blood sugar is more likely to go up and down, up and down. The mechanisms for healing and repair don't have all the energy they need because it's being diverted to the digestive tract. Too-frequent eating is also a really good way to take in a lot more calories than you need. People eat for stress relief, out of boredom, for entertainment, and as a social activity. It's like we've completely forgotten about the real reason to eat: TO LIVE.

Our ancestors never had the kind of 24/7 access to high-calorie food that we have now. They had to go out and work hard to get food, so while they might have been snacking on a few berries, nuts, or leafy greens here and there while gathering food, most of their calories probably came from one or two prepared meals shared with their families or tribes. This is a good model for us now. We just happen to call it "intermittent fasting."

It's easy to do. Instead of eating all day long, try going for longer periods of time without eating by tuning in to your body for signs of real hunger—not boredom, not anxiety, not habit, but actual stomach hunger. Are you really hungry the second you wake up? Are you really hungry right before you go to bed? We all fast when we sleep, but eating right before bed and first thing when you wake up doesn't give your body a chance to fall asleep easily or wake up gradually. Chances are that if you have been eating well enough throughout the day, you aren't hungry at either of those times anyway. This is a way to begin thinking about intermittent fasting.

To put it into practice, most experts recommend that the minimum time you should go without eating overnight is 12 hours. For example, if you finish your last bite of dinner by 7 pm, the earliest you should eat breakfast is at 7 am. Proponents of intermittent fasting say that 14, 16, or even 18 hours of fasting is even better, which can amount to only two or just one meal a day. One nice thing about this method is that you can eat more at each meal because you need to fit in all your day's calories and nutrients into fewer eating sessions, and that's fine.

Since blood sugar tends to be more reactive in the evening, the old adage that you should eat breakfast like a king, lunch like a prince, and dinner like a pauper is good advice. Front-load your calories for best effect. It's probably better to skip dinner than breakfast, although if that really doesn't work for you, it's also fine to wait until lunch to eat, then stop eating after dinner. Waiting to eat can help you remember what it really feels like to be hungry. It can increase your sensitivity and awareness of your body's cues for when it really needs food.

Wonderful as all that sounds, there are cases where I don't recommend intermittent fasting at all, beyond maybe a 12-hour fast overnight. If you have blood sugar balance issues, you may do better eating three small meals and two small snacks per day. The problem with doing this is that it's easy to eat too much. It takes some practice and mindfulness to eat small portions. If you eat just enough to keep your blood sugar stable, with fat and protein at every meal, it can help with blood sugar spikes as well as hypoglycemia, in those prone to such problems.

I don't recommend intermittent fasting during times of extreme stress, either. When you are pumping out cortisol and feeling stressed, you need more regular food intake to calm your adrenals and nourish your organs, sending your body the message that everything is fine. Don't try fasting until you are in a calm, parasympathetic mode.

The last scenario that isn't a good fit with intermittent fasting is for those who have an eating disorder and don't have a good sense of natural hunger, or who can get triggered to binge eat by skipping meals.

But you don't have to be so regimented about it. You may find that "intuitive eating" works well for you. This is the practice of listening to your body and eating when you are hungry, rather than at prescribed times. That's what I do. Before you eat, ask yourself if you are really hungry. If you aren't, then don't eat, or have a light vegetable salad or soup. Both intuitive eating and intermittent fasting can help you eliminate mindless snacking, especially after dinner, when many people snack their way to the calories of another complete meal.

If you try intermittent fasting and/or intuitive eating for a while and you like the results—people often report more energy, less chronic pain, and easier weight loss—you could take fasting a bit further. Some people skip a day of eating once every week, or go 24 hours without food. For example, if you finished dinner at 7 pm one night, you would not start dinner until 7 pm the next night.

If this is appealing to you, start with intermittent fasting first, and gradually increase the time you go without food over the course of a few weeks or longer so your body can adjust to what you are doing and get the most out of the fast, without causing excessive hunger or anxiety. Going a whole day without food can help your body clean out those drawers, cupboards, and closets where it has stuffed all those toxins, but in an easy, less aggressive way. It contributes to organ reserve and rests your digestive tract so your energy can go to other parts of your body where it's needed for repair, rejuvenation, and yes, detoxification.

Many cultures fast without anxiety or drama. Give your body a break, drink plenty of water to help flush out toxins your body releases, and take it easy on fast days. If you aren't taking in food, you won't have spare energy for high-intensity exercise or stress. Take a relaxing walk outside, breathe deeply, and let your body power down. Pay close attention to how your body responds. Fasting can raise cortisol and make you feel a bit nervous, so make allowances for that and dial up your stress management.

If you don't like the idea or the very thought stresses you out, don't worry about a day of fasting. Even a 12-hour fast overnight will make a difference and give your body a chance to focus on detoxification. Fasting is not for everyone, but some people swear by it. Don't take it too far, though. I never recommend that anyone go longer than two or three days without food unless under direct medical supervision. This is more like starvation, which can concentrate toxins and cause muscle wasting, as I've mentioned.

• • •

Detoxification can seem technical, and it certainly is a complex process, but you don't have to understand every single detail to support it. All you really have to remember about detoxification is that you don't have to make it happen, but you certainly can help it happen. Here are your three primary detox takeaways:

1. You can relax and forget about that punishing cleanse program. Your body is already on the job, all day every day.

2. You can help your body take out the garbage with a daily bowel movement. Do what it takes but keep things moving.

3. You can clean up your environment and eat organic food. Reduce your toxic exposure as much as you can.

DETOXIFICATION WINS

To start you on your way, try one or more of these detoxification wins today.

BATHROOM TIME. Make it your goal to move your bowels once a day. Most people don't spend enough time in the bathroom (except perhaps your husband?). Don't give up unless you've been sitting there for at least 15 minutes. It can take some time to relax enough to get things moving, especially if you've been holding it in all day long. Think of it as a break from your family! Try different strategies to see what works best for you. Everyone is different, so what works for someone else might not be what works for you. Increase your daily fiber intake, take magnesium citrate before bed, try a triphala supplement, or do some yoga twisting poses. When you find something that works, stick with it.

○ *I tried it! Here's how it felt:* _____

_____

_____

_____

EAT YOUR BROCCOLI. Add at least one serving of raw cruciferous vegetables to your meals every day, for detoxification (broccoli, Brussels sprouts, cauliflower, kale, cabbage, bok choy). Make some fresh coleslaw, have a kale salad, or snack on raw broccoli florets dipped in delicious hummus.

○ *I tried it! Here's how it felt:* _____

_____

_____

_____

RULE OF HALVES RENOVATION. You don't have to detoxify your entire household at once. Remember the Rule of Halves. Start by going through your cleaning supplies or your personal care products and see if you can replace half of them with natural versions.

○ *I tried it! Here's how it felt:* _____

_____

_____

_____

CHAPTER 9

The Sustainer: How to Build a Truly Resilient Immune System

Your immune system is your first responder, your protector, and the always-active system constantly seeking out the things that can hurt you. It sustains you in times of crisis, and it is a smart system with many layers and approaches to personal protection. In a perfect world, it would kill off all viruses and bacteria before they could infect and harm you, root out all cancerous cells before they could form tumors or spread, and always be able to distinguish your healthy cells and nontoxic food proteins from dangerous pathogens.

Even in our imperfect world, your immune system works hard and does a pretty good job. You are exposed to pathogens and your cells mutate all the time, and your immune system quickly takes down most of these invaders and solves most of these issues before you ever know you had them. However, viruses, cancer cells, and other pathogens want to survive and proliferate, so they try to trick your immune system with clever evasion strategies. They disguise themselves as your own healthy cells. They go to parts of your body that aren't well patrolled by your immune system. They block various immune system actions so they can proceed undetected. They mutate quickly so the immune system doesn't have a chance to mark them. It's like an ongoing chess game inside of you: your immune system versus the things that would take it (and you) down.

There are some genetic reasons why your immune system may not work as well as it could, but many of the problems with the immune system have to do with you and (you know the drill by now) your lifestyle: what you eat, how much exercise you get, and how you manage your stress. Inflammation is a healthy response your immune system triggers to protect you from invaders like viruses and bacteria. It sends white blood cells (and other substances they manufacture, like histamine and inflammatory prostaglandins) to where a perceived invader may be—bacteria entering through a break in the skin, inhaled viruses, fungi, or pathogens from your own microbiome that overgrow or go where they shouldn't. These white blood cell products surround and fight off the invaders.

However, sometimes inflammation can become chronic, meaning it doesn't go away when the threat is gone, or it isn't able to fully eliminate the threat so it just keeps trying. Chronic inflammation can also be triggered or aggravated by a high-stress life, a diet full of high-fat, high-sugar food, or even a lack of exercise (since many of the biological processes that happen because of exercise help to calm chronic inflammation). When inflammation becomes chronic, your body's natural immune processes can get confused. This can inhibit the ability of your immune system to recognize what is dangerous and what is safe. If you live an inflammatory lifestyle, you will essentially be choosing to inhibit the effectiveness of your own immune system, and that can result in a weakened, less intelligent immune response to infectious diseases and cancer cells, or an overzealous, also less intelligent immune response that attacks your own healthy tissue, thinking it is "helping." A recent theory is that the immune system attacks proteins that look abnormal because they've been bound by toxins. Makes sense to me!

YOUR TWO IMMUNE SYSTEMS

You have two types of immune system: the innate immune system and the adaptive immune system. You are born with your innate immune system, which includes all the basic, nonspecific ways your body tries to keep bad things out. Some are simple barriers to entry, like skin, earwax, mucus, stomach acid, hair, and enzymes in saliva and tears. Others are chemical, like macrophages and natural killer cells that seek out viruses, bacteria, and cancer cells and destroy them.

Your adaptive immune system is more complex and able to recognize specific proteins or antigens that look dangerous or foreign. Simply put, this immune response adapts to what it encounters to more specifically target and destroy dangerous cells. It has the capacity to respond to all of the many billions of foreign proteins it is exposed to in your lifetime. It also remembers what it sees, so if you are exposed to a virus, for example, then if you are ever exposed to that virus again, your immune system remembers and responds more quickly and aggressively to take down that familiar foe. It is also able to differentiate between what is you and what is not you, as well as what is healthy you and what is non-normal you (such as a cancer cell).

Essentially, your innate immune system is like locking up your house with dead bolts and alarm systems. It keeps out intruders of all types in the same way. Your adaptive immune system is a much more sensitive and stronger system that changes its response according to the nature of the threat, like a team of special forces surrounding your home, searching all possible ways clever criminals might try to find a way in and outsmarting them as they appear.

The two primary ways your immune system can fail are in some ways opposite problems. One is due to immune underactivity, and the other is due to overactivity, but both share the problem of an immune system that is not properly assessing the internal situation. If your immune system isn't working, it needs to get smarter, and you can help. Remember the Big Six, from chapter two? Those common chronic diseases—heart disease, cancer, type 2 diabetes, obesity, autoimmunity, and dementia—all involve a failure of the immune system, so let's get yours online and working at capacity.

WHEN INFLAMMATION INTERFERES WITH IMMUNITY

If you are exposed to a virus, a bacterium, a fungus, or any other potential infectious agent, your immune system should jump into action and, most of the time, it will. However, there are a few things that can slow and confuse your immune system's response. One is an extra-clever pathogen that evades the normal defense system, but a more common problem is a body that isn't healthy and, in particular, is suffering from chronic inflammation.

Inflammation is a healthy survival response by your immune system, but it is meant to be temporary. If you cut yourself or break a bone, the injured area will get red, sore, hot, and swollen, which are all signs of inflammation. As your immune system mobilizes to prevent infection and mop up any invaders that could have come into the body (such as through a break in the skin), part of the collateral damage is a little bit of tissue destruction, but this is not as bad as a serious infection and is essentially a necessary price to pay. After the wound is closed and the job is done, the inflammation should subside.

Sometimes, though, it doesn't subside, or it proliferates due to a longer-term exposure to something that continually mobilizes the immune system but is never resolved.[1] A wound that won't heal, that keeps getting re-infected, could cause chronic inflammation. Exposure to toxins, from cigarette smoke to pollutants to chemical exposures, can cause inflammation, as the body is constantly trying to protect you and never gets a rest. Obesity can cause inflammation because excessive fat stores can release inflammatory chemicals as well as excess hormones that can confuse your system as it tries to process out excessive estrogen, for example. (Fat can act like an endocrine gland and actually produce its own hormones.) We also know that those same old lifestyle factors we've been talking about in this book can increase inflammation: a poor diet, especially one high in saturated fat, refined sugar and flour, fried food, and red meat; a sedentary lifestyle; isolation and loneliness or unhappy relationships; and the stress that all of these lifestyle habits generate in the body.

It may seem ironic that the immune system creates inflammation, but can also be hindered by inflammation. It's the chronic part that causes the problem in an otherwise well-designed system. Imagine driving a beautiful new race car. If the car has been built well and is well maintained, you can run it hard and fast. Afterward, you turn off the engine and do maintenance. You would never just leave it running. But imagine if you did. Imagine if you never turned off that race car. It would wear down a lot faster because it never gets a chance to cool off, even if you kept a steady flow of fuel coming in. The parts would wear out, the oil would get dirty, and it would not last as long or run as well.

In the same way, your body can handle acute inflammation as long as it's over when the problem is solved, but chronic inflammation causes much more wear and tear and will eventually interfere with all the systems. If you are chronically inflamed, then when you are exposed to a pathogen like a virus, your immune system may not notice, or may not be able to mount its normal full-scale attack because it is too distracted and worn out trying to manage the chronic inflammation that has been going on for weeks or months or years. That makes you more vulnerable to infectious disease as well as to chronic diseases in which inflammation is a primary component, including heart disease,[2] cancer,[3] and dementia.[4]

WHEN YOUR IMMUNE SYSTEM IS OVERZEALOUS: AUTOIMMUNITY

Autoimmunity is a condition in which the immune system attacks healthy tissue because it mis-identifies it as something foreign or harmful. This shouldn't happen, but in the last few years there has been a disturbing rise in autoimmune conditions. Something in our environments or lifestyles is confusing our immune systems into thinking the cells in our healthy joints, thyroids, skin, or other organs are the enemies.

Earlier in this chapter, I mentioned that one of the skills of the adaptive immune system is the ability to distinguish foreign cells and damaged cells from your own healthy cells. To get just a bit more technical, as the adaptive immune system cells are developing and waiting to be called on for duty, some of those cells (T-cells and B-cells) can be overzealous. Adaptive immune cells are supposed to know, via a complex signaling process, which cells they are supposed to kill and which cells they are supposed to ignore. These overly excitable immune cells show early signs of lacking this natural discernment between "self" and "other." The immune system detects these imprudent, self-reactive cells and destroys them before they can get into your system and cause trouble by mistakenly attacking your own healthy cells. Or, it should. However, sometimes the immune system doesn't catch these unrestrained troublemakers. When they are released, they can be a trigger for autoimmune diseases, which are, in essence, self attacking self.

There are other reasons this can happen, and inflammation can play a part, too. Some viruses, as well as some food proteins, resemble our own natural cells, so when the immune system is not 100 percent focused, due to chronic inflammation, it may mistake your own cells for a virus or errant food protein and attack. You probably know how much easier it is to make mistakes when you have been working too hard for too long. Exposure to toxins, an inflammatory diet, obesity, chronic tobacco or alcohol use, unresolved infections—all of those inflammatory contributors create a perfect storm for autoimmunity, which is then, disastrously, self-fueling because as the body attacks its own tissues, inflammation becomes worse and the chronic cycle continues in a destructive downward spiral.

There are many different autoimmune diseases, which are generally divided according to where the tissue destruction is occurring. In rheumatoid arthritis, healthy joints are targeted. In multiple sclerosis, it's the brain and spinal cord. In lupus, it's connective tissue, blood vessels, and skin. In celiac disease, it's the lining of the small intestine where nutrients are absorbed, although the skin, joints, and organs including the brain can all be affected. In Hashimoto's thyroiditis and Graves' disease, it's the thyroid. In Addison's, it's the adrenals. In type 1 diabetes, it's the pancreas. In Crohn's disease, it's the colon. There are over 100 autoimmune diseases,[5] and scientists are discovering autoimmune action in many other common diseases not thought of as autoimmune, like atherosclerosis[6] and heart disease,[7] and also linking autoimmunity with conditions like cancer that are due to immune surveillance failure, since inflammation from autoimmunity can make people more susceptible to cancer.[8]

What these conditions all have in common is that the immune system is working hard, not smart. If you want to minimize your chances for developing an infectious disease or an autoimmune disease, the most powerful intervention is to un-confuse your immune system as much as you can by eliminating inflammation. And how do you do it? I'm sure you know this by now: Implement the Vibrant Triad. Power your immune system with nutrition and inflammation-fighting foods, support your immune system with stress-reducing, circulation-promoting exercise, and increase your chances of avoiding illness and healing more quickly by fostering supportive relationships. All three approaches reduce chronic stress and chronic inflammation that are interfering with your immune function, confusing your immune responses, and basically lowering your immune system's natural intelligence and discernment.

DISEASES OR PHANTOMS?

I'd like to take a pause here, while we are on the subject of your immune system, to talk about an issue that has been bothering me for years. It's another one of my soapbox speeches, but I think it might help you if you have a disease diagnosis, especially for a chronic disease your doctor says has no cure. It's about the very notion of disease.

What is a disease, really? The technical definition of disease is a disorder of the structure or function of a living organism, especially when it produces specific symptoms or affects a specific system or area of the body and is not just the result of an injury. That definition does describe infectious diseases and also autoimmune diseases, as these are disorders of function, as well as chronic diseases like cancer and heart disease, which are disorders of both structure and function. But my quibble with the idea of "dis-ease" is more in how our culture uses this term.

It might be controversial to say, but when it comes to disease diagnosis, things are not as they appear. When people don't feel well or know something is wrong with them, they often desire a diagnosis. They want to know what they have. Giving something a name may make it feel more manageable, but the names we have given to the diseases doctors diagnose are somewhat arbitrary. Diseases don't exist in a vacuum. They are usually the end-stage result of a long process of health deterioration that starts long before you ever notice any symptoms.

Diseases are really just names based on collections of symptoms we have decided to categorize, which makes them seem like they are distinct, but really, they aren't. We are naming the tail end of a long, complex process that is different in each person. Imagine ten different snakes in different colors who all have a similar tail tip. Naming a disease is like saying all those snakes are the same because they have the same tail. This thinking doesn't take into account that the initial trigger and the cascade of dysfunction that followed is often completely different in different people. For example, a symptom, such as a headache or high blood sugar or stomach cramps, can be caused by very different dysfunctional pathways.

In other cases, we have pathologized totally natural life transition stages, like puberty or perimenopause, which also manifest differently in different people, depending on their health status. Yet, people buy into the system enthusiastically—so much so that, once they have their sought-after diagnosis, they may think of themselves as helpless victims of that disease. I've said this before, but: They buy the T-shirt. They punch the card. They go to the meetings. The so-called disease becomes part of their very identity.

Let's take a breath—I agree 100 percent that knowledge about your condition is a good thing. It allows you to be more proactive and empowered in seeking healing and reestablishing wellness. If it helps you to wear the T-shirt and attend the seminar, great. I don't mean to make fun, just to make a point. I also want to confirm that your symptoms and suffering are real. Those, I do not doubt.

What I object to is the labeling. As soon as you label yourself as someone with a disease, aligning your identity with that diagnosis, you become, consciously or not, a victim of an outside force. It's that *disease* that's ruined your life. It's that *disease* that is causing you so much suffering. It's that *disease* that has lost you your job, your relationship, your happiness. You see it as a thing, not a process. A noun, not a verb. But you are only looking at the tail of the snake, and blaming the tail for the whole animal.

You could argue this is all a matter of semantics, but words are powerful and how you think about things can mean the difference between feeling like a victim and feeling empowered. Pinning down chronic diseases is like trying to pin down a phantom. Instead of trying to systemize and name and treat these supposedly isolated "diseases," I believe we must focus on the root cause of health dysfunction in a broader sense with an awareness that all chronic diseases are individual manifestations of sub-optimal health.

What if there were no diseases, only a spectrum of health? What if, instead of focusing on a disease, you focused on how well your body is working? When you are vibrantly healthy, your immune system will take care of pathogens and won't mistakenly attack you. What people often forget is that they can control (at least mostly) where they are on the spectrum of health, and their position is never fixed. It is always shifting.

I propose that you see your "dis-ease" more as a call from your body that you need to intervene. If your symptoms, i.e., your body messages, are severe and painful, you are on the wrong end of that spectrum, but every lifestyle choice you make can push you back in the right direction.

What is type 2 diabetes, after all, but a call from your body to eat better and exercise more? What is perimenopause but a natural hormonal transition, whose side effects are more uncomfortable if you are under a lot of stress and not living a healthy lifestyle? What is an autoimmune disease (Hashimoto's, rheumatoid arthritis, multiple sclerosis, etc.), other than a misguided immune system that might just need a dietary anti-inflammatory intervention? What is "adult ADHD" but a brain that needs better support? What is adrenal fatigue, but a stress-response system that is overtaxed?

I'll say again that your symptoms are real, your discomfort is real, and the dangers of the many manifestations of poor health are very, very real. But the real question is: *What can you do about it?* You can do a lot, and that starts by stepping back and looking at the big picture of your health, not the microscopic virus or the end-stage joint pain or the rash or the hair loss or the cognitive impairment.

Intervene now, before you get to that end-stage state. You can make every single food choice about what will support your health rather than tear it down. You can make every single exercise decision about what your body needs: strength, flexibility, better circulation, or more relaxation. You can choose to increase your stress or manage it. You can choose to sleep more, answer your body's requests with supplement support, ask for help.

If you can do all that and still think of yourself as someone with a disease, if that helps to motivate you, then that's up to you, not me. I only want to say that the concept of a disease sweeping in from somewhere and taking you down is a drastic oversimplification and reductionist view of how the body works. You are not a helpless victim. You have a full battalion at the ready, to defend you. How will you train them?

HOW TO BUILD A SMARTER IMMUNE SYSTEM

What you want to do for your immune system is not necessarily to make it stronger, or to suppress it when it is overreactive, but to restore its natural ability to find and destroy legitimate threats, and ignore what is benign and what is your own healthy tissue. You don't need to understand immunology to do this. Your body already knows how to do this innately. The primary reason why it's not working as well as it should is because something is interfering, like a guest that won't leave.

Your immune system is naturally smart, but it is easily distracted, especially by influences it wouldn't naturally encounter. Advocates of ancestral health often say there is an evolutionary mismatch between our bodies and the world we live in. We were designed for an environment in which we evolved over millions of years, not the environment that has only recently changed significantly. There are so many influences on our bodies nowadays that it can be confusing for the immune system to know exactly what really poses a threat and what doesn't. We've already talked about those influences: processed food, inflammatory food, a sedentary lifestyle, a toxic environment, chronic stress, loss of meaningful relationships, poor sleep quality, and distraction by digital devices. You've already been working on all of that, and you are already on the right track.

But since the most destructive influence on immunity is inflammation, the best way to help your immune system get smart again is to target inflammation.

Eating for Optimized Immunity

The Vibrant Food List is full of anti-inflammatory foods, but there are a few foods that are particularly good at quelling inflammation. According to a study that reported the antioxidant content of more than 3,000 foods, beverages, spices, herbs, and supplements,[9] the foods below are the superstars. If your immune system is your priority right now, these are the foods to eat more of.

See if you can include at least some of them in your diet every day.

- Berries, especially blueberries but also raspberries, blackberries, and strawberries, all of which have high cellular antioxidant activity[10]
- Nuts, especially walnuts[11] and pecans[12]
- Pomegranates[13]
- Coffee, especially dark[14]
- Tea, especially green tea[15]
- Chocolate, extra dark or raw cacao only[16]

AMLA BERRY

The berry with the highest antioxidant content by far is amla, aka Indian gooseberry, but this popular Indian berry is not widely available in the United States to my knowledge, except in supplement form. You can buy amla supplements or triphala, which is a supplement containing three different berries, one of which is amla (triphala was one of my supplement recommendations in the detoxification chapter). These supplements are often used in Ayurvedic medicine for digestive support. Both have a much higher antioxidant content than any fresh berries we have available to us in the United States.

Many common dried kitchen herbs and herbal teas have much higher antioxidant content than most foods or even the fresh versions of the herbs because drying concentrates the antioxidant content. The herbs and herbal teas with the highest antioxidant content[17] (I only listed those I know to be widely available) include:

- Allspice, dried and ground
- Basil, dried
- Bay leaves, dried
- Chervil, dried
- Chilis, dried
- Chives, dried
- Cinnamon, dried and ground
- Cloves, dried and ground
- Cumin, dried and ground
- Curry powder
- Dill, dried
- Ginger, dried and ground
- Green mint leaves, dried
- Juniper berries, dried
- Lavender, leaves and flowers, dried
- Lemon balm leaves, dried
- Mint leaves, all types, dried
- Mustard seed, ground
- Nutmeg, dried and ground
- Oregano, dried

- Peppers, dried, all types
- Raspberry leaves, dried
- Rosemary, dried
- Saffron, dried and ground
- Sage, dried
- Thyme, dried
- Turmeric powder
- Wild marjoram leaves, dried

THE BEST SUPPLEMENTS FOR A SMART IMMUNE SYSTEM

Food is always the best way to get bioavailable nutrients into your system, but when it comes to immunity, there are likely some gaps you need to fill. First of all, if I haven't already convinced you to start taking vitamin C, vitamin D3, and a B-complex supplement, it's time. These may be the three most influential vitamins for immune support. (For dosage information, see page 31.) But you can go even further in helping your body recognize what requires a vigorous immune attack and what is actually just a harmless food protein. Here are my smart immunity supplement recommendations:

- **Prebiotics, probiotics, postbiotics:** Your microbiome produces most of the signaling necessary for a healthy immune response, so that requires a healthy microbiome rich in beneficial bacteria. Taking probiotics, which help to infuse your digestive tract with beneficial microbes, along with prebiotics, which feed beneficial microbes, can support that process. A recent trend is something called postbiotics, which is really just a short chain fatty acid (SCFA) supplement. I've been recommending that people take these for years, but they've only recently become trendy. SCFAs are fermentation products that your microbiome makes when it digests the fiber and resistant starch you eat, and they are key players in regulating immune cell function.[18] SCFAs also help to keep the intestinal barrier sealed against "leaks." Taking these in supplement form can add to what your microbiome is already doing for you, like sending in extra troops.

- **Zinc (and selenium):** Zinc is an old standby for immune support, and research backs this up. Many studies have shown that zinc enhances immune response against viruses.[19] Selenium, which I mentioned in chapter four, shows similar ability to enhance immunity.[20]

> • **Elderberry:** Whenever a new virus pops up, everybody starts talking about taking elderberry. There is research showing that supplementing with elderberry does decrease the duration of the common cold,[21] so it couldn't hurt and it might help support your body's ability to fight off other viruses.

Exercise and Your Immune System

For many years, there was a belief that strenuous exercise actually suppressed immune function,[22] at least temporarily (they were studying marathon runners). While it's true that vigorous exercise is a stressor, albeit one that results in increased strength and resilience, I always found it suspect that exercise could make you more susceptible to illness. A couple of years ago, a study came out finally debunking the notion that exercise suppresses immunity.[23] The exhaustive study showed that exercise, over the course of a lifetime, improves immune function and can also delay the slow decline of immune function that happens with aging. This is just one more in a long list of reasons to exercise regularly.

Social Bonds, Disease Risk, and Recovery

Over the past few decades, many studies have reviewed the impact of social relationships on immunity, and the results have been mostly consistent.[24] The wider the social network, the stronger the immunity. Those who are happily married, have more emotional support, and those who attend church also all generally show superior immune function compared to those with smaller social networks and those who report more loneliness. A few studies have shown better immunity in those people who not only have broader social networks but also report low stress, but since more emotional support from friends and family is also a stress-reducer, it's hard to tease out the separation. If you haven't already done so, start today to refresh and build your healthy human connections. Who is a friend or relative you haven't called in a while who would love to hear from you?

• • •

By this point in the book, none of what I'm saying should be a surprise. Better food, more exercise, and more social support all reduce stress, improve brain function, make the detoxification system more efficient and effective, and improve immune intelligence. That summarizes this entire book, and my thesis on health. To put it more succinctly:

> # WHEN YOU LIVE IN THE CENTER OF THE VIBRANT TRIAD, YOU WILL LIVE A VIBRANT LIFE.

It's really not so complicated, after all.

• • •

IMMUNITY WINS

A strong and smart immune system will engage when it should and not when it shouldn't. It will help you become more impervious to infections and maintain your vital force so that you feel vibrant even when everyone else is down with whatever virus is going around. It can take out cancer cells, bacteria, pathogenic fungi, and parasites, and help you heal from injuries faster and better. And it won't attack you by mistake. Are you ready to support yours? Let's wrap up this chapter with our final wins.

REMOVE GLUTEN AND CASEIN. If you haven't already, try going one week without gluten and/or casein, to see if you feel any different. Certain food proteins tend to be more inflammatory than others, and gluten (a protein in wheat, rye, and barley) and casein (a protein in dairy products) are two of the most notorious. You won't know if you feel better without them until you take them out of your diet for a while, so give it a try and pay attention to how your body responds. It may be that you feel better without one, but the other responds. After a week, do a "challenge"—eat a bunch of gluten and see how you feel the next morning. Then try it with dairy. How does it make you feel? This is a good way to determine your sensitivity. For many, eliminating them both can significantly reduce inflammation.

○ *I tried it! Here's how it felt:* _____

_____

UP YOUR C. You may already be taking vitamin C, but for maximum immune support, calibrate up gradually to 5,000 mg per day, divided between three doses in the morning, afternoon, and evening.

○ *I tried it! Here's how it felt:* _____

_____

ADD A PROBIOTIC. Many of the critical components of your immune system are manufactured in your digestive tract by the microbes that make up your gut microbiome. To support their efforts on your behalf, start taking a probiotic every day, along with fiber-rich foods (or a prebiotic supplement), to feed those beneficial microbes and help them strengthen their numbers and crowd out the more pathogenic intestinal microbes like inflammatory bacteria and yeasts. I recommend rotating between a few different formulas of probiotics from reputable companies, for maximum diversity. A more diverse microbiome is a stronger microbiome.

○ *I tried it! Here's how it felt:* _____

_____

PART IV

Surfacing

Together we have gone deep, deeper, and deepest in your quest to further understand your body's amazing and complex systems and what you need to live a thriving, vital, and vibrant life. Now that you've explored how working the Vibrant Triad can empower you to set sustainable health goals with true insight about where you are now and where you want to be, and gotten granular about what is going on inside of you, how your organs and systems work, and how you can best take care of them, I bet you are feeling pretty good. I hope I have inspired you to keep going in a way that will be transformative and meaningful for your quality of life.

Now let's come back up to the surface, roll up our sleeves, and really dig into your habit makeover. In this section, I'm going to give you even more tools for success, which you can remember like this:

> ## 30 HABITS · 40 RECIPES · 50-YEAR CHALLENGE

- **30 VIBRANT HABITS:** your 30-day Vibrant Habit Makeover Plan based on the "wins" throughout this book (you've been practicing, so you already have a head start);

- **40 RECIPES:** easy-to-make recipes for meals and snacks your body will love;

- **50-YEAR CHALLENGE:** a send-off and call to embrace your vibrant future.

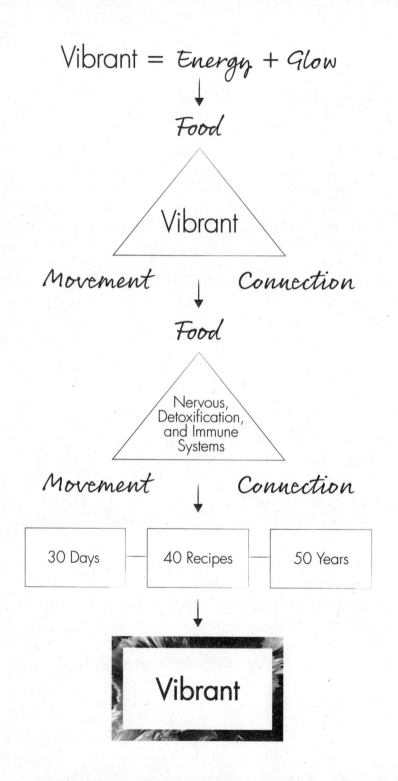

CHAPTER 10

30 Vibrant Habits to Cultivate

I n every chapter in this book, I've given you three "wins" that you can try to begin shifting your habits. Now it's time to really invest in those habits, and more, to begin the necessary transformation of your lifestyle from "good enough" (or not so much) to "vibrant." I'm not going to give you some rigorous diet and exercise plan to follow for a few weeks until you get tired of it. Instead, I've always found with myself and my patients that gradual changes are more likely to stick. That is why I am giving you a 30-day plan to make over your habits.

Each day, I'll give you just one thing to do and one thing to think about, along with space to note one thing you appreciated, enjoyed, or are grateful for, and any other notes of things you want to remember. This is a great place to jot down how your body responds to each new habit and to your gradually changing lifestyle. You don't have to keep this habit forever. I just want you to try it for one day. You might like it more than you think you will. If you do, then keep it. If you don't, move on to the next day.

You might already be doing some of the "wins," and that's great. You can pick something else, or skip that day. Or maybe you tried some of them for a while but stopped. This is a chance to give those good habits another chance, or kick those bad habits to the curb again. Just keep moving forward and trying new things. By the end of 30 days, you will know for sure which habits you like and can integrate into your life, and which habits just aren't going to work for you.

It's all up to you. Remember, you are the CEO of your body. You are empowered to decide how you want to change your lifestyle. I'm just giving you options, but just like your mother used to tell you: "How do you know you don't like it unless you try it?" These 30 days are your chance to try out lots of different ways to bring more vibrancy into your life every day.

Before you start, let's rate your energy. Look back to chapter one, where you rated your energy before trying any of the wins. How is your energy now, compared to then?

On a scale of 1 to 10—with 1 being "exhausted" and 10 being "I feel like I could do anything right now!"—what is your energy today? Circle your level.

VIBRANT ENERGY RATING

1   2   3   4   5   6   7   8   9   10

If it's better, that's great. You are already moving in the right direction. If it's the same, or even worse, and you really haven't been doing any of the wins yet, that's okay, too. Sometimes people need to spend time thinking about and mentally preparing for change before they do anything different.

This 30-day plan is just a kick-start. I hope you will continue to move in the right direction, becoming ever more vibrant with each passing day. Little changes are easy, but with consistency, they can cause huge shifts in your life, your health, how you look, and how you feel. So let's do this! Pick a day to begin, then check this chart every morning to see what to do that day, and every evening to make your notes. Make a commitment to see where it will get you, and remain ever-alert to your body's messages. Your body will tell you better than I ever could when you are on the right track.

Are you ready for a vibrant month? Let's get started.

YOUR 30-DAY VIBRANT HABIT MAKEOVER

BEFORE YOU BEGIN: *Remember to note your Vibrant Energy Rating on a scale of 1–10.*

DAY 1: Try a mirror evaluation and practice self-love.

DO THIS TODAY

Spend five minutes in front of the mirror with an eye for what you can do to help yourself feel better. Be honest and evaluate the signs of health and the signs of health dysfunction that you see in front of you. Check your skin, posture, expression, signs of energy or fatigue, signs of happiness or sadness, areas that could use more muscle or a bit less fat.

THINK ABOUT THIS TODAY

Your body is doing the best it can with what you give it. Have compassion for yourself and your body, rather than judgment. It's never too late to be kinder to yourself and make changes that you will feel on the inside and that will show on the outside.

DAILY MOMENT OF APPRECIATION, JOY, OR GRATITUDE

NOTES FOR THE DAY

DAY 2: Listen to and try to decipher your body's signals.

DO THIS TODAY

Notice your body's signals today. Don't try to control them. Just notice how your body responds to the things you eat, the way you move, how long you sit, how well you sleep. Notice when you feel a good feeling or a bad one. Pay attention to your moods. Every ache, every twinge, every cramp, every itch, every mood change is a message to you about what you are doing. Tune in to the subtle signs that mean your body is talking to you.

THINK ABOUT THIS TODAY

Try to decipher your body's signals. Why do you think you have that stomachache? Why does your knee hurt? Why are you suddenly so tired in the middle of the day? Why are you feeling a bit blue? Whatever you notice, ask yourself "Why?" You may not always have the answer, but asking the question is the first step.

DAILY MOMENT OF APPRECIATION, JOY, OR GRATITUDE

NOTES FOR THE DAY

DAY 3: Walk, and notice how it feels.

DO THIS TODAY

Take a brisk 15-minute walk today, or add 15 minutes to your regular walk. Pick up the pace and breathe!

THINK ABOUT THIS TODAY

Notice how it feels to move a little bit more than usual. Good? Worth it?

DAILY MOMENT OF APPRECIATION, JOY, OR GRATITUDE

NOTES FOR THE DAY

DAY 4: Scale down those energy crutches and turn up the fountain.

DO THIS TODAY

Pick an energy crutch—that thing you do when your energy is lagging that you know isn't great for your health (more coffee, sugar, alcohol, nicotine?)—and have half what you would normally have today. Does it still help? Are the side effects less?

THINK ABOUT THIS TODAY

You know how to create energy, so why do you choose to seek energy from something you know will ultimately deplete you? Think about better ways to build your energy. Review chapter two and work to turn up your energy fountain.

DAILY MOMENT OF APPRECIATION, JOY, OR GRATITUDE

NOTES FOR THE DAY

DAY 5: Sleep in the dark and limit screen time.

DO THIS TODAY

Make your room completely dark tonight. Block all window light and cover or remove all signs of light, including all light from electronics. Put your phone in another room. Go to bed early enough to get eight hours of sleep and see what happens. Notice how you feel in the morning.

THINK ABOUT THIS TODAY

Think about the role electronics play in your life. Would you be less stressed if you spent less time looking at your phone? What if you had less electronic exposure overall? Could you set time limits? Move the TV out of the bedroom? Turn things all the way off more often? In our modern world, you obviously can't turn off completely, but think about some shifts that might make you feel more free.

DAILY MOMENT OF APPRECIATION, JOY, OR GRATITUDE

NOTES FOR THE DAY

DAY 6: Look for signs of dehydration; drink more water.

DO THIS TODAY

Hydration is critical for your health at the cellular level. Today, drink half your body weight number in ounces of water.

THINK ABOUT THIS TODAY

Might you be chronically dehydrated? If you have dry skin, dry mouth, dark urine, and low energy, you probably are. Think about how easy it is to fix this problem.

DAILY MOMENT OF APPRECIATION, JOY, OR GRATITUDE

NOTES FOR THE DAY

DAY 7: Try Beauty Breathing and notice how it affects you.

DO THIS TODAY

Once in the morning and once in the evening, do the Beauty Breathing exercise on page 79.

THINK ABOUT THIS TODAY

Deep breathing can lower your blood pressure, slow your heart rate, slow your breathing, and stop an anxiety attack in its tracks. Is this worth doing more often? It's so easy and it only takes a few minutes.

DAILY MOMENT OF APPRECIATION, JOY, OR GRATITUDE

NOTES FOR THE DAY

DAY 8: Try the Triple Oil Treatment, inside and out.

DO THIS TODAY

Look and feel better inside and out with my Triple Oil Treatment today:

1. If you aren't allergic, rub unrefined coconut oil on your lips and cuticles. (PSST: IT'S ALSO LUBRICATING FOR YOUR LADY PARTS.)
2. Take an EPA/DHA supplement (see page 175).
3. Have a salad with a tablespoon of extra-virgin olive oil and a squeeze of lemon for dressing.

THINK ABOUT THIS TODAY

Some oil is good for your insides, like fish oil and olive oil. Some is better for your outsides only, like coconut oil. Due to its high saturated fat content, it's not good for your heart or arteries (despite the fad). Think about how you might continue to use the right oils in the right places.

DAILY MOMENT OF APPRECIATION, JOY, OR GRATITUDE

NOTES FOR THE DAY

DAY 9: Max out on veggies!

DO THIS TODAY

Have 3 cups of green vegetables today, raw or cooked. Lettuce, kale, collards, chard, microgreens, sprouts, broccoli, Brussels sprouts, cabbage, green beans, asparagus, and artichokes are all good options.

THINK ABOUT THIS TODAY

It's easy to overeat, but green vegetables are the one food you can eat as much of as you want. You never need to limit them because they contain maximum nutrition for minimum calories, and nobody binges on broccoli. Remember that the next time you want second helpings.

DAILY MOMENT OF APPRECIATION, JOY, OR GRATITUDE

NOTES FOR THE DAY

"I DON'T LIKE VEGETABLES!"

Every so often, somebody says this to me, and my answer is similar to the answer I give when somebody tells me they don't like to exercise. I say: "Do it anyway!" I grew up in the central Midwest and there were a lot of foods I wasn't exposed to until I was an adult. For example, my family never ate fish, so I was suspicious of it at first. But children have sensitive palates, and you are not a child. There are plenty of things we do in life that we don't particularly like, but we do them anyway because we know they will have a good result. Vegetables do so much good for you that they are worth getting used to—and you will get used to them. It doesn't take long to start developing a taste for vegetables once you find ways to prepare them that you like, and the more you eat something, the more it will appeal to you (most of the time). This is an opportunity to expand your palate. There are also hundreds of vegetables out there in the world, so if you don't like a few of them, try some other ones. Variety is the spice of life. (And spices also make vegetables more delicious!)

DAY 10: Find a protein shake you like and try it for breakfast or a snack.

DO THIS TODAY

Have a pea-protein- or rice-protein-based shake today. See page 102 for guidance on how to choose a high-quality protein shake.

THINK ABOUT THIS TODAY

I don't normally recommend any processed food, but protein shakes are an exception because they have condensed nutrition and can fill in nutrient gaps, especially when you don't feel like eating a whole meal. When you find one you like, can it be your go-to when you need a quick breakfast or snack?

DAILY MOMENT OF APPRECIATION, JOY, OR GRATITUDE

NOTES FOR THE DAY

DAY 11: Go gluten-free today and notice how it feels.
Can you go longer?

DO THIS TODAY

If you haven't eliminated gluten, see if you can go for an entire day without it. If you already have eliminated it, see if you can go an entire day without any grains of any kind, including gluten-free grains like brown rice, quinoa, and corn. See pages 96–99 for information on what contains gluten.

THINK ABOUT THIS TODAY

Depending on who you ask, most or even all people have trouble digesting gluten, even if they don't necessarily feel it. There is nothing with gluten that contains anything you can't get from some other food, and going gluten-free can really help with cutting back on empty carbs and junk food. Considering all that, would it be worth trying to go for a week or more without it, to see how you react?

DAILY MOMENT OF APPRECIATION, JOY, OR GRATITUDE

NOTES FOR THE DAY

DAY 12: Start scaling back on sitting time and move more instead.

DO THIS TODAY

Figure out how much you normally sit during the day. Cut that amount of time in half today by standing more while working, taking more breaks to walk around, and maybe doing some exercises while watching television or listening to a podcast.

THINK ABOUT THIS TODAY

One of the things I often say to people trying to move more is that any amount of exercise is better than no exercise. Start small, but keep increasing, and your fitness and health benefits will increase steadily, too.

DAILY MOMENT OF APPRECIATION, JOY, OR GRATITUDE

NOTES FOR THE DAY

DAY 13: Push yourself a little harder.

DO THIS TODAY

Whatever exercise you do now (or don't do), see if you can push yourself a little bit today. Don't go overboard, but do try to go a little bit farther, faster, harder, or heavier than you normally would.

THINK ABOUT THIS TODAY

When you push yourself with exercise, your muscle cells respond by making more mitochondria to produce more energy. When exercise feels hard, just remember that you are getting stronger with every push!

DAILY MOMENT OF APPRECIATION, JOY, OR GRATITUDE

NOTES FOR THE DAY

DAY 14: Take care of your own needs.

DO THIS TODAY

Do something good for yourself today—something you really enjoy. Learning to meet your own needs is essential if you want to be in a healthy relationship between two whole people.

THINK ABOUT THIS TODAY

When you feel tapped out, remember the saying: "You have to fill up your own cup before you can fill up someone else's."

DAILY MOMENT OF APPRECIATION, JOY, OR GRATITUDE

NOTES FOR THE DAY

DAY 15: Challenge yourself to communicate without any criticism.

DO THIS TODAY

See if you can go for the entire day without criticizing anyone you love. It might be harder than you think, but remember that criticizing is just a habit. You can break this one!

THINK ABOUT THIS TODAY

People often criticize unintentionally in order to prove they are right. The real challenge is to explain your point without any low blows. Are you up for the challenge?

DAILY MOMENT OF APPRECIATION, JOY, OR GRATITUDE

NOTES FOR THE DAY

DAY 16: Reach out to a friend.

DO THIS TODAY

No one person can ever meet all your needs, so make a date with a friend today to talk about your feelings. It feels good to spread your emotional needs around to a few close friends, and to be able to help meet theirs, too.

THINK ABOUT THIS TODAY

Each person has their own set of skills and their own brand of emotional intelligence. Give some thought to what you are good at, and what your partner is good at. Where do you intersect? Are you good at talking, or better at touching? Are you good at helping each other do things, or better at sharing in the pride at what you each did on your own? Contemplate the ways you and your partner interact best.

DAILY MOMENT OF APPRECIATION, JOY, OR GRATITUDE

NOTES FOR THE DAY

DAY 17: Improve your sleep hygiene.

DO THIS TODAY

Stop eating three hours before you go to sleep. See if you sleep better or have more energy the next day. If you get too hungry to sleep, have a glass of almond milk or a small handful of raw nuts, which will be unlikely to impact your blood sugar. Night eating is usually just a habit, so, with practice, you will stop being hungry at night.

THINK ABOUT THIS TODAY

Think about some other ways you could improve your sleep hygiene. Which would you be most likely to be able to keep up? Review page 178 for ideas.

DAILY MOMENT OF APPRECIATION, JOY, OR GRATITUDE

NOTES FOR THE DAY

DAY 18: Try diaphragmatic breathing.

DO THIS TODAY

Do 10 minutes of diaphragmatic breathing, as described on page 181.

THINK ABOUT THIS TODAY

Some smartphones and fitness watches can be set to cue you when to do a minute of deep breathing. This can be a good reminder. If you have this capability, try turning it on and see if it helps your stress level.

DAILY MOMENT OF APPRECIATION, JOY, OR GRATITUDE

NOTES FOR THE DAY

DAY 19: Meditation Day!

DO THIS TODAY

Try meditating today. Use the visualization exercise on page 185. How do you feel afterward?

THINK ABOUT THIS TODAY

There are many ways to meditate. Do a bit of research and see if you find techniques that appeal to you. Research has proven time and again that meditation benefits your health in many ways, so it's worth finding the style that you will actually do.

DAILY MOMENT OF APPRECIATION, JOY, OR GRATITUDE

NOTES FOR THE DAY

DAY 20: Take 1,000 mg of vitamin C.

DO THIS TODAY

If you aren't already taking vitamin C, start taking 1,000 mg per day, ideally divided between two or three daily doses. If you are already taking vitamin C, try going up to 3,000 or even 5,000 mg per day, if your stomach tolerates that dose. You'll be supercharging your immune system!

THINK ABOUT THIS TODAY

Spend some time researching Linus Pauling and vitamin C for an interesting history lesson and some useful information about why vitamin C is so valuable for a healthy immune system.

DAILY MOMENT OF APPRECIATION, JOY, OR GRATITUDE

NOTES FOR THE DAY

DAY 21: Digital detox day!

DO THIS TODAY

Try a digital detox today. See if you can go the whole day with your phone, computer, and television turned off. Instead, focus on listening to music, reading, and spending time with the people who you are actually physically with. Notice how you feel at the end of the day.

THINK ABOUT THIS TODAY

Some people have no problem going without their devices, but for others, it can feel like torture. Digital devices encourage shortened attention spans and reduced focus and concentration, and they can distract us from the real world around us. It's not healthy, so if a digital detox is very difficult for you, it's a sign that you should probably do it more often. Food for thought!

DAILY MOMENT OF APPRECIATION, JOY, OR GRATITUDE

NOTES FOR THE DAY

DAY 22: Go a whole day without dairy products. Can you go longer?

DO THIS TODAY

If you still haven't ditched the dairy, see if you can go an entire day without any dairy products. No milk, cheese, yogurt, cream, ice cream, or anything else made from the milk of an animal. Notice if you have any changes in how you feel, especially digestively. Do you have less bloating, less reflux, less gas, or less stomach pain?

THINK ABOUT THIS TODAY

Fortunately, there are a lot of non-dairy products that mimic dairy products and they are better tasting than ever. Try milks, cheeses, yogurts, creamers, or ice cream made from almonds, cashews, coconut, rice, oats, hemp, flax, hazelnuts, or peas. If you find some favorites, giving up dairy will be a lot easier.

DAILY MOMENT OF APPRECIATION, JOY, OR GRATITUDE

NOTES FOR THE DAY

DAY 23: Take a probiotic. Rotate brands.

DO THIS TODAY

If you aren't already taking probiotics, take one today. If you already take a probiotic, look for a different brand with different strains of friendly flora. If you rotate the types of probiotics you take, you will expose your gut to a wider variety of beneficial microbes.

THINK ABOUT THIS TODAY

There is some controversy about whether the microbes from probiotics actually stay in your gastrointestinal tract, but we do know they are beneficial, at least while passing through. To help encourage colonization, be sure to eat fiber with your probiotics. Fiber is your gut bacteria's favorite food.

DAILY MOMENT OF APPRECIATION, JOY, OR GRATITUDE

NOTES FOR THE DAY

DAY 24: Toss old medication and supplements.

DO THIS TODAY

Go through your medicine cabinet today and get rid of all the old expired medication and supplements. Most pharmacies will take your expired medication off your hands, or there may be a community drop-off spot.

THINK ABOUT THIS TODAY

The FDA has a Q&A page on their website explaining how to safely dispose of different kinds of medications. Some are flushable, some are disposable, some should be dropped off at an authorized disposal site. Visit fda.gov to learn more.

DAILY MOMENT OF APPRECIATION, JOY, OR GRATITUDE

NOTES FOR THE DAY

DAY 25: Go a whole day without any added sweetener. Can you go longer?

DO THIS TODAY

If you haven't already, try going for an entire day without any sugar or added sweetener of any kind, including honey, maple syrup, coconut sugar, agave, stevia, and especially artificial sweeteners, which damage your microbiome. If you really need something sweet, have some mint or cinnamon herbal tea, or fresh fruit (not dried).

THINK ABOUT THIS TODAY

Some people have an extremely difficult time giving up sugar. If this is too hard for you, remember the Rule of Halves. See if you can cut your sugar intake in half today. This is a more gradual, less harsh way to ease this addictive substance with no nutritional value out of your diet. If you can get to the point where you only have one square of extra dark chocolate each day, I would call that a success.

DAILY MOMENT OF APPRECIATION, JOY, OR GRATITUDE

NOTES FOR THE DAY

DAY 26: Try a grain-free breakfast.

DO THIS TODAY

Have a cup of fresh berries with ½ cup unsweetened vanilla almond or coconut yogurt for breakfast today. See if this keeps you full longer than a breakfast of grains (like oatmeal or toast).

THINK ABOUT THIS TODAY

Many people who rely on grain-based breakfasts like cereal, oatmeal, toast, pancakes, waffles, or breakfast burritos and think it's fine are amazed at how much better they feel with a grain-free breakfast. Could you be one of those people?

DAILY MOMENT OF APPRECIATION, JOY, OR GRATITUDE

NOTES FOR THE DAY

DAY 27: Have a clean whole-food day with no grain, dairy, sugar, or processed food. You can do it!

DO THIS TODAY

Here's a real dietary challenge, but I believe you are ready! Weigh yourself in the morning, then go for the whole day eating nothing but fresh vegetables (including lots of leafy greens), fresh fruit, nuts (including unsweetened almond or coconut milk), seeds, grilled or broiled seafood, and legumes (including hummus) with only olive oil and lemon juice as a dressing or sauce. No grains, no dairy, no sugar, no processed food. Drink lots of water throughout the day. You can have one cup of black coffee and two cups of green tea if you need them. Weigh yourself the next morning. Do you like the results?

THINK ABOUT THIS TODAY

Your day might look like this:

Breakfast could be a bowl of fresh berries and raw nuts and seeds with half a cup of unsweetened almond milk or coconut yogurt.

Snack is a piece of fresh fruit or some raw veggies with hummus.

Lunch could be a big salad full of fresh veggies with a piece of grilled salmon, dressed with olive oil and lemon juice.

Dinner could be a big bowl of chunky lentil veggie soup, or a stir-fry with lots of fresh veggies and some scallops or shrimp over cauliflower "rice" or spaghetti squash.

Need dessert? How about a small spoonful of almond butter with some raw cacao nibs sprinkled on top, or some apple slices with cinnamon and chopped pecans?

DAILY MOMENT OF APPRECIATION, JOY, OR GRATITUDE

NOTES FOR THE DAY

DAY 28: Exercise for an hour! Go, you!

DO THIS TODAY

Let's up the exercise ante today! Commit to one full hour of continuous moving. You can walk, you can run, you can lift weights, you can do yoga, but whatever you do, do it for an hour.

THINK ABOUT THIS TODAY

Think how great you could feel if you did this six days a week. This would be a great goal.

DAILY MOMENT OF APPRECIATION, JOY, OR GRATITUDE

NOTES FOR THE DAY

DAY 29: Be vulnerable with somebody you love.

DO THIS TODAY

Have an honest talk with your partner or a friend today. Tell them what they mean to you. Tell them how important they are in your life. Commit to loving them better. Being vulnerable in front of another person feels hard but it also feels great.

THINK ABOUT THIS TODAY

In an entitlement culture where people tend to think they deserve everything but shouldn't have to work for it, admitting you need someone and that you value them can feel scary. It opens a door to a new level of intimacy, though, so if you really want to feel closer to someone, vulnerability is what it takes.

DAILY MOMENT OF APPRECIATION, JOY, OR GRATITUDE

NOTES FOR THE DAY

DAY 30: Consider what has worked for you and what hasn't, and pat yourself on the back. Great job! I'm so proud of you!

DO THIS TODAY

Today, look back over the past 30 days. Which habits are you still doing? Which do you want to pick back up? Which are not going to work for you? Make a list of what you want to incorporate into your life and keep going. We all slip up now and then. Nobody's perfect. But if you can stick with your new good habits and leave most of your old bad habits behind you most of the time, you will become more and more vibrant.

THINK ABOUT THIS TODAY

What did you learn about yourself over the last 30 days? Let's rank your energy level one more time, on a scale of 1 to 10. How is your energy fountain *now*?

DAILY MOMENT OF APPRECIATION, JOY, OR GRATITUDE

NOTES FOR THE DAY

Visit
vibrantdoc.com
for a printable
version.

CHAPTER 11

The Vibrant Kitchen: 40 Recipes for Vitality and Glow

Are you ready to cook for the new you? Maybe you already love to cook, in which case, these recipes will be a snap to make and you'll be thinking of your own healthy variations as you try them. I encourage you to get creative, within the generous boundaries of the Vibrant Food List. If you haven't turned on the stove recently (like me—cooking is not my favorite thing), these easy-to-make recipes will help coax you back into the kitchen. When I cook, I want it to be simple. That's exactly what I confided to Chef Quenby Schuyler, who created these recipes for me, and for you. I've tried them all, and I can assure you they are clean, easy, and delectable. We've got 10 breakfasts, 10 lunches, 10 snacks, and 10 dinners designed to support your vibrant life!

> **KITCHEN NOTES**
> These recipes all serve four people, except for the snacks, desserts, and drinks, which indicate servings on each recipe. If you are cooking

for one or two, you will have leftovers, which can be great for the next day, or for freezing for later. However, these recipes are ultimately scalable. If you would rather make one or two servings, just cut the ingredients to one-quarter or one-half. If you want to serve eight, just double the recipe. Everything should still work out just fine.

Also, whenever possible, I encourage you to use fresh organic ingredients. They are the cleanest and will nourish your liver without also requiring it to detoxify your meal.

A few more things for you to know:

- For meat, poultry, and fish, use grass-fed, pastured, or wild-caught whenever possible.

- For all yogurt and milk, use any unsweetened plant-based alternatives, such as coconut, almond, cashew, rice, or oat.

- When using tofu or tempeh, use non-GMO organic only.

- If you don't have or like a particular vegetable, fruit, nut, or seed called for in a recipe, you can always swap out for a different one, such as broccoli for green beans, peaches for apples, almonds for pecans, or sunflower seeds for pumpkin seeds. I encourage you to try different combinations and new vegetables whenever you have the opportunity.

- You can always swap out olive, avocado, and grapeseed oil, depending on what you have on hand, but do not use any other type of oil or fat.

NOTE: FOR PHOTOS OF SOME OF THESE DELICIOUS DISHES, FLIP TO THE INSERT.

BREAKFAST

Do you like your breakfasts sweet? Savory? Are you all about the eggs? Or do you prefer a quick smoothie to take with you as you rush out the door? I've got all your options covered here, and I hope you'll try them all. On those days when you really don't have time to prepare anything, I hope you will at least blend up a protein shake before you hit the road. When you do have time, start your morning out right with these nutrient-dense, quick breakfasts.

274 BERRY BEAUTIFUL PARFAITS

275 MERMAID BOWL WITH BLUE BUTTERFLY PEA POWDER

276 TROPIC GREEN SMOOTHIE

277 CHOCOLATE CHERRY BOMB SMOOTHIE

278 QUINOA BREAKFAST BOWL WITH SAUTÉED APPLES

279 CHICKEN SAUSAGE BREAKFAST SKILLET

280 SUMMER PATTY PAN EGG CUPS

281 MEDITERRANEAN CRUSTLESS QUICHE

282 SMOKED SALMON AND VEGGIE BREAKFAST PLATTER WITH CHIVE-YOGURT SAUCE

283 TURMERIC TOFU SCRAMBLE

BERRY BEAUTIFUL PARFAITS

PREP TIME: 5 MINUTES   *SERVES 4*

2 cups mixed raspberries, blueberries, blackberries, divided

4 cups unsweetened coconut (or other non-dairy) yogurt of choice, divided

4 teaspoons slivered or sliced almonds

2 teaspoons unsweetened coconut shavings (optional)

Honey for drizzle

1. Divide ⅓ of the berries between 4 glasses. Divide half the yogurt between the glasses, spooning it on top of the berries. Repeat with another layer of berries, another layer of yogurt, and a final layer of berries.
2. Top with almonds and coconut, if using, and drizzle with honey if you like.

NOTE: *You can make this recipe ahead and refrigerate it, but wait until you are ready to serve to add the nuts, coconut, and honey.*

MERMAID BOWL WITH BLUE BUTTERFLY PEA POWDER

PREP TIME: 10 MINUTES   *SERVES 4*

4 cups unsweetened vanilla coconut yogurt (or other plant-based yogurt)
4 teaspoons butterfly pea powder (see Note)
1 cup strawberries, sliced
1 cup blueberries
1 cup blackberries

4 teaspoons shelled roasted pistachios
4 teaspoons shaved unsweetened coconut
4 teaspoons hemp seeds (optional)
Honey for drizzle (optional)
Mint leaves for garnish

1. In a large mixing bowl, combine the yogurt and butterfly pea powder. Stir until fully combined without any chunks. (You can also combine them in a blender.)
2. Divide the yogurt between 4 bowls.
3. Divide the berries between the bowls, arranging them on top of the yogurt.
4. Top with the pistachios, coconut, and hemp seeds and honey, if using.
5. Garnish with fresh mint leaves.

NOTE: *You can find butterfly pea powder readily available online.*

TROPIC GREEN SMOOTHIE

PREP TIME: 20 MINUTES   *SERVES 4*

You will need 4 (16-ounce) mason jars or other glasses of choice.

4 cups unsweetened vanilla or
plain coconut milk

2 cups pineapple, chopped
(frozen or fresh)

1 cup mango, chopped
(frozen or fresh)

2 cups fresh spinach or greens
of choice

1 tablespoon fresh ginger,
chopped

2 sprigs mint

1. Place all ingredients in a high-powered blender (such as a Vitamix or Ninja). Blend on high until all ingredients are fully mixed and smooth.
2. Evenly distribute in glasses and serve immediately.

CHOCOLATE CHERRY BOMB SMOOTHIE

PREP TIME: 20 MINUTES *SERVES 4*

4 cups unsweetened vanilla almond milk (or other non-dairy milk)
2 cups frozen dark sweet cherries
½ cup unsweetened raw almond butter

1 tablespoon raw organic cacao powder
1 teaspoon vanilla extract
Extra cacao powder and/or cinnamon for sprinkle

1. Place all ingredients (except the sprinkle) in a high-powered blender. Blend until all ingredients are fully mixed and smooth.
2. Divide between 4 glasses.
3. Sprinkle with the cacao powder and/or cinnamon.
4. Serve immediately.

NOTE: *If you have leftovers, you can freeze this smoothie in a freezer-safe bowl, then scoop it out for a delicious, chocolate-y "nice cream" dessert.*

QUINOA BREAKFAST BOWL WITH SAUTÉED APPLES

PREP TIME: 15 MINUTES *SERVES 4*

1 tablespoon olive oil
2 cups apples, sliced
1 teaspoon cinnamon
4 cups cooked organic quinoa
  of choice

1 cup organic unsweetened
  oat milk
4 tablespoons walnuts, chopped
4 tablespoons raisins or chopped
  dried apricots
Honey for drizzle (optional)

1. Heat the olive oil in a medium soup pot or saucepan over medium heat.
2. Add the apples and sauté until semi-soft, about 5 minutes.
3. Add cinnamon and stir until it evenly coats the apples.
4. Stir in the cooked quinoa and oat milk at the same time. Add more oat milk if you like a thinner consistency.
5. Divide the quinoa mixture between 4 bowls.
6. Divide the walnuts and dried fruit between the bowls.
7. Drizzle each bowl with honey, if using.

CHICKEN SAUSAGE BREAKFAST SKILLET

PREP TIME: 20 MINUTES *SERVES 4*

1 package organic gluten-free chicken sausage
¼ cup avocado oil
½ white onion, diced
1 green bell pepper, diced
4 cups cubed butternut squash or squash of choice (acorn, kabocha)

1 tablespoon garlic, minced
4 cage-free organic eggs
¼ cup non-dairy unsweetened milk of choice
½ teaspoon sea salt
½ teaspoon black pepper
Chopped spinach or cherry tomato for garnish

1. Slice chicken sausages on the bias, about ½-inch-thick pieces.
2. Heat large nonstick skillet over medium heat and add the avocado oil.
3. Once the avocado oil is heated, add the sausage, onion, bell pepper, and squash and begin to sauté until all ingredients are slightly browned. (If ingredients are looking too dry, add a splash of water or bone broth to continue to soften the veggies.)
4. Once the chicken and veggies are sautéed through, stir in the garlic until fragrant.
5. Crack the 4 eggs into the skillet and add the non-dairy milk. Stir until the eggs begin to scramble.
6. Just before finishing, add the salt and pepper.
7. Garnish with fresh spinach or sliced cherry tomatoes.

SUMMER PATTY PAN EGG CUPS

PREP TIME: 40 MINUTES *SERVES 4*

4 large patty pan squash
4 tablespoons olive oil
4 teaspoons garlic, minced
4 dashes of salt
4 dashes of pepper

4 large organic eggs
4 tablespoons fresh spinach,
   chopped
4 tablespoons fresh cherry
   tomatoes, chopped

1. Preheat oven to 350 degrees.
2. Line a standard cookie sheet or 9-by-12-inch glass pan with parchment paper.
3. While oven is preheating, slice off the knobs on the bottom of the squash so they lie flat on a surface.
4. With a spoon, scoop an egg-size hole out from the top of each squash, 2–3 inches deep and around, depending on size of the squash.
5. Using 1 tablespoon of oil for each squash, oil the inside of the squash and lightly season with 1 teaspoon of garlic and a dash of salt and pepper.
6. Place squash in oven for 10–15 minutes to soften.
7. Remove from oven, crack 1 egg into each cup, and return to oven to bake for 10 minutes or until the egg is cooked through and the whites are no longer translucent.
8. Garnish with the spinach and tomatoes and serve immediately.

NOTE: *For those who can tolerate dairy, this recipe is good with a little bit of goat cheese sprinkled on top.*

MEDITERRANEAN CRUSTLESS QUICHE

PREP TIME: 1 HOUR *SERVES 4*

12 egg whites (about 1½ cups)
½ red pepper, diced (plus 2 tablespoons, minced, for garnish)
1 medium zucchini, diced
1 yellow squash, diced
½ onion, minced
1 tablespoon minced garlic

2 tablespoons minced fresh basil, plus extra for garnish
1 teaspoon dried oregano
½ teaspoon salt
½ teaspoon pepper
Fresh chopped oregano for garnish
Sea salt for garnish

1. Preheat oven to 350 degrees.
2. Spray a round pie pan, glass or nonstick, with avocado or coconut oil.
3. Whip egg whites in a nonreactive glass bowl and set aside.
4. Spray a medium nonstick skillet with avocado or coconut oil and heat over medium flame.
5. Once heated, add the red pepper, zucchini, yellow squash, and onion. Sauté until firm yet slightly browned.
6. Add the garlic and cook until fragrant.
7. Pour the veggie mixture into the egg white mixture, along with the 2 tablespoons basil and the dried oregano, salt, and pepper. Stir to evenly distribute.
8. Pour mixture into the pie pan and bake for 25–30 minutes, until fork comes out clean or eggs are firm.
9. Remove from oven and let sit for 10–15 minutes to set.
10. Slice into 4 large pie pieces, or 8 for smaller portions.
11. Garnish with fresh basil, fresh oregano, minced red pepper, and sea salt.

SMOKED SALMON AND VEGGIE BREAKFAST PLATTER WITH CHIVE-YOGURT SAUCE

PREP TIME: 10 MINUTES *SERVES 4*

Platter

4 cups fresh field greens (or other mixed greens)
1 (8-ounce) package Norwegian smoked salmon
4 hard-boiled eggs, halved
1 medium cucumber, sliced on the bias
1 avocado, sliced
½ cup Kalamata olives
½ cup quartered cherry tomatoes
½ cup microgreens
¼ cup capers
4 tablespoons high-quality balsamic vinegar
1 lemon, sliced, for garnish
Fresh dill for garnish

Sauce

1 cup unsweetened almond milk (or other non-dairy) yogurt of choice
3 tablespoons minced chives
½ teaspoon minced garlic
⅛ teaspoon salt
⅛ teaspoon pepper

To make the platter:
1. Put the field greens on a platter or divide between individual plates.
2. Arrange the salmon, eggs, cucumber, avocado, olives, tomatoes, microgreens, and capers over the greens.
3. Drizzle with the balsamic vinegar.
4. Garnish with lemon slices and fresh dill.

To make the sauce:
1. In a small mixing bowl, mix all the sauce ingredients together until fully combined.
2. Serve the sauce on the side.

TURMERIC TOFU SCRAMBLE

PREP TIME: 15 MINUTES   *SERVES 4*

1 tablespoon olive oil
½ white onion, diced
1 medium yellow or orange bell
  pepper, chopped
1 fresh tomato, chopped
4 cups fresh spinach

1 (14-ounce) package organic
  extra firm tofu, drained and
  dried with paper towels
2 tablespoons minced garlic
2 teaspoons ground turmeric
½ teaspoon salt
¼ teaspoon pepper
Fresh cilantro for garnish

1. Heat the olive oil in a large skillet over medium heat.
2. Add the onion and sauté until translucent, about 3 minutes.
3. Add the chopped bell pepper and sauté for an additional 5 minutes.
4. Stir in the tomato and spinach and continue to sauté until the spinach wilts, about 2 more minutes.
5. Crumble the block of tofu into the skillet. Add the garlic, turmeric, salt, and pepper. Sauté until everything is combined and the tofu is fully coated in the turmeric and just beginning to brown.
6. Garnish with cilantro and serve hot.

LUNCH

Keep your lunch light but nutritious. Lunch is especially important if you've had a very light breakfast, or if you are a breakfast-skipper because you aren't hungry first thing, or you are intermittent fasting (see page 208). Make sure it's got plenty of protein and isn't too high on the carbs, so you aren't wishing for a nap at 3:00 pm. Salads are my go-to and we've got some good ones here, plus a few other tasty meals for variety, because sometimes you just want a creamy soup or something a bit more substantial.

285 GROUND TURKEY TACO SALAD BOWLS

286 CREAMY ROASTED CAULIFLOWER SOUP

287 DETOX SALAD WITH KALE, POMEGRANATE SEEDS, AND FORBIDDEN RICE

288 ROASTED BEETS OVER LEAFY GREENS

289 GINGERY SESAME TUNA POKE BOWLS

290 SIMPLE MASSAGED KALE CAESAR SALAD WITH PROTEIN-PACKED ANCHOVY DRESSING

291 GREEK ROASTED SALMON POWER BOWL

292 SMOKED SALMON NIÇOISE SALAD WITH DIJON TARRAGON DRESSING

293 EASY 30-MINUTE ROASTED CHICKEN AND KALE SOUP WITH BONE BROTH

294 ROASTED ATHENIAN CHICKEN COBB SALAD

GROUND TURKEY TACO SALAD BOWLS

PREP TIME: 1 HOUR *SERVES 4*

Bowls

1 pound lean ground turkey
½ white onion, diced
½ teaspoon salt
½ teaspoon pepper
1 small can green chilies
1 tablespoon chili powder
1 teaspoon cumin
1 tablespoon garlic, minced
2 packages organic field greens

1 red bell pepper, diced
1 green bell pepper, diced
½ can corn, rinsed and drained
1 can black beans, rinsed and drained
1 avocado, diced
1 tomato, diced
2 green onions, chopped
3 sprigs cilantro, chopped

Aioli

1 cup vegan mayo (see Note)
3 tablespoons chipotle adobo sauce

½ teaspoon garlic, minced
2 cilantro sprigs, chopped

To make the bowls:
1. Spray a medium skillet with avocado oil or grapeseed oil.
2. Heat skillet over medium heat.
3. Add the ground turkey and onion.
4. Season with salt and pepper.
5. As onions begin to turn translucent, add the green chilies, chili powder, cumin, and garlic.
6. Cook 10 minutes or until thoroughly cooked through.
7. Set aside to cool.
8. In a large salad bowl, lay down the bed of greens.
9. Arrange the turkey mixture, bell peppers, corn, beans, avocado, and tomato in pockets or separate piles over the greens.
10. Top with the green onions and cilantro.

To make the aioli:
1. In a small food processor, blender, or simple bowl, mix all the ingredients together.
2. Drizzle over salad and enjoy.

NOTE: *For a less spicy dressing, use less adobo and more mayo.*

CREAMY ROASTED CAULIFLOWER SOUP

PREP TIME: 40 MINUTES   *SERVES 4*

2 heads cauliflower, rustic chopped in large pieces
6 cloves garlic
4 tablespoons avocado or olive oil, divided
1 leek, sliced and rinsed

1 bay leaf
3 sprigs thyme, destemmed
5 cups chicken or veggie bone broth
1 teaspoon salt
1 teaspoon pepper

1. Preheat oven to 415 degrees.
2. Line a baking sheet with parchment paper or tinfoil, and spray down with oil of choice.
3. In a large mixing bowl, toss the cauliflower, garlic, and 3 tablespoons of the olive oil.
4. Season with a sprinkle of salt and pepper.
5. Place the oiled cauliflower and garlic in an even layer on the baking pan and bake for 15–20 minutes, until the garlic appears "charred."
6. Remove from oven and set aside.
7. In a large soup pot, heat the remaining tablespoon of oil over medium heat.
8. Begin to sauté the leek until it becomes translucent.
9. Add the entire sheet pan of roasted cauliflower, bay leaf, thyme, and broth to the pot.
10. Bring to a boil, then reduce to a slow simmer for 15–20 minutes.
11. Remove the bay leaf and allow to cool a bit before blending.
12. Add ingredients in batches to a high-powered blender. (Do not fill the blender, as the heat may create steam burns.)
13. Pour blended batches into a separate large bowl until all the ingredients are blended.
14. Ladle into soup bowls.
15. Add salt and pepper to taste, and enjoy!

DETOX SALAD WITH KALE, POMEGRANATE SEEDS, AND FORBIDDEN RICE

PREP TIME: 1 HOUR *SERVES 4*

Salad

2 cups cooked Forbidden Black Rice (or wild rice or brown rice)

Two bunches lacinato (dinosaur) kale, destemmed and chopped (or mixed baby kale, spinach, or arugula)

1 cucumber, sliced in rounds

10 cherry tomatoes, halved

2 green onions, chopped

¼ cup sunflower seeds, roasted or raw

¼ cup pomegranate seeds

¼ cup pumpkin seeds

2 tablespoons hemp seeds

Vinaigrette

½ cup avocado oil

Juice of one orange (plus optional juice of an additional orange for added sweetness)

1 clove garlic, minced

5 fresh basil leaves

¼ teaspoon sea salt

¼ teaspoon pepper

To make the salad:

1. Prepare the rice according to the package directions.
2. Massage the kale with your hands until it turns bright green and releases some of its juice.
3. Divide the kale between 4 plates or put it on a platter.
4. Arrange the rice, cucumber slices, and tomatoes over the greens and sprinkle with the remaining salad ingredients.

To make the vinaigrette:

1. In a small food processor or blender, blend the dressing ingredients together.
2. Drizzle over the salad.

ROASTED BEETS OVER LEAFY GREENS

PREP TIME: 1 HOUR *SERVES 4*

8 beets (mixed colors), peeled
3 tablespoons olive oil
1 teaspoon sea salt
1 teaspoon pepper
¼ cup Dijon mustard
3 sprigs fresh tarragon, chopped

1 package leafy greens (power greens, field greens)
1 cucumber, diced
1 avocado, chopped (optional)
2 tablespoons fig balsamic or regular balsamic vinegar

1. Preheat oven to 415 degrees.
2. Line a cookie sheet with parchment or foil.
3. Toss the beets in the olive oil, salt, and pepper, and place in an even layer on the cookie sheet.
4. Roast the beets for 20–30 minutes until soft and fragrant.
5. Remove the beets, place in a mixing bowl, and toss with Dijon mustard and tarragon.
6. Allow to cool to room temperature.
7. Lay a bed of greens down in a large salad bowl or large platter.
8. Place the beets evenly over the greens.
9. Top with the cucumber and avocado, if using.
10. Drizzle with balsamic as the final touch.

GINGERY SESAME TUNA POKE BOWLS

PREP TIME: 1 HOUR   *SERVES 4*

18 ounces fresh sashimi-grade ahi tuna, diced into 1-inch cubes
¼ cup tamari
3 tablespoons toasted sesame oil
1 tablespoon ginger, minced
½ tablespoon garlic, minced
2 tablespoons black sesame seeds (plain is a fine substitute)

4 cups cauliflower rice
1 cup mango, diced
1 cup pineapple, diced
1 cup cucumber, diced
1 avocado, diced
4 tablespoons pickled ginger
5 sprigs cilantro, chopped
4 lime wedges

1. In a nonreactive mixing bowl, lightly mix the tuna, sesame oil, tamari, ginger, garlic, and sesame seeds.
2. Set aside to marinate in fridge for 20 minutes.
3. In the meantime, equally distribute 1 cup each of the cauliflower rice (you can sauté or serve raw) into decorative soup bowls.
4. Arrange the mango, pineapple, and cucumber in pockets over the cauliflower rice.
5. Remove the tuna from the fridge and place in the bowls in pockets as well.
6. Add the avocado and pickled ginger either in pockets or sprinkled on top.
7. Garnish with cilantro and lime wedges, and enjoy!

SIMPLE MASSAGED KALE CAESAR SALAD WITH PROTEIN-PACKED ANCHOVY DRESSING

PREP TIME: 30 MINUTES *SERVES 4*

Dressing

1 clove garlic, minced
1 teaspoon anchovy paste
1 tablespoon lemon juice
1 teaspoon Dijon mustard

½ teaspoon Worcestershire
 sauce
½ cup vegan mayonnaise
¼ cup nutritional yeast

Salad

3 bunches lacinato (dinosaur)
 or red kale, destemmed and
 chopped
1 tomato, diced
1 cucumber, sliced

2 hard-boiled eggs, quartered
1 can chickpeas, rinsed and
 drained
Fresh-chopped anchovies
 (optional)

To make the dressing:

1. In a mixing bowl, whisk all the dressing ingredients together.
2. Cover and set in fridge for at least 1 hour or up to a few days prior to making the salad.

To make the salad:

1. In a large mixing bowl, massage the kale with your hands until the kale wilts and the oils start to extract from the leaves.
2. Remove the kale from the mixing bowl and place in a large decorative salad bowl.
3. Arrange the remaining ingredients on top of the salad.
4. You can use fresh-chopped anchovies for added omega-3s if you like.
5. Drizzle the dressing over the salad, starting sparingly and adding to taste.
6. Toss the salad and enjoy!

GREEK ROASTED SALMON POWER BOWL

PREP TIME: 1 HOUR *SERVES 4*

Dressing

¼ cup lemon juice
¼ cup olive oil

1 tablespoon chopped fresh oregano
1 tablespoon chopped fresh basil
1 clove garlic, minced

Bowl

24 ounces boneless salmon fillets, cubed in 1-inch pieces
3 tablespoons olive oil
1 teaspoon oregano
1 teaspoon basil
4 cups cooked quinoa

20 Kalamata olives
1 cucumber, chopped
1 jar roasted red peppers, drained and diced (no seeds)
2 cups spinach, chopped
Salt and pepper to taste

To make the dressing:

1. In a high-powered blender, add all dressing ingredients and blend until smooth.
2. Remove and place in small bowl.

To make the bowl:

1. Preheat oven to 375 degrees.
2. Line a cookie sheet with parchment paper and spray with a little olive oil.
3. In a nonreactive bowl, toss the salmon cubes with the olive oil, oregano, and basil.
4. Roast the salmon for 15–20 minutes for lightly pinker salmon.
5. Remove the salmon from the oven and set aside.
6. In a large mixing bowl, mix the quinoa, olives, cucumbers, roasted peppers, and spinach together.
7. Add salt and pepper to taste.
8. Spoon out evenly into 4 decorative bowls.
9. Arrange cubed salmon on top.
10. Drizzle the bowls with the dressing.
11. You can garnish with fresh basil, lemon zest, and oregano.

SMOKED SALMON NIÇOISE SALAD WITH DIJON TARRAGON DRESSING

PREP TIME: 30 MINUTES *SERVES 4*

Dressing

6 sprigs fresh tarragon (4 sprigs chopped for the dressing and 2 sprigs for garnish)
½ cup Dijon mustard

2 tablespoons avocado oil
1 teaspoon honey
¼ teaspoon black pepper

Salad

2 packages (or 8 cups) spring mix or power greens
2 cups fresh blanched green beans
2 hard-boiled eggs, quartered
1 large tomato, chopped
1 seedless cucumber, sliced

12 green or black olives
1 cup shredded carrots
16 ounces Norwegian smoked salmon
1 tablespoon avocado oil
4 lemon wedges, deseeded

To make the dressing:

1. Mix the chopped tarragon in with the Dijon, avocado oil, honey, and black pepper.
2. Set aside.

To make the salad:

1. Arrange the spring greens in a bed in a large salad bowl.
2. Place the beans, eggs, tomato, cucumber, olives, and carrots in arranged pockets over the greens.
3. Lay the salmon decoratively in the top center of the salad. Drizzle with avocado oil. Arrange the lemon wedges in the corners.
4. Drizzle the prepared dressing over the salad or serve in ramekins on the side.
5. Use the remaining sprigs of tarragon as a garnish.

EASY 30-MINUTE ROASTED CHICKEN AND KALE SOUP WITH BONE BROTH

PREP TIME: 30 MINUTES   *SERVES 4 PLUS*

1 roasted chicken (white
  meat only)
¼ cup avocado oil
1 cup diced organic carrots
1 white onion, diced
1 cup diced celery
4 cloves garlic, chopped

5 sprigs fresh thyme
1 tablespoon oregano
2 bay leaves
1 teaspoon sea salt
1 teaspoon black pepper
2 quarts organic bone broth or
  organic chicken stock

1. Shred roasted chicken, being careful to leave out any bones and using white meat only (although you can use dark meat as well if preferred). Set aside in a mixing bowl.
2. In a large soup pot, heat the avocado oil over medium to high heat.
3. Add the carrots, onion, and celery.
4. Sweat the vegetables, stirring frequently to avoid burning.
5. Once the onions are translucent, add the garlic and cook until fragrant.
6. Tie the thyme sprigs into a knot and throw into the pot with the oregano, bay leaves, salt, and pepper.
7. Stir lightly.
8. Add the bone broth or stock and bring to a boil.
9. Once the soup is boiling, reduce to medium-low and simmer.
10. Add the shredded chicken and allow to cook for 20-plus minutes. (You will render deeper flavor the longer the soup cooks.)
11. Season to taste with salt and pepper once finished.
12. Remove bay leaves and thyme sprigs before serving.

ROASTED ATHENIAN CHICKEN COBB SALAD

PREP TIME: 1 HOUR 30 MINUTES *SERVES 4*

Salad

2 (8-ounce) organic chicken breasts

1 red bell pepper, chopped into 1-inch pieces

1 yellow bell pepper, chopped into 1-inch pieces

½ red onion, chopped into 1-inch pieces

½ cup halved cherry tomatoes

1 teaspoon fresh chopped oregano

1 teaspoon fresh chopped marjoram

1 teaspoon fresh chopped basil

1 teaspoon garlic powder

3 tablespoons olive oil

2 packages (or 8 cups) field greens or power greens

½ cup diced cucumber

2 green onions, diced

¼ cup minced olives (any type you like)

4 lemon wedges

Dressing

¼ cup fresh-squeezed lemon juice

¼ cup olive oil

1 teaspoon oregano

1 teaspoon basil

¼ teaspoon sea salt

¼ teaspoon black pepper

To make the salad:

1. Preheat oven to 400 degrees.
2. Line a baking sheet with parchment paper or aluminum foil.
3. Mix the chicken, bell peppers, onions, tomatoes, herbs, and garlic powder in a large mixing bowl. Drizzle with the olive oil and toss to coat.
4. Spread the chicken-vegetable mixture evenly over the baking sheet and roast for 35 minutes or until veggies are turning golden and just getting crispy along the edges, and chicken is cooked through. (If the chicken cooks to an interior temperature of 165 degrees before the veggies are finished roasting, remove the chicken, set aside, and continue to roast the vegetables until they are golden and crispy.)
5. Set the chicken and vegetables aside to cool.
6. While the chicken is cooling, arrange the field greens in a bed on a large platter or in a large decorative salad bowl.

7. Dice the chicken into 1-inch cubes.
8. Arrange the roasted veggies, cucumbers, green onions, and olives decoratively over the greens.
9. Sprinkle the chicken on top, then drizzle with the dressing and garnish with the lemon wedges.

To make the dressing:
1. In a small food processor or blender, blend the dressing ingredients together.
2. Drizzle over the salad and serve.

SNACKS/DESSERTS/MOCKTAILS

Sometimes you just need a little something extra. A snack in the afternoon, a bite of something sweet after dinner, or a refreshing mocktail you can celebrate with, without regretting it the next morning. This is the section for all that deliciousness. These are super quick and easy to put together, but with an air of something special. I hope you'll dip into this section often.

297 SLICED BLOOD ORANGES WITH SHAVED DARK CHOCOLATE

298 FROZEN BANANA "NICE CREAM" WITH MADAGASCAR VANILLA

299 FROZEN BERRY BEAUTY "NICE CREAM"

300 CLEAN TURMERIC AND PAPRIKA ROASTED KALE CHIPS

301 SIMPLE FAMILY FUN CHOCOLATE STACKERS

302 EASY APPLES WITH CINNAMON RAISIN ALMOND BUTTER

303 DATE AND PECAN POWER TRUFFLES

304 REFRESHING SLICED CUCUMBER WITH HAND-SMASHED GUACAMOLE

305 ROSEMARY RELEASE MOCKTAIL

306 RUBY-THROATED DRAGON MOCKTAIL

SLICED BLOOD ORANGES WITH SHAVED DARK CHOCOLATE

PREP TIME: 10 MINUTES *SERVES 4*

4 large blood oranges or regular Cara Cara oranges, wedged

4 teaspoons shaved dark chocolate

Pinch of cinnamon if preferred

1. Place orange wedges on a large decorative platter, or in individual bowls.
2. Evenly sprinkle the dark chocolate over the oranges.
3. Add cinnamon if you wish. Enjoy!

FROZEN BANANA "NICE CREAM" WITH MADAGASCAR VANILLA

PREP TIME: 6 HOURS   *SERVES 4*

8 ripe bananas, sliced into discs
1 tablespoon high-quality Madagascar vanilla extract, or any organic vanilla extract
1 tablespoon maple syrup
1 cup nut milk of choice (unsweetened vanilla coconut preferred), plus more as needed

Slivered almonds (for optional topping)
Shaved unsweetened coconut (for optional topping)
Honey (for optional drizzle)

1. Line a large cookie sheet with parchment paper and arrange the banana discs on the sheet.
2. Place the sheet in the freezer and freeze for at least 6 hours.
3. Once the banana discs are frozen, remove from the cookie sheet and place in a high-powered blender with the vanilla extract, maple syrup, and nut milk.
4. Blend on high, adding more nut milk a little at a time if necessary to create a soft-serve ice cream texture.
5. Evenly distribute into ice cream bowls.
6. Top with preferred toppings and optional drizzle of honey, and enjoy immediately.

FROZEN BERRY BEAUTY "NICE CREAM"

PREP TIME: 10 MINUTES   *SERVES 4*

24 ounces of organic mixed berries of choice

1 cup orange juice

1 cup nut milk of choice (unsweetened vanilla coconut preferred)

Shaved orange rind (optional topping)

Green shelled pistachios (optional topping)

Fresh mint (optional topping)

Honey (optional drizzle)

1. Place the berries, orange juice, and nut milk in a high-powered blender and blend until smooth, adding more nut milk if necessary to create a soft-serve ice cream texture.
2. Once blended and smooth, ladle out into ice cream bowls.
3. Top with preferred toppings and optional drizzle of honey, and serve immediately.

CLEAN TURMERIC AND PAPRIKA ROASTED KALE CHIPS

PREP TIME: 45 MINUTES *SERVES 4*

1 head curly red kale, or
  green kale
2 tablespoons olive oil

1 teaspoon turmeric
½ teaspoon paprika
Sea salt for seasoning

1. Preheat oven to 275 degrees.
2. Remove the ribs from the kale and cut into 2-inch pieces.
3. Lay kale on a cookie sheet and toss with the olive oil, spices, and sea salt.
4. Bake until the kale crisps up, about 20 minutes, making sure to turn the kale over halfway through.
5. Sprinkle with more salt if preferred and enjoy!

SIMPLE FAMILY FUN CHOCOLATE STACKERS

PREP TIME: 15 MINUTES *SERVES 4*

16 (1-inch) organic dark
  chocolate squares

16 large dried apricots
16 almonds

1. Arrange the dark chocolate squares on a large serving platter.
2. Place one apricot flat on each piece.
3. Press the almond gently into the apricot and enjoy as a quick and sweet energy boost!

EASY APPLES WITH CINNAMON RAISIN ALMOND BUTTER

PREP TIME: 20 MINUTES   *SERVES 4*

⅓ cup smooth raw almond butter
1 tablespoon honey
3 tablespoons chopped walnuts
2 tablespoons raisins

2 large Honeycrisp apples,
or apples of choice, cut
into wedges
1 teaspoon Saigon cinnamon

1. Place the almond butter in a small soup or cereal bowl.
2. Top with honey, walnuts, and raisins.
3. In a mixing bowl, toss the apple wedges with the cinnamon.
4. Place the almond butter bowl in the center of a large platter.
5. Arrange apple wedges around the bowl and serve immediately!

DATE AND PECAN POWER TRUFFLES

PREP TIME: 30 MINUTES *SERVES 4 PLUS*

12 pitted large Medjool dates, plus more as needed
4 tablespoons chopped roasted pecans

1 teaspoon raw cocoa powder
½ teaspoon Saigon cinnamon
1 cup shaved unsweetened coconut

1. Place the ingredients, minus the coconut, into a food processor or high-powered blender. Blend until evenly mixed and slightly sticky. (If the mixture is too dry to roll into balls with your fingers, add a few more dates until you reach the right consistency.)
2. Scoop out the mixture into a mixing bowl.
3. Place the coconut shavings in a separate small mixing bowl.
4. Roll the date mixture into 1- to 2-inch balls and roll in the coconut shavings. Continue until mixture is finished or you have made the desired amount for your snack.
5. Place the truffles on parchment-lined plates and keep refrigerated until serving. Enjoy!

REFRESHING SLICED CUCUMBER WITH HAND-SMASHED GUACAMOLE

PREP TIME: 20 MINUTES *SERVES 4*

3 large chilled Hass avocados, deseeded and scooped from skin
10 cherry tomatoes, quartered
¼ white onion, diced
2 cloves garlic, minced
½ teaspoon sea salt
½ teaspoon pepper
½ teaspoon avocado oil
6 sprigs cilantro (4 sprigs chopped with stems and 2 sprigs for garnish)
½ lime for fresh-squeezed juice
2 large English cucumbers, sliced on the bias

1. In a large mixing bowl, while wearing gloves, smash the avocado to desired texture (slightly chunky).
2. Combine the avocados with the tomatoes, onion, garlic, salt, pepper, oil, 4 chopped cilantro sprigs, and juice of the lime squeezed into the mixture.
3. Place the guacamole in a small decorative bowl and garnish with the 2 remaining cilantro sprigs.
4. Arrange the sliced cucumbers around the bowl and enjoy immediately.

ROSEMARY RELEASE MOCKTAIL

PREP TIME: 20 MINUTES *SERVES 4*

32 ounces sparkling
unsweetened lemon water
(or Perrier)
1 cup Seedlip Citrus Non-
Alcoholic Herbal Elixir

1 blood orange or regular
orange, deseeded and sliced
into discs
4 sprigs fresh rosemary

1. Combine ingredients in a large pitcher and give it a few stirs.
2. Cover with plastic wrap and place in fridge for 15–20 minutes to meld flavors before serving.
3. Remove from fridge and pour into glasses.
4. Top glasses with ice to keep the fruit and rosemary at the bottom. To your health!

RUBY-THROATED DRAGON MOCKTAIL

PREP TIME: 30 MINUTES *SERVES 4*

32 ounces brewed and
chilled hibiscus tea (such as
Tazo Passion)
2 cups sparkling lime water
(or Perrier)

1 lime, cut into discs
4 sprigs mint
2 tablespoons minced ginger

1. Mix ingredients in a large pitcher.
2. Cover with plastic wrap.
3. Refrigerate for 20 minutes and pour into beautiful glasses.
4. Top with ice and enjoy!

DINNER

It's what we all look forward to, at the end of a long day—that moment when we can let everything else go and sit down with family, friends, or in peaceful solitude, for a really good meal. If you're used to getting take-out or ordering in—or worse, eating in your car on the way home from work—it's time to give dinner the respect it needs. These recipes make it easy. Whip up a mocktail (see options on pages 305 and 306) and take your time lovingly preparing the evening meal with fresh whole-food ingredients. Make your plate look pretty. Sit down, relax, and savor every delicious, vibrant bite. This meal has to carry you all the way through to breakfast, so let it be an event every night, as part of your vibrant life. Here are the delicious dinner recipes you have to choose from.

308 MACKEREL WITH ZUCCHINI WRAPPED IN PARCHMENT

309 ROASTED SALMON WITH BLUEBERRY COMPOTE

310 SUMMER TURMERIC CHICKEN OVER SAUTÉED PURPLE KALE AND MUSHROOMS

311 MEDITERRANEAN AHI STEAKS WITH ROASTED RED PEPPER COMPOTE

312 SLOW COOKER BISON STEW

313 CAST IRON VENISON STEAKS

314 DIJON-ENCRUSTED LAMB LOIN CHOPS WITH CAULIFLOWER SMASH

315 ALL-DAY ELK BOLOGNESE WITH ZUCCHINI NOODLES

316 ROASTED BUTTERNUT SQUASH AND KALE HASH

317 TEMPEH TACO LETTUCE CUPS

MACKEREL WITH ZUCCHINI WRAPPED IN PARCHMENT

PREP TIME: 45 MINUTES   *SERVES 4*

You will need 4 (8-by-10-inch) parchment squares to make this dish.

4 (6-ounce) skinless, boneless
  mackerel fillets
1 teaspoon salt
1 teaspoon pepper

2 lemons, sliced thin in rounds
1 zucchini, sliced thin on the bias
12 sprigs of thyme
4 teaspoons olive oil

1. Preheat oven to 400 degrees.
2. Place one fillet in the center of each piece of parchment paper.
3. Sprinkle salt and pepper evenly over each fillet.
4. Layer the lemons and zucchini over each fillet in a pattern (lemon slice, then zucchini, then repeat).
5. Place three sprigs of thyme over each fillet.
6. Drizzle each fillet with 1 teaspoon olive oil.
7. Fold each fillet into a parchment square, envelope style. Once completely folded, crumple the edges with your hands so as not to allow any air out.
8. Place on a baking sheet and cook in oven for 20–30 minutes.
9. Remove from oven and serve on a plate, with the packets closed until time to eat. Enjoy!

ROASTED SALMON WITH BLUEBERRY COMPOTE

PREP TIME: 45 MINUTES   *SERVES 4*

This dish can be served with fresh blanched green beans or on a bed of sautéed kale.

1 cup fresh blueberries
¼ cup orange juice
4 (6-ounce) wild salmon fillets,
   no skin, deboned

1 teaspoon salt
1 teaspoon pepper

1. Preheat oven to 350 degrees.
2. In a small saucepan, heat the blueberries with the orange juice on medium-low until the mixture starts to simmer.
3. When juice begins to evaporate, mash the blueberries with a fork or spoon, remove from heat, and set aside.
4. Spray a cookie sheet or glass pan with olive oil and place each fillet in the sheet or pan.
5. Season each fillet with equal amounts of salt and pepper.
6. Bake the fillets for 20 minutes for medium rare, 30 minutes for well done.
7. Remove the fillets and place on a platter.
8. Drizzle the compote over the fillets and serve with fresh blanched green beans or on a bed of sautéed kale.

SUMMER TURMERIC CHICKEN OVER SAUTÉED PURPLE KALE AND MUSHROOMS

PREP TIME: 45 MINUTES *SERVES 4*

12 medium-sized chicken tender cutlets or 4 (6-ounce) chicken breasts
2 teaspoons turmeric
1 teaspoon garlic powder
½ teaspoon smoked paprika
½ teaspoon salt
½ teaspoon pepper

5 tablespoons olive oil, divided
1 package sliced baby bella mushrooms
2 heads destemmed red curly kale or dinosaur kale
2 cloves garlic, chopped
Avocado topping (optional)

1. Place the chicken, turmeric, garlic powder, paprika, salt, and pepper in a nonreactive mixing bowl and mix with 2 tablespoons of olive oil so the chicken is equally seasoned and marinating.
2. While the chicken is marinating, heat a medium-sized skillet on medium.
3. Pour 2 tablespoons of olive oil into the skillet and allow to heat for 2 minutes.
4. Stir in the baby bella mushrooms until they begin to brown slightly. (If the pan is too dry, you may splash a few tablespoons of water or chicken stock to deglaze the pan.)
5. Once the mushrooms have softened, stir in the kale until it is wilted yet maintains its bright color.
6. At the very end, add the garlic and cook until fragrant. Set aside.
7. Heat a cast iron skillet or nonstick skillet over medium-high heat and add the remaining tablespoon olive oil, spread equally over the pan.
8. Once the skillet is hot, add the chicken and sear each side for 4–6 minutes, until it is browned on both sides. (To expedite cooking, you may place a lid over the skillet after you brown the chicken.)
9. Place the kale mixture on plates or platters and serve the chicken over the kale and mushrooms.
10. An optional avocado topping is a great addition to this earthy dish.

MEDITERRANEAN AHI STEAKS WITH ROASTED RED PEPPER COMPOTE

PREP TIME: 30 MINUTES   *SERVES 4*

This dish goes well with fresh greens and a lemon zest garnish.

4 (6-ounce) high-quality sashimi-grade ahi tuna fillets
1 teaspoon salt
1 teaspoon pepper
6 teaspoons olive oil, divided
16 Kalamata olives

1 jar of roasted red peppers, drained
1 garlic clove, minced
Leaves from 4 sprigs of fresh oregano
Juice of 1 lemon

1. Place the tuna fillets in a nonreactive dish and season with salt and pepper.
2. Pour 4 teaspoons of oil into the dish and mix until tuna is completely covered.
3. In a glass bowl, mix the remaining 2 teaspoons olive oil, the olives, red peppers, garlic, oregano leaves, and lemon juice, and set aside.
4. Heat a cast iron or nonstick skillet to high heat and spray with a good amount of olive or grapeseed oil until the pan is covered.
5. Sear each fillet for 2 minutes per side for rare, 4 minutes per side for medium rare. Remove from heat and place on a platter.
6. Spoon the red pepper mixture on top of each fillet and enjoy with fresh greens and a lemon zest garnish if you like.

SLOW COOKER BISON STEW

PREP TIME: 6–8 HOURS *SERVES 4*

1 pound bison or elk or grass-fed beef, cubed small
⅔ cup finely chopped celery
⅔ cup finely chopped white onion
⅔ cup finely chopped carrots
½ cup red wine
1 red bell pepper, chopped
3 cups bone broth
2 tablespoons chopped fresh rosemary
2 teaspoons chopped fresh thyme
4 cloves garlic, minced
1 can organic diced tomatoes
2 teaspoons salt
2 teaspoons pepper
Any fresh-chopped herbs for garnish (basil, oregano, thyme, etc.)

1. Heat a cast iron skillet or nonstick skillet to medium-high.
2. Sear the cubed meat until browned on all sides.
3. Remove the meat and place in a slow cooker set to low.
4. In the same skillet, add the celery, onion, and carrots and sauté until they are soft.
5. Add the red wine and scrape to remove any brown bits from the bottom of the pan.
6. Add the vegetables and remaining ingredients, except the garnish, to the slow cooker, pouring the mixture over the beef.
7. Cover the slow cooker and cook on low for 6–8 hours.
8. Serve hot, garnished with fresh-chopped herbs.

CAST IRON VENISON STEAKS

PREP TIME: 30 MINUTES *SERVES 4*

4 (4-ounce) venison or
   bison steaks
2 teaspoons salt

2 teaspoons pepper
3 tablespoons olive or
   grapeseed oil

1. Preheat the oven to 400 degrees.
2. Season each steak with equal amounts of salt and pepper. (This works best when steaks are at room temperature.)
3. Heat a cast iron skillet over stove on high. Once the skillet is hot, add the oil.
4. Sear the steaks 2 by 2, or all 4 at once, for 4 minutes on each side.
5. Using an oven mitt, transfer the cast iron skillet with steaks to the oven and allow to cook 5 more minutes for rare, or 12–15 minutes for medium.
6. Remove and serve.

NOTE: *This dish pairs beautifully with sautéed mushrooms and a salad or steamed veggies.*

DIJON-ENCRUSTED LAMB LOIN CHOPS WITH CAULIFLOWER SMASH

PREP TIME: 45 MINUTES *SERVES 4*

Cauliflower Smash

1 head of cauliflower, chopped into medium chunks
2 cloves garlic
2 tablespoons olive oil
½ teaspoon salt
½ teaspoon pepper
½ cup bone broth

Lamb Loin Chops

1 pound lamb loin chops, or 4 large chops
2 tablespoons Dijon mustard
1 clove garlic, chopped
½ teaspoon salt
½ teaspoon pepper
5 tablespoons olive oil, divided
1 tablespoon chopped fresh rosemary plus 4 small rosemary sprigs for garnish

To make the cauliflower smash:

1. Preheat oven to 400 degrees.
2. Toss the smash ingredients (except the bone broth) together in a mixing bowl and lay them out flat on a cookie sheet.
3. Roast the cauliflower for 10–15 minutes until browned and fragrant.
4. Remove from oven and place in a mixing bowl.
5. Add the bone broth and use a hand mixer to create a cauliflower smash that resembles a mashed potato consistency.
6. Set aside.

To make the lamb loin chops:

1. In a nonreactive bowl, mix the chops with the mustard, garlic, salt, pepper, 1 tablespoon of the olive oil, and the chopped rosemary to coat the lamb.
2. Heat a large cast iron skillet with the remaining 4 tablespoons of olive oil or grapeseed oil.
3. When oil is hot, sear the chops for 3 minutes on each side.
4. Place the chops in the cast iron skillet in the oven and bake at 400 degrees for 15 minutes for medium rare.

(continued)

5. Smear the cauliflower on a platter or individual plates and place the chops on top.
6. Garnish with the rosemary sprigs.

ALL-DAY ELK BOLOGNESE WITH ZUCCHINI NOODLES

PREP TIME: 3 HOURS *SERVES 4*

1 tablespoon olive oil
1 pound ground elk, bison, venison, or grass-fed beef (even a mixture is fine)
1 cup mirepoix (chopped carrot, celery, and white onion)
½ cup plain nut milk of choice (almond recommended)
1 (4-ounce) can tomato paste

1 tablespoon minced garlic
1 teaspoon chopped fresh rosemary
1 teaspoon chopped fresh thyme
1 teaspoon salt
1 teaspoon pepper
2 pounds spiraled zucchini "noodles," fresh (see Note)

1. In a large soup pot or Dutch oven, add the olive oil and ground meat and sauté until slightly browned.
2. Add the mirepoix and sauté over medium heat for 10 minutes.
3. Add the nut milk and sauté for another 10 minutes.
4. Add the rest of the ingredients (minus the zucchini noodles) and stir.
5. Cover and cook on low for 1–3 hours. (The longer the cook time, the deeper the flavor. Stir occasionally to avoid burning the bottom.)
6. If sauce appears too thick, you may add a splash of bone broth.
7. Place the zucchini noodles in four separate bowls.
8. Ladle out the Bolognese sauce on top of the noodles.
9. Garnish with fresh herbs and enjoy!

NOTE: *If you don't have a spiralizer, you can cut zucchini the long way with a vegetable peeler to make the "noodles."*

ROASTED BUTTERNUT SQUASH AND KALE HASH

PREP TIME: 45 MINUTES   *SERVES 4*

1 large butternut (or kombucha
  or acorn) squash, deseeded
  and cubed, or 1 (1-pound)
  package cubed squash
3 tablespoons olive oil
½ teaspoon salt
½ teaspoon pepper

1 teaspoon turmeric
½ teaspoon cumin
1 head kale of choice,
  destemmed and chopped
4 green onions, diced
1 clove garlic, chopped
½ cup tahini

1. Preheat oven to 400 degrees.
2. In a large mixing bowl, toss the squash, olive oil, salt, pepper, turmeric, and cumin together.
3. Place on a large cookie sheet lined with parchment and roast for 20 minutes until the squash is soft and browned.
4. Remove the squash from the oven and place hot in a mixing bowl.
5. Add the rest of the ingredients, slightly mashing the squash as you mix, until the kale has softened.
6. Season with extra salt and pepper if needed and enjoy!

TEMPEH TACO LETTUCE CUPS

PREP TIME: 30 MINUTES   *SERVES 4*

1 pound organic gluten-free
tempeh
1 tablespoon avocado oil or
grapeseed oil
1 can organic black beans,
drained and rinsed (see Notes)
½ white onion, chopped
1 green bell pepper, chopped
½ red bell pepper, chopped
1 (12-ounce) can diced
fire-roasted tomatoes

2 cloves garlic
1 tablespoon chili powder
1 teaspoon cumin
1 teaspoon salt
1 teaspoon pepper
1–2 heads Bibb lettuce or
romaine for wrapping
Chopped cilantro for garnish
Avocado (optional)

1. In a large mixing bowl, crumble the tempeh to resemble a ground
   beef texture.
2. In a large skillet over medium-high heat, add the oil and heat for
   1 minute.
3. Add the tempeh, black beans, onion, and bell peppers and sauté for
   5 minutes.
4. Add the tomatoes, garlic, chili powder, cumin, salt, and pepper.
5. Stir and continue to sauté until onions become translucent.
   Alternatively, cover and simmer for 15–20 minutes on low.
6. Meanwhile, wash the lettuce and remove leaves, picking out the
   bigger leaves for wrapping.
7. Spoon the taco mixture into the lettuce cups.

NOTES: *You can prepare dried beans quickly using an instant
pressure cooker, if you prefer these to canned, or you can soak them
overnight and prepare them in a slow cooker or on the stove the
old-fashioned way, but this takes more time. If you prepare your own
beans, use 1½ cups cooked beans to replace 1 can of beans.*

*Enjoy this dish with cilantro as a garnish, add avocado or the
Hand-Smashed Guacamole (page 304), or turn this into a salad by
chopping the lettuce and using the chipotle dressing from the Ground
Turkey Taco Salad recipe (page 285)!*

CHAPTER 12

The 50-Year Challenge: Toward a More Vibrant World

Now that we have come to the end of our vibrant journey, I want to emphasize to you that this is not really the end. It is just the beginning. Before I send you on your way, I want to issue a challenge.

Can you live 50 more years, feeling vibrant until the end?

I believe you can. Whether you are 20, 30, 40, 50 years old, or more, I don't think 50 additional years is too lofty a goal. Not if you are vibrant! I can't prove what the maximum human life span is, but what's to stop us from pushing those boundaries and moving as far into the future as we can?

Let's take a quick look back at how far you have come. Flip back to chapter one. Take a look at those detailed checklists of positive health habits and negative health habits. See what you checked then, and what you can check now. Then go down to those three habits you wanted to focus on adding, and the three you wanted to focus on conquering. How have you done with those?

Now, look back at your very first energy rating. What was it then and what is it now? Finally, take a good, close look at that picture you took of yourself when you did your very first mirror assessment. Can you tell the difference? I bet you're looking and feeling much more vibrant today than you were when we began our vibrant journey.

Let's recap a few of the key concepts so you can tuck them into your memory:

Vibrant = Energy + Glow

Food

Vibrant

Movement   Connection

Food

Nervous, Detoxification, and Immune Systems

Movement   Connection

Your tools:

1. 30 days of wins, which is to say, a structure for helping you to establish more healthful habits, including the best ways to incorporate anti-inflammatory, nutrient-dense foods; movement that will build strength and resilience; more supportive and fulfilling relationships; improved sleep hygiene; effective stress management; a high-quality supplement protocol; and better self-care.

2. 40 recipes, based on the Vibrant Food List, that are easy to prepare, delicious, and nourishing, along with a two-week suggested meal plan to get you started.

3. 50-year challenge: Can you live for 50 more years? Take this idea with you as you move ahead into your increasingly vibrant and fulfilling life.

By using the Vibrant Triad and these supportive tools to strengthen your complex and astounding self, you can achieve vibrancy in its fullest and most radiant aspect. You will be filled with energy and you will glow with it, from the inside out. You will understand what your body is telling you, and you will know how to give it what it needs. You will feel good. You will feel happy, and more importantly, fulfilled. You will be beautiful and busy, full of purpose and love. You will be committed to all that is good in your life, and you will let go of all that is holding you back. This is the life you have dreamed of, and it can be yours.

What will you do with it? What do you hope to accomplish by feeling your best? What will you do with more energy? Who will you be with more glow? What will you do with your many more years of life?

The final secret I want to tell you before you go is that when you are truly vibrant, you will be fully equipped to find your passion and live with purpose and meaning. What is the point of a long life if you don't know what to do with it? We are all here for a reason. I believe that. We all have something to offer the world, and to each other, but when you don't feel good, it's a lot more difficult to live your purpose, or even discover what it is. That is why it is so important to take care of yourself first.

I want to offer you a vision for the future.

When you are fulfilled, you will be able to take that final step toward finding your passion and living your purpose. You will be able to help, to serve, to support, to love, and you will know how to be loved. It takes hard work and a lot of self-reflection and self-knowing to change your life, but when you do, it's good to turn that lens outward again and see who else needs a helping hand. In my life, I have found that the greatest gift of health has been to have the energy and capacity to help other people. Personally, I devote a lot of resources to philanthropy, but everyone will find their own calling. What out there needs to be done that you might be great at doing? Who needs a listening ear? Who in your community is suffering? What speaks to your heart and cries out to you that you are the one to help?

I hope you are well past any notion that self-care is selfish. Instead, you know it is perhaps the least selfish thing you can do, to take care of yourself, because only when you are full do you have anything to offer. When you have the energy, the clarity of mind, and the sense of self to know where your talents lie and what you can do to participate fully in life and give back to the world, you will enjoy a fullness and feeling of satisfaction and meaning you could never get if you only looked inward. So, embrace the vibrant life by looking within and building your inner resources, and then, look around you with fresh eyes and see what the world needs that you can give. When your mind is clear, your body is strong, and your psyche is supported, you will know what it is you need to do in this life, and that will give your time on this earth richness and meaning. That is my parting advice.

Go forth, my vibrant friend, into the miraculous and surprising world. You have much to gain, and much to give. You have a light inside of you, waiting to shine brightly. You have the knowledge you need to be fully and completely vibrant. It's time to become the best possible you. Welcome back! Your life, and the world, are waiting.

APPENDIX: INTEGRATIVE MEDICINE 101

Here is a list of common integrative and holistic healing methodologies. (This list is by no means inclusive—a truly complete list would fill an entire book.)

INTEGRATIVE/ALTERNATIVE/HOLISTIC/COMPLEMENTARY/LIFESTYLE MEDICINE: These are all similar terms for a philosophy of healthcare that looks at the whole person and the person's lifestyle and environment to discover the cause of health dysfunction, rather than focusing on symptoms and medications to relieve them. Integrative medicine, and its close counterparts, use information and techniques from many systems of care, including both Eastern and Western medicine and ancient as well as modern therapies, to support the body's natural healing ability by adjusting lifestyle. If needed, integrative practitioners will use or advise medication or surgery, but the least invasive, most naturally supportive therapies are the first intervention. Although some forms of holistic medicine are not based in Western science, many do rely on science-based therapies, as many aspects of lifestyle have been well studied (such as nutrition, exercise, certain herbal remedies, meditation, acupuncture, chiropractic care, yoga, massage, and stress reduction techniques like deep breathing), as have the threats to health from environmental toxins, poor nutrition, a sedentary lifestyle, and stress.

CONVENTIONAL/MODERN/MAINSTREAM/ALLOPATHIC MEDICINE: This is the type of healthcare most people use. It is what is taught in mainstream medical schools in Western culture and is the type of training most doctors have. It is modern, science-based medicine that is symptom-focused and tends to rely on medications and surgeries rather than lifestyle interventions as primary modes of treatment.

FUNCTIONAL MEDICINE: This is a specific type of integrative/lifestyle medicine that is based in systems biology and focuses on discovering and addressing the root causes of health dysfunction, rather than focusing on symptoms. It was developed by Dr. Jeffrey S. Bland. Functional medicine doctors are becoming more numerous, but many do not take insurance. They should be a valid expense for a health savings account, however. For more information or to find a practitioner, visit the Institute for Functional Medicine website (ifm.org).

NATUROPATHY: One of the oldest Western types of holistic, alternative medicine that uses food, herbs, and other nature-based traditional as well as some modern techniques for preventing disease and supporting natural healing rather than intervening with drugs and surgery. Naturopathic doctors may or may not take health insurance, or you may need to get preauthorization to visit one. To learn more or to find a naturopathic physician, consult the American Association of Naturopathic Physicians website (naturopathic.org).

OSTEOPATHY: Osteopathic doctors have the designation "DO" (Doctor of Osteopathy) instead of "MD," but they are fully licensed physicians. They have special training in the manipulation of the musculoskeletal system (similar to chiropractors), but they are also able to provide comprehensive medical care to patients, including prescribing drugs if necessary. Like other forms of integrative medicine, the primary focus is on prevention and the whole person. Most osteopathic doctors accept regular health insurance. To find a Doctor of Osteopathy near you, consult the American Academy of Osteopathy Advanced Physician Search tool (academyofosteopathy.org/find-an-osteopathic-physician).

CHIROPRACTIC CARE: Chiropractors are also doctors but with the designation "DC" (Doctor of Chiropractic). Their training is specifically about noninvasive spinal and other musculoskeletal manipulation and may include guidance for other natural treatments, from massage to supplements. Chiropractors are widely available and many take insurance. I recommend asking around in your community to find the ones with the most experience and best reputation.

NUTRITION THERAPY: This is a system of healthcare focused on what you eat, which operates based on the philosophy that food is the primary influence on health. You can get great food guidance from a Certified Nutrition Specialist (CNS—that is one of my degrees), who has advanced nutrition training and is credentialed. You could also work with any nutritionist, but know that anyone can call themselves a nutritionist. I advise looking for someone who is credentialed. You may be curious about dietitians. These practitioners have advanced training and must be licensed to use the RD (Registered Dietitian) designation, but they are typically trained in a conventional approach to nutrition. If you want to work with someone, I advise finding a practitioner who shares your views about healthcare, especially if you are seeking someone with a more holistic, integrative view of diet. For more information or to find a CNS, check out The American Nutrition Association (I am a board member) at theana.org. Their website includes a Practitioner Finder tool.

TRADITIONAL CHINESE MEDICINE (TCM): This ancient Chinese system of healing and wellness uses herbal formulas (often personalized for the individual), acupuncture, cupping, and other techniques to balance energy (chi) in the body, according to an energy system of meridians that exist within the human body. I talk about TCM in the energy chapter. It's something I use frequently, consulting with my genius TCM doctor, Dr. Jing Liu. I have also trained in acupuncture myself.

ACUPUNCTURE: This ancient Eastern healing technique is a part of TCM, but many practitioners only practice acupuncture. It involves the insertion of very fine needles into points along energy meridians in the body. It is based in Eastern rather than Western anatomy, but has proven to be so effective that many insurance companies cover acupuncture treatments. You don't have to be a doctor to practice acupuncture, although some integrative doctors (myself included) study acupuncture so they can use it as an additional therapy with their clients. Others specialize only in acupuncture, and many have learned it in China and now practice in the United States. There is no one central directory of all the people who are qualified to practice acupuncture, but most cities have at least several choices. I suggest asking for recommendations from your integrative doctor or knowledgeable friends who have had good experiences with certain practitioners. A variation is acupressure, which uses deep pressure instead of needles.

AYURVEDA: This is India's ancient system of health and wellness, and like TCM, it utilizes herbal formulas, but different ones native to India, as well as certain massage techniques, yoga, specific dietary interventions, and cleansing techniques. Ayurvedic practitioners diagnose your essential energy type (*dosha*) and your imbalances through pulse diagnosis, among other methods. Instead of meridians and points, Ayurveda views energy in the body as moving through channels called nadis and energy centers called chakras. Many people who get serious about yoga end up learning a lot about Ayurvedic medicine and living by its principles. I talk about Ayurveda in the energy chapter.

ENVIRONMENTAL MEDICINE: This form of medicine focuses on the impact of the environment—air, water, soil, and food—on health and disease. It considers things like pollution, allergens, mold, radiation, bacteria, heavy metals, pesticides, and also the effects of family dynamics, trauma, and other psychosocial factors. To learn more or to find an environmental medicine practitioner, consult the American Academy of Environmental Medicine website (aaemonline.org).

HERBAL MEDICINE: Just as it sounds, herbal medicine treats symptoms and underlying conditions using natural herbs rather than pharmaceutical drugs. The term "herbalist" is not regulated in the United States, however, so if you want to work with an herbalist, be sure it is someone experienced and trustworthy. You can learn herbalism while also training to be an integrative practitioner, but others are herbalists only.

REIKI: Pronounced RAY-kee, this is a type of Eastern energy medicine. Trained practitioners manipulate energy with their hands hovering over or touching the patient, in order to balance and free it within the body, for physical and emotional healing. Reiki is not based in Western science but it is aligned with the Eastern view of the body and many people swear by it.

BIOFEEDBACK: This is a technology that gives you information about what is going on inside your body so you can become aware of it and learn to control it. Practitioners attach electrical sensors to you and then you see the feedback on a screen. You are then taught how to control your heart rate, blood pressure, breathing rate, muscle tension, brain waves, and other aspects of what is going on inside your body, by becoming aware of how they feel as you see how they change on the screen. You learn how to manipulate these functions by making subtle changes to your muscles, breath, and brain, to influence them. It is most often used to help people self-treat their anxiety, headaches, or other chronic issues that are otherwise difficult to treat. To find a practitioner, visit the website for Applied Psychophysiology & Biofeedback (biofeedback.org).

HOMEOPATHY: Homeopathy is a gentle way to treat health imbalances. It uses very diluted substances thought to cause certain symptoms in order to treat those same symptoms, operating on the principle of "like cures like." The substances, usually made from plants or minerals, are so diluted that they cannot harm, but are thought to stimulate healing as needed. Homeopathic remedies are available in most health-food and supplement stores or online and do not require a practitioner, although you can visit one for personalized guidance. Homeopathy is more popular in Europe than in the United States.

AROMATHERAPY: This pleasant therapy uses essential oils to treat physical as well as emotional conditions. Different scents are thought to address different issues. Anyone can buy essential oils and use them as needed, but never ingest them unless you get a food-grade formula. They are not all ingestible.

MASSAGE THERAPY: Do you need an excuse to get a massage? I'm happy to provide one! There is a lot of research supporting the health, circulation, relaxation, healing, and stress relief of different kinds of massage. There are also many forms of massage, both Eastern and Western, such as Swedish massage, Shiatsu, deep tissue, trigger point, sports massage, Thai massage, reflexology, and massages that utilize hot stones and/or essential oils. There are also variations on the massage theme, such as Rolfing, an intense deep tissue technique; Therapeutic Touch, which is a gentler laying on of hands; and craniosacral therapy, which is a gentle manipulation of the skull, spine, and pelvis.

MOVEMENT THERAPIES/SOMATIC THERAPIES: There are so many movement therapies, I won't list them all, but they address posture and the body in motion for easier healing and improved health. There are both Eastern and Western movement therapies, including things you can do on your own or in a class, like yoga, Pilates, tai chi, chi kung, qi gong, and techniques that require a practitioner, like dance therapy, the Alexander Technique, Feldenkrais, and other somatic therapies.

ANTI-AGING MEDICINE is an exciting new field that focuses on what causes aging and on the so-called "diseases of aging" with the goal of prevention, longevity, and increased health span, which is the period of life during which you remain healthy. It uses advanced techniques not always supported by conventional medicine, such as human growth hormone injections and other hormonal manipulation, chelation therapy, and supplements, but it is becoming increasingly popular and many doctors (myself included) have added this training to their integrative arsenal. To learn more or to find a practitioner, visit the American Academy of Anti-Aging Medicine website (a4m.com).

REGENERATIVE MEDICINE: Similar to anti-aging medicine (they used to share an organization but have since separated), regenerative medicine is about helping to regenerate, renew, reengineer, or replace the materials of the body that are aging or have been damaged or destroyed through disease or injury. It often works at the cellular level and includes the study and practice of soft tissue regeneration, tissue engineering, stem cell therapy, artificial organs, and more. For example, a popular regenerative medicine practice is the injection of stem cells into injured areas of the body to facilitate self-repair.

ORTHOMOLECULAR MEDICINE: Linus Pauling established the term "orthomolecular medicine" in 1968. The focus of this type of medicine is to slow aging and regenerate the body through the use of supplements. Linus Pauling is most famous for his championing of high-dose vitamin C, and I am a fan of both him and vitamin C to combat the effects of aging and increase the intelligence of the immune system. Orthomolecular medicine also uses other supplements such as other vitamins, minerals, essential fatty acids, and amino acids to optimize function.

POSITIVE PSYCHOLOGY: Alfred Adler was a student of Sigmund Freud, but broke away to form his own school of psychology called Individual Psychology. It is today more often called Adlerian Psychology or Positive Psychology (although some people distinguish the two, they are quite similar), and it is at its essence about the study of what is good in life, what makes life worth living, and what creates happiness. It focuses on strengths, not weaknesses, and positive life goals and emotions rather than psychological problems.

SHAMANIC HEALING: Ancient but also trendy, shamanic healing uses the Native American system of healing and wellness. Like TCM and Ayurveda, it is energy-based and works to heal blockages and improve energy flow, but there is also a definite spiritual component to shamanic healing.

NOTES

INTRODUCTION

1. Martin A. Makary, Michael Daniel, "Medical error—the third leading cause of death in the US," *BMJ* 353(i2139) (2016), http://doi.org/10.1136/bmj.i2139; "Study Suggests Medical Errors Now Third Leading Cause of Death in the U.S.," Johns Hopkins Medicine, News Release Archive, May 3, 2016, https://www.hopkinsmedicine.org/news/media/releases/study_suggests_medical_errors_now_third_leading_cause_of_death_in_the_us.

2. Tait D. Shanafelt, MD, Charles M. Balch, MD, Gerald Bechamps, MD et al., "Burnout and Medical Errors Among American Surgeons," *Annals of Surgery* 251(6) (2010): 995–1000, https://doi.org/10.1097/SLA.0b013e3181bfdab3.

3. Institute of Medicine (US) Committee on Quality of Health Care in America, LT Kohn, JM Corrigan, MS Donaldson, editors, *To Err Is Human: Building a Safer Health System*. Washington (DC): National Academies Press, 2000. 2, Errors in Health Care: A Leading Cause of Death and Injury, https://www.ncbi.nlm.nih.gov/books/NBK225187/#:~:text=Total%20national%20costs%20(lost%20income,billion%20for%20preventable%20adverse%20events.&text=Health%20care%20costs%20account%20for,half%20of%20the%20total%20costs.

4. Ibid.

5. "Painkillers Driving Addiction, Overdose," National Safety Council, 2020, https://www.nsc.org/home-safety/safety-topics/opioids.

6. "Medication Errors and Adverse Drug Events," PSNet, Primers, September 2019, https://psnet.ahrq.gov/primer/medication-errors-and-adverse-drug-events.

7. "About Chronic Diseases," CDC, October 23, 2019, https://www.cdc.gov/chronicdisease/about/index.htm.

CHAPTER 1

1. Elizabeth Landau, "Studies clash on vitamin benefits," CNN Health, April 19, 2010, https://www.cnn.com/2010/HEALTH/04/19/vitamins.cancer.heart/index.html; "Multivitamin/mineral Supplements," National Institutes of Health Office of Dietary Supplements, October 17, 2019, https://ods.od.nih.gov/factsheets/MVMS-HealthProfessional/.

2. Michael F. Holick, MD, PhD, "Vitamin D Deficiency," *New England Journal of Medicine* 357 (2007): 266–281, https://www.nejm.org/doi/full/10.1056/NEJMra070553.

3. Ranjani R. Starr, MPH, "Too Little, Too Late: Ineffective Regulation of Dietary Supplements in the United States," *American Journal of Public Health* 105(3) (2015): 478–485, https://www.ncbi.nlm.nih.gov/pmc/articles/PMC4330859/#bib9.

4. Pieter A. Cohen, MD, "The FDA and Adulterated Supplements—Dereliction of Duty," JAMA Network Open 1(6)(e183329) (2018): 1–3, https://jamanetwork.com/journals/jamanetworkopen/fullarticle/2706489.

5. Denise Mann, MS, "Half of all multivitamins don't do what they claim—here's how to pick the right one," Reader's Digest, January 8, 2018, https://www.businessinsider.com/half-of-all-multivitamins-dont-do-what-they-claim-2018-1.

CHAPTER 2

1. Timothy W. Puetz, "Physical Activity and Feelings of Energy and Fatigue," *Sports Medicine* 36 (2006): 767–780, https://doi.org/10.2165/00007256-200636090-00004.

2. Giovanni Maciocia, *The Foundations of Chinese Medicine: A Comprehensive Text for Acupuncturists and Herbalists* (London: Churchill Livingstone, 1989), 137.

3. Romain Meeusen, Martine Duclos, Carl Foster, et al., "Prevention, Diagnosis, and Treatment of the Overtraining Syndrome: Joint Consensus Statement of the European College of Sport Science and the American College of Sports Medicine," *Medicine & Science in Sports & Exercise* 45(1) (2013): 186–205, https://doi.org/10.1249/MSS.0b013e318279a10a; Dianna Purvis, Stephen Gonsalves, and Patricia A. Deuster, "Physiological and Psychological Fatigue in Extreme Conditions: Overtraining and Elite Athletes," *PM&R* 2(5) (2010): 442–450, https://doi.org/10.1016/j.pmrj.2010.03.025.

4. Jaw-Chyun Chen, Chien-Yun Hsiang, Yung-Chang Lin, et al., "Deer Antler Extract Improves Fatigue Effect through Altering the Expression of Genes Related to Muscle Strength in Skeletal Muscle of Mice," *Evidence-Based Complementary and Alternative Medicine* 2014(540580) (2014), https://doi.org/10.1155/2014/540580.

CHAPTER 3

1. Aris P. Agouridis, Moses S. Elisaf, Devaki R. Nair, et al., "Ear lobe crease: a marker of coronary artery disease?" *Archives of Medical Science* 11(6) (2015): 1145–1155, https://doi.org/10.5114/aoms.2015.56340.

2. Hongdong Song, Siqi Zhang, Ling Zhang, et al., "Effect of Orally Administered Collagen Peptides from Bovine Bone of Skin Aging in Chronically Aged Mice," *Nutrients* 9(11) (2017), https://doi.org/10.3390/nu9111209.

3. Liane Bolke, Gerrit Schlippe, Joachi Gerß, et al., "A Collagen Supplement Improves Skin Hydration, Elasticity, Roughness, and Density: Results of a Randomized, Placebo-Controlled, Blind Study," *Nutrients* 11(10) (2019), https://doi.org/10.3390/nu11102494.

4. Alexander G. Schauss, Jerome Stenehjem, Joosang Park, et al., "Effect of the Novel Low Molecular Weight Hydrolyzed Chicken Sternal Cartilage Extract, BoiCell Collagen, on Improving Osteoarthritis-Related Symptoms: A Randomized, Double-Blind, Placebo-Controlled Trial," *Journal of Agricultural and Food Chemistry* 60(16) (2012): 4096–4101, https://doi.org/10.1021/jf205295u.

5. Shanika Samarasinghe, Farah Meah, Vinita Singh, Arshi Basit, Nicholas Emanuele, Mary Ann Emanuele, Alaleh Mazhari, and Earle W Holmes, "Biotin Interference with Routine Clinical Immunoassays: Understand the Causes and Mitigate the Risks," National Library of Medicine, https://pubmed.ncbi.nlm.nih.gov/28534685.

6. Ibid.

7. Murad Alam, MD, MSCI, MBA, Anne J. Walter, MD, MBA, Amelia Geisler, BS, et al., "Association of Facial Exercise with the Appearance of Aging," *JAMA Dermatology* 154(3) (2018): 365–367, https://jamanetwork.com/journals/jamadermatology/article-abstract/2666801?redirect=true.

8. Leonardo Barbosa Barreto de Brito, Djalma Rabelo Ricardo, Denise Sardinha Mendes Soares de Araújo, et al., "Ability to sit and rise from the floor as a predictor of all-cause mortality," *European Journal of Preventive Cardiology* 21(7) (2012): 1–7, https://geriatrictoolkit.missouri.edu/srff/deBrito-Floor-Rise-Mortality-2012.pdf.

CHAPTER 4

1. Jessica M. Yano, Kristie Yu, Gregory P. Donaldson, et al., "Indigenous bacteria from the gut microbiota regulate host serotonin biosynthesis," *Cell* 161(2) (2015): 264–276, https://doi.org/10.1016/j.cell.2015.02.047.

2. Yasmine Belkaid, Timothy Hand, "Role of the Microbiota in Immunity and Inflammation," *Cell* 157(1) (2014): 121–141, https://doi.org/10.1016/j.cell.2014.03.011.

3. Knvul Sheikh, "How Gut Bacteria Tell Their Hosts What to Eat," Mind, *Scientific American*, April 25, 2017, https://www.scientificamerican.com/article/how-gut-bacteria-tell-their-hosts-what-to-eat/.

4. Lawrence A. David, Corinne F. Maurice, Rachel N. Carmody, et al., "Diet Rapidly and Reproducibly Alters the Human Gut Microbiome," *Nature* 505(7484) (2014): 559–563, https://pubmed.ncbi.nlm.nih.gov/24336217/.

5. Aleksandra Tomova, Igor Bukovsky, Emilie Rembert, et al., "The Effects of Vegetarian and Vegan Diets on Gut Microbiota," *Frontiers in Nutrition* 6(47) (2019), https://doi.org/10.3389/fnut.2019.00047.

6. "Low-Carbohydrate Diets," Harvard T.H. Chan School of Public Health, 2020, https://www.hsph.harvard.edu/nutritionsource/carbohydrates/low-carbohydrate-diets/.

7. Tingting Dong, Man Guo, Peiyue Zhang, et al., "The effects of low-carbohydrate diets on cardiovascular risk factors: A meta-analysis," *PLoS ONE* 15(1) (2020), https://journals.plos.org/plosone/article?id=10.1371/journal.pone.0225348.

8. Alice H. Lichtenstein, Linda Van Horn, "Very Low Fat Diets," *Circulation* 98(9) (1998): 935–938, https://doi.org/10.1161/01.CIR.98.9.935; Dean Ornish, MD, Larry W. Scherwitz, PhD, James H. Billings, PhD, et al., "Intensive Lifestyle Changes for Reversal of Coronary Heart Disease," *JAMA* 280(23) (1998): 2001–2007, https://www.ornish.com/wp-content/uploads/Intensive-lifestyle-changes-for-reversal-of-coronary-heart-disease1.pdf.

9. Peter R. Huttenlocher, "Ketonemia and Seizures: Metabolic and Anticonvulsant Effects of Two Ketogenic Diets in Childhood Epilepsy," *Pediatric Research* 10 (1976): 536–540, https://www.nature.com/articles/pr197666.pdf?origin=ppub.

10. Tanya J. Williams, Mackenzie C. Cervenka, "The role for ketogenic diets in epilepsy and status epilepticus in adults," *Clinical Neurophysiology Practice* 2 (2017): 154–160, https://doi.org/10.1016/j.cnp.2017.06.001.

11. Jocelyn Tan-Shalaby, MD, "Ketogenic Diets and Cancer: Emerging Evidence," *Federal Practitioner* 34(1) (2017): 37S–42S, https://www.ncbi.nlm.nih.gov/pmc/articles/PMC6375425/.

12. Diane Mapes, "Keto, fat and cancer: It's complicated," Fred Hutch, October 24, 2019, https://www.fredhutch.org/en/news/center-news/2019/10/keto-fat-cancer-its-complicated.html.

13. Stewart Rose, Amanda Strombom, "A Plant-Based Diet Prevents and Treats Prostate Cancer," *Cancer Therapy & Oncology International Journal* 11(3) (2018): 1–7, https://doi.org/10.19080/CTOIJ.2018.11.555813.

14. Bob Barnett, "A Low-Fat, Plant-Based Diet Cuts the Risk of Dying of Breast Cancer," *Cancer Health*, Treatment News, May 16, 2019, https://www.cancerhealth.com/article/low-fat-plant-based-diet-cuts-breast-cancer-mortality.

15. Miguel A. Martinez-Gonzales, Nerea Martin-Calvo, "Mediterranean diet and life expectancy; beyond olive oil, fruits, and vegetables," *Current Opinion in Clinical Nutrition and Metabolic Care* 19(6) (2016): 401–407, https://www.ncbi.nlm.nih.gov/pmc/articles/PMC5902736/.

16. Roddy Scheer, Doug Moss, "Dirt Poor: Have Fruits and Vegetables Become Less Nutritious?" EarthTalk, *Scientific American*, Environment, April 27, 2011, https://www.scientificamerican.com/article/soil-depletion-and-nutrition-loss/.

17. "Celiac Disease," National Center for Advancing Translational Sciences, Diseases, February 5, 2014, https://rarediseases.info.nih.gov/diseases/11998/celiac-disease/cases/43805.

18. "Alessio Fasano—Spectrum of Gluten-Related Disorders: People Shall Not Live by Bread Alone," YouTube video, 57:07, posted by "The IHMC," January 21, 2014, https://www.youtube.com/watch?v=VvfTV57iPUY.

19. Anna Sapone, Julio C. Bai, Carolina Ciacci, et al., "Spectrum of gluten-related disorders: consensus on new nomenclature and classification," *BMC Medicine* 10(13) (2012), https://bmcmedicine.biomedcentral.com/articles/10.1186/1741-7015-10-13.

20. "Exclusive Interview with Alessio Fasano, MD," YouTube video, 25:22, posted by "The Institute for Functional Medicine," April 10, 2018, https://www.youtube.com/watch?v=bczElP7RP0s.

21. Alessio Fasano, "Zonulin, regulation of tight junctions, and autoimmune diseases," *Annals of The New York Academy of Sciences* 1258(1) (2012): 25–33, https://www.ncbi.nlm.nih.gov/pmc/articles/PMC3384703/.

22. "Exclusive Interview with Alessio Fasano, MD," YouTube video, 25:22, posted by "The Institute for Functional Medicine," April 10, 2018, https://www.youtube.com/watch?v=bczElP7RP0s.

23. Ellie Chen, MD, Nadime Ajami, PhD, Liang Cheng, MD, et al., "Dairy Intake and Mucosa-Associated Gut Microbiome in Healthy Individuals: Presidential Poster Award," *American Journal of Gastroenterology* 113 (2018): S137, https://journals.lww.com/ajg/Fulltext/2018/10001/Dairy_Intake_and_Mucosa_Associated_Gut_Microbiome.235.aspx#:~:text=Conclusion%3A%20Higher%20total%20dairy%20product,cancer%20risk%20through%20gut%20microbiome.

24. Sonia González, T. Fernández-Navarro, Silvia Arboleya, et al., "Fermented Dairy Foods: Impact on Intestinal Microbiota and Health-Linked Biomarkers," *Frontiers in Microbiology* (May 24, 2019), https://www.frontiersin.org/articles/10.3389/fmicb.2019.01046/full.

25. Jean-Philippe Drouin-Chartier, Yanping Li, Andres V. Ardisson Korat, et al., "Changes in Dairy Product Consumption and Risk of Type 2 Diabetes among U.S. Men and Women," American Diabetes Association 79th Scientific Sessions, June 9, 2019, https://plan.core-apps.com/tristar_ada19/abstract/911b3311d835ee268a64bdcae1b03f11.

26. "Shrimp Recommendations," Monterey Bay Aquarium Seafood Watch, Seafood Recommendations, 1999–2020, https://www.seafoodwatch.org/seafood-recommendations/groups/shrimp.

CHAPTER 5

1. JE Manson, FB Hu, JW Rich-Edwards, et al., "A prospective study of walking as compared with vigorous exercise in the prevention of coronary heart disease in women," *New England Journal of Medicine* 341(9) (1999): 650–658.

2. Frank W. Booth, Christian K. Roberts, and Matthew J. Laye, "Lack of exercise is a major cause of chronic diseases," *Comprehensive Physiology* 2(2) (2012): 1143–1211, https://www.ncbi.nlm.nih.gov/pmc/articles/PMC4241367/.

3. IM Lee, PJ Skerrett, "Physical activity and all-cause mortality: what is the dose-response relation?" *Medicine and Science in Sports and Exercise* 33(6) (2001): S459–S471.

4. JE Manson, P Greenland, AZ LaCroix, et al., "Walking compared with vigorous exercise for the prevention of cardiovascular events in women," *New England Journal of Medicine* 347(10) (2002): 716–725.

5. American College of Cardiology, "Higher fitness level can determine longer lifespan after age 70," ScienceDaily, March 6, 2019, https://www.sciencedaily.com/releases/2019/03/190306081829.htm#:~:text=%22We%20found%20fitness%20is%20an,fit%2C%22%20said%20Seamus%20P; Lauren Sharkey, "Exercise levels predict lifespan better than smoking, medical history," *Medical News Today*, November 9, 2019, https://www.medicalnewstoday.com/articles/326958#:~:text=Share%20on%20Pinterest%20New%20research,help%20them%20prolong%20their%20lives; European Society of Cardiology, "Women, exercise and longevity," ScienceDaily, December 7, 2019, https://www.sciencedaily.com/releases/2019/12/191207073534.htm.

6. P Boström, J Wu, MP Jedrychowski, et al., "A PGC1-α-dependent myokine that drives brown-fat-like development of white fat and thermogenesis," *Nature* 481(7382) (2012): 463–468.

7. Vincent Gremeaux, Mathieu Gayda, Romuald Lepers, et al., "Exercise and longevity," *Maturitas* 73 (2012): 312–317, https://www.centreepic.org/wp-content/uploads/2015/04/2012_Gremeaux_V_et_al_Maturitas.pdf.

8. Peter Kokkinos, "Physical Activity, Health Benefits, and Mortality Risk," *ISRN Cardiology* 2012 (2012), https://doi.org/10.5402/2012/718789.

9. JN Morris, JA Heady, PAB Raffle, et al., "Coronary heart-disease and physical activity of work," *Lancet* 262(6796) (1953): 1111–1120.

10. P Kokkinos, J Myers, "Exercise and physical activity: clinical outcomes and applications," *Circulation* 122(16) (2010): 1637–1648; SN Blair, HW Kohl, CE Barlow, et al., "Changes in physical fitness and all-cause mortality: a prospective study of healthy and unhealthy men," *JAMA* 273(14) (1995): 1093–1098.

11. "Are gym memberships worth the money?" *Hustle*, January 5, 2019, https://thehustle.co/gym-membership-cost#:~:text=A%20Statistic%20Brain%20survey%20%5Bpaywall,than%201%20time%20per%20week.

12. "Health Risks of an Inactive Lifestyle," Medline Plus, Health Topics, January 9, 2020, https://medlineplus.gov/healthrisksofaninactivelifestyle.html.

13. "Obesity and Cancer," National Cancer Institute at the National Institutes of Health, About Cancer, January 17, 2017, https://www.cancer.gov/about-cancer/causes-prevention/risk/obesity/obesity-fact-sheet#what-is-known-about-the-relationship-between-obesity-and-cancer-.

14. American Friends of Tel Aviv University, "Obesity plays major role in triggering autoimmune diseases,"ScienceDaily, November 10, 2014, https://www.sciencedaily.com/releases/2014/11/141110110722.htm#:~:text=According%20to%20the%20research%2C%20obesity,progression%20and%20hinder%20its%20treatment.

15. "The Health Effects of Overweight and Obesity," Centers for Disease Control and Prevention, Healthy Weight, April 10, 2020, https://www.cdc.gov/healthyweight/effects/index.html.

CHAPTER 6

1. "The Holmes-Rahe Stress Inventory," The American Institute of Stress, 2020, http://www.stress.org/holmes-rahe-stress-inventory/.

2. Debra Umberson, Jennifer Karas Montez, "Social Relationships and Health: A Flashpoint for Health Policy," *Journal of Health and Social Behavior* 51(Suppl) (2010): S54–S66, https://doi.org/10.1177/0022146510383501.

3. Julianne Holt-Lunstad, Timothy B. Smith, J. Bradley Layton, "Social Relationships and Mortality Risk: A Meta-analytic Review," *PLoS Medicine* 7(7) (2010), https://doi.org/10.1371/journal.pmed.1000316.

4. Ibid.

5. Harvard Women's Health Watch, "The health benefits of strong relationships," Harvard Health Publishing, August 6, 2019, https://www.health.harvard.edu/newsletter_article/the-health-benefits-of-strong-relationships.

6. Alvin Powell, "When love and science double date," *Harvard Gazette*, February 13, 2018, https://news.harvard.edu/gazette/story/2018/02/scientists-find-a-few-surprises-in-their-study-of-love/.

7. Ibid.

8. Michael S. Rendall, Margaret M. Weden, Melissa M. Favreault, et al., "The Protective Effect of Marriage for Survival: A Review and Update," *Demography* 48(2) (2011): 481–506, https://doi.org/10.1007/s13524-011-0032-5; Lamberto Manzoli, Paolo Villari, Giovanni M. Pirone, et al., "Marital Status and Mortality in the Elderly: A Systematic Review and Meta-Analysis," *Social Science & Medicine* 64(1) (2007): 77–94, https://doi.org/10.1016/j.socscimed.2006.08.031.

9. Philip Donald St John, Patrick Roy Montgomery, "Marital Status, Partner Satisfaction, and Depressive Symptoms in Older Men and Women," *Canadian Journal of Psychiatry* 54(7) (2009): 487–492, http://doi.org/10.1177/070674370905400710.

10. Alan W. Shindel, MD, Zhong-Chen Xin, MD, Guiting Lin, MD, PhD, et al., "Erectogenic and Neurotrophic Effects of Icariin, a Purified Extract of Horny Goat Weed (Epimedium spp.) In Vitro and In Vivo," *Journal of Sexual Medicine* 7 4(Pt 1): 1518–1528, https://www.ncbi.nlm.nih.gov/pmc/articles/PMC3551978/.

11. "Key Statistics for Prostate Cancer," American Cancer Society, Cancer A–Z, January 8, 2020, https://www.cancer.org/cancer/prostate-cancer/about/key-statistics.html.

12. Zhigang Cui, MD, Dezhong Liu, MD, Chun Liu, MD, et al., "Serum selenium levels and prostate cancer risk: A MOOSE-compliant meta-analysis," *Medicine (Baltimore)* 96(5) (2017): e5944, http://doi.org/10.1097/MD.0000000000005944.

13. David F. Jarrard, MD, "Does Zinc Supplementation Increase the Risk of Prostate Cancer?" *Archives of Ophthalmology* 123(1) (2005): 102–103, https://jamanetwork.com/journals/jamaophthalmology/fullarticle/416806#:~:text=Zinc%20has%20been%20found%20to,factor%20%CE%BAB%2C%20an%20antiapoptotic%20protein.&text=Tissue%20levels%20of%20zinc%20are,when%20compared%20with%20normal%20specimens.

CHAPTER 7

1. Amy F.T. Arnsten, "Stress signalling pathways that impair prefrontal cortex structure and function," *Nature Reviews Neuroscience* 10(6) (2009): 410–422, https://www.ncbi.nlm.nih.gov/pmc/articles/PMC2907136/.

2. Britta K. Hölzel, James Carmody, Karleyton C. Evans, et al., "Stress reduction correlates with structural changes in the amygdala," *Social Cognitive and Affective Neuroscience* 5(1) (March 2010): 11–17, https://doi.org/10.1093/scan/nsp034.

3. Harvard Women's Health Watch, "Protect your brain from stress," Harvard Health Publishing, Harvard Medical School, August 2018, https://www.health.harvard.edu/mind-and-mood/protect-your-brain-from-stress.

4. CL Bender, X Sun, M Farooq, et al., "Emotional Stress Induces Structural Plasticity in Bergmann Glial Cells via an AC5-CPEB3-GluA1 Pathway," *Journal of Neuroscience* 40(17) (April 2020): 3374–3384, https://doi.org/10.1523/JNEUROSCI.0013-19.2020.

5. "Heavy Metal Detoxification," National Integrated Health Associates, Medical Programs, 2020, https://www.nihadc.com/health-programs/heavy-metal-detoxification-removal.html.

6. Ranna Parekh, MD, MPH, "Warning Signs of Mental Illness," American Psychiatric Association, Patients & Families, July 2018, https://www.psychiatry.org/patients-families/warning-signs-of-mental-illness.

7. Walter R. Boot, PhD, Arthur F. Kramer, PhD, "The Brain-Games Conundrum: Does Cognitive Training Really Sharpen the Mind?" Cerebrum 2014 (November 3, 2014): 15, https://www.ncbi.nlm.nih.gov/pmc/articles/PMC4445580/.

8. Abdulrahman Al-Thaqib, Fahad Al-Sultan, Abdullah Al-Zahrani, et al., "Brain Training Games Enhance Cognitive Function in Healthy Subjects," *Medical Science Monitor Basic Research* 24 (2018): 63–69, https://www.ncbi.nlm.nih.gov/pmc/articles/PMC5930973/.

9. Amanda MacMillan, "Yes, Brain Games Improve Memory, but Only Under Some Circumstances," Alzheimer's Disease, *Health*, November 17, 2016, https://www.health.com/condition/alzheimers/brain-games-improve-memory.

10. Nikhil Swaminathan, "Why Does the Brain Need So Much Power?" Mind, *Scientific American*, April 29, 2008, https://www.scientificamerican.com/article/why-does-the-brain-need-s/.

11. Daniel G. Amen, William S. Harris, Parris M. Kidd, et al., "Quantitative Erythrocyte Omega-3 EPA Plus DHA Levels Are Related to Higher Regional Cerebral Blood Flow on Brain SPECT," *Journal of Alzheimer's Disease* 58(4) (2017): 1189–1199, https://doi.org/10.3233/JAD-170281.

12. A. David Smith, Stephen M. Smith, Celeste A. de Jager, et al., "Homocysteine-Lowering by B Vitamins Slows the Rate of Accelerated Brain Atrophy in Mild Cognitive Impairment: A Randomized Controlled Trial," PLoS ONE 5(9): e12244, https://doi.org/10.1371/journal.pone.0012244.

13. Arizona State University, "Essential nutrient may help fight Alzheimer's across generations," ScienceDaily, January 8, 2018, https://www.sciencedaily.com/releases/2019/01/190108084424.htm#:~:text=Choline%20is%20used%20by%20the,role%20in%20regulating%20gene%20expression.

14. Crystal N. Holick, Edward L. Giovannucci, Bernard Rosner, et al., "Prospective study of intake of fruit, vegetables, and carotenoids and the risk of adult glioma," *American Journal of Clinical Nutrition*, 85(3) (2007): 877–886, https://doi.org/10.1093/ajcn/85.3.877.

15. Ross S. Mancini, Yanfei Wang, Donald F. Weaver, "Phenylindanes in Brewed Coffee Inhibit Amyloid-Beta and Tau Aggregation," *Frontiers in Neuroscience* 12 (2018): 735, https://doi.org/10.3389/fnins.2018.00735.

16. Samina Salim, "Oxidative Stress and the Central Nervous System," *Journal of Pharmacology and Experimental Therapeutics* 360(1) (January 2017): 201–205, https://doi.org/10.1124/jpet.116.237503.

17. DH Chui, M Marcellino, F Marotta, et al., "A Double-Blind, RCT Testing Beneficial Modulation of BDNF in Middle-Aged, Life Style-Stressed Subjects: A Clue to Brain Protection?" *Journal of Clinical and Diagnostic Research* 8(11) (November 2014): MC01–MC06, https://doi.org/10.7860/JCDR/2014/10301.5141.

18. R Molteni, RJ Barnard, Z Ying, et al., "A High-Fat, Refined Sugar Diet Reduces Hippocampal Brain-Derived Neurotrophic Factor, Neuronal Plasticity, and Learning," *Neuroscience* 112(4) (2002): 803–814, https://doi.org/10.1016/s0306-4522(02)00123-9.

19. University of California–Irvine, "Learning keeps brain healthy: Mental activity could stave off age-related cognitive and memory decline," ScienceDaily, March 3, 2010, https://www.sciencedaily.com/releases/2010/03/100302151242.htm.

20. T Ngandu, E von Strauss, E-L Helkala, et al., "Education and dementia: What lies behind the association?" *Neurology* 69(14) (October 2007): 1442–1450, https://doi.org/10.1212/01.wnl.0000277456.29440.16.

21. Daniel Eriksson Sörman, Michael Rönnlund, Anna Sunström, et al., "Social Relationships and Rise of Dementia: A Population-Based Study," *International Psychogeriatrics* 27(8) (2015): 1391–1399, https://doi.org/10.1017/S1041610215000319.

22. Brigid MacCarthy, Richard Brown, "Psychosocial factors in Parkinson's disease," *British Journal of Clinical Psychology* 28(1) (1989): 41–52, https://doi.org/10.1111/j.2044-8260.1989.tb00810.x.

23. David Castro Costa, Maria José Sá, José Manuel Calheiros, "Social support network and quality of life in multiple sclerosis patients," *Arquivos de Neuro-Psiquiatria* 75(5) (2017): 267–271, https://doi.org/10.1590/0004-282x20170036.

24. Shivani Ghaisas, Joshua Maher, and Anumantha Kanthasany, "Gut microbiome in health and disease: linking the microbiome-gut-brain axis and environmental factors in the pathogenesis of systemic and neurodegenerative diseases," *Pharmacology & Therapeutics* 158 (2016): 52–62, https://www.ncbi.nlm.nih.gov/pmc/articles/PMC4747781/.

25. Kuan-Pin Su, MD, PhD, Ping-Tao Tseng, MD, Pao-Yen Lin, MD, PhD, "Association of Use of Omega-3 Polyunsaturated Fatty Acids with Changes in Severity of Anxiety Symptoms: A Systematic Review and Meta-analysis," *JAMA Network Open* 1(5) (2018): e182327, https://doi.org/10.1001/jamanetworkopen.2018.2327.

26. Gregory C. Shearer, Olga V. Savinova, William S. Harris, "Fish oil—how does it reduce plasma triglycerides?" *Biochimica et Biophysica Acta* 1821(5) (2012): 843–851, https://www.ncbi.nlm.nih.gov/pmc/articles/PMC3563284/.

27. Elham Rajaei, Karim Mowla, Ali Ghorbani, "The Effect of Omega-3 Fatty Acids in Patients with Active Rheumatoid Arthritis Receiving DMARDs Therapy: Double-Blind Randomized Controlled Trial," *Global Journal of Health Science* 8(7) (2016): 18–25, https://www.ncbi.nlm.nih.gov/pmc/articles/PMC4965662/.

28. Carol J. Fabian, Bruce F. Kimler, Stephen D. Hursting, "Omega-3 fatty acids for breast cancer prevention and survivorship," *Breast Cancer Research* 17(1) (2015): 62, https://doi.org/10.1186/s13058-015-0571-6.

29. Narendra Singh, Mohit Bhalla, Prashanti de Jager, et al., "An Overview on Ashwagandha: A Rasayana (Rejuvenator) of Ayurveda," *African Journal of Traditional, Complementary and Alternative Medicines* 8(5) (2011): 208–213, https://www.ncbi.nlm.nih.gov/pmc/articles/PMC3252722/.

30. Rammohan V. Rao, Olivier Descamps, John Varghese, et al., "Ayurvedic medicinal plants for Alzheimer's disease: a review," *Alzheimer's Research & Therapy* 4(3) (2012): 22, https://doi.org/10.1186/alzrt125.

31. Sultan Zahiruddin, Parakh Basist, Abida Parveen, et al., "Ashwagandha in Brain Disorders: A Review of Recent Developments," *Journal of Ethnopharmacology* 257 (2020), https://doi.org/10.1016/j.jep.2020.112876.

32. Dale E. Bredesen, MD, *The End of Alzheimer's: The First Program to Prevent and Reverse Cognitive Decline* (New York: Penguin Random House, 2017), https://www.amazon.com/End-Alzheimers-Program-Prevent-Cognitive/dp/0735216207.

33. Navneet Kumar, L.G. Abichandani, Vijay Thawani, et al., "Efficacy of Standardized Extract of *Bacopa monnieri* (Bacognize) on Cognitive Functions of Medical Students: A Six-Week, Randomized Placebo-Controlled Trial," *Evidence-Based Complementary and Alternative Medicine* 2016(4103423) (2016), https://doi.org/10.1155/2016/4103423.

34. Ibid.

35. Office of Dietary Supplements, "Choline Fact Sheet for Health Professionals," National Institutes of Health, Health Information, June 3, 2020, https://ods.od.nih.gov/factsheets/Choline-HealthProfessional/.

36. Rüdiger Hardeland, S.R. Pandi-Perumal, Daniel P. Cardinali, "Molecules in focus: Melatonin," *International Journal of Biochemistry & Cell Biology* 38(3) (2006): 313–316, https://doi.org/10.1016/j.biocel.2005.08.020.

37. Nadia Aalling Jessen, Anne Sofie Finmann Munk, Iben Lundgaard, et al., "The Glymphatic System: A Beginner's Guide," *Neurochemical Research* 40(12) (2015): 2583–2599, https://www.ncbi.nlm.nih.gov/pmc/articles/PMC4636982/#:~:text=The%20glymphatic%20system%20is%20a,from%20the%20central%20nervous%20system.

38. Sarah Laxmi Chellappa, Roland Steiner, Peter Blattner, et al., "Non-Visual Effects of Light on Melatonin, Alertness and Cognitive Performance: Can Blue-Enriched Light Keep Us Alert?" *PLoS One* 6(1) (2011): e16429, https://doi.org/10.1371/journal.pone.0016429.

39. Kyungah Choi, Cheong Shin, Taesu Kim, et al., "Awakening effects of blue-enriched morning light exposure on university students' physiological and subjective responses," *Scientific Reports* 9(1) (January 23, 2019): 345, https://doi.org/10.1038/s41598-018-36791-5.

40. Mariana G. Figueiro, Andrew Bierman, Barbara Plitnick, et al., "Preliminary evidence that both blue and red light can induce alertness at night," *BMC Neuroscience* 10(105) (2009), https://doi.org/10.1186/1471-2202-10-105.

41. "Brain Basics: Understanding Sleep," National Institute of Neurological Disorders, Disorders, Patient & Caregiver Education, August 13, 2019, https://www.ninds.nih.gov/Disorders/Patient-Caregiver-Education/Understanding-Sleep.

42. Office of Communications and Public Liaison, "Brain Basics: Understanding Sleep," National Institute of Neurological Disorders and Stroke, Disorders, Patient & Caregiver Education, August 13, 2019, https://www.ninds.nih.gov/Disorders/Patient-Caregiver-Education/Understanding-Sleep.

43. Robert Sapolsky, *Why Zebras Don't Get Ulcers* (New York: Henry Holt and Company, 2004), https://www.amazon.com/Why-Zebras-Dont-Ulcers-Third/dp/0805073698/ref=tmm_pap_title_0?_encoding=UTF8&qid=&sr=.

44. Amy F.T. Arnsten, "Stress signalling pathways that impair prefrontal cortex structure and function," *Nature Reviews Neuroscience* 10 (2009): 410–422, https://www.ncbi.nlm.nih.gov/pmc/articles/PMC2907136/.

45. PA Adlard, CW Cotman, "Voluntary exercise protects against stress-induced decreases in brain-derived neurotrophic factor protein expression," *Neuroscience* 124(4) (2004): 985–992, https://doi.org/10.1016/j.neuroscience.2003.12.039.

46. Ibid.

47. Zsolt Radak, Haie Y. Chung, Erika Kotai, et al., "Exercise, oxidative stress and hormesis," *Ageing Research Reviews* 7(1) (2007): 34–42, http://tf.hu/wp-content/uploads/2009/08/Rad%C3%A1k-Zsolt-NTK-56.pdf.

48. "Physical Activity Reduces Stress," Anxiety and Depression Association of America, For the Public, Understand the Facts, 2018, https://adaa.org/understanding-anxiety/related-illnesses/other-related-conditions/stress/physical-activity-reduces-st#:~:text=Scientists%20have%20found%20that%20regular,can%20stimulate%20anti%2Danxiety%20effects.

49. Steven Rosenzweig, Diane K. Reibel, Jeffrey M. Greeson, et al., "Mindfulness-based stress reduction lowers psychological distress in medical students," *Marcus Institute of Integrative Health* 1 (2003), https://jdc.jefferson.edu/cgi/viewcontent.cgi?article=1000&context=jmbcimfp.

50. G. Sunil Naik, G.S. Gaur, and G.K. Pal, "Effect of Modified Slow Breathing Exercise on Perceived Stress and Basal Cardiovascular Parameters," *International Journal of Yoga* 11(1) (2018): 53–58, https://www.ncbi.nlm.nih.gov/pmc/articles/PMC5769199/.

51. Xiao Ma, Zi-Qi Yue, Zhu-Qing Gong, et al., "The Effect of Diaphragmatic Breathing on Attention, Negative Affect and Stress in Healthy Adults," *Frontiers in Psychology* 8 (2017), https://doi.org/10.3389/fpsyg.2017.00874.

52. Kristen E. Riley, Crystal L. Park, "How does yoga reduce stress? A systematic review of mechanisms of change and guide to future inquiry," *Health Psychology Review* 9(3) (2015): 379–396, https://spiritualitymeaningandhealth.uconn.edu/wp-content/uploads/sites/2598/2019/03/How-does-yoga-reduce-stress-A-systematic-review-of-mechanisms-of-change-and-guide-to-future-inquiry.pdf.

53. Alice G. Walton, "7 Ways Meditation Can Actually Change The Brain," Innovation, *Forbes*, February 9, 2015, https://www.forbes.com/sites/alicegwalton/2015/02/09/7-ways-meditation-can-actually-change-the-brain/#4fcadd601465.

54. "Meditation: In Depth," National Center for Complementary and Integrative Health, Health Information, April 2016, https://www.nccih.nih.gov/health/meditation-in-depth.

55. Laurent Valosek, "Effect of Meditation on Emotional Intelligence and Perceived Stress in the Workplace: A Randomized Controlled Case Study," *Permanente Journal* 22 (October 29, 2018): 17–172, http://www.thepermanentejournal.org/issues/2018/fall/6884-workplace-study.html.

56. Emma Seppälä, PhD, "20 Scientific Reasons to Start Meditating Today," *Psychology Today*, September 11, 2013, https://www.psychologytoday.com/us/blog/feeling-it/201309/20-scientific-reasons-start-meditating-today.

57. Patricia A. Tun, Margie E. Lachman, "The Association Between Computer Use and Cognition Across Adulthood: Use It so You Won't Lose It?" *Psychology and Aging* 25(3) (2010): 560–568, https://www.ncbi.nlm.nih.gov/pmc/articles/PMC3281759/.

58. Sandee LaMotte, "MRIs show screen time linked to lower brain development in preschoolers," CNN Health, November 4, 2019, https://www.cnn.com/2019/11/04/health/screen-time-lower-brain-development-preschoolers-wellness/index.html.

59. Melinda Smith, MA, Lawrence Robinson, Jeanne Segal, PhD, "Smartphone Addiction," HelpGuide, October 2019, https://www.helpguide.org/articles/addictions/smartphone-addiction.htm.

60. SA Bahrainian, KH Alizadeh, MR Raeisoon, et al., "Relationship of Internet addiction with self-esteem and depression in university students," *Journal of Preventive Medicine and Hygiene* 55(3) (2014): 86–89, https://www.ncbi.nlm.nih.gov/pmc/articles/PMC4718307/.

CHAPTER 8

1. Rachel Morello-Frosch, Lara J. Cushing, Bill M. Jesdale, et al., "Environmental Chemicals in an Urban Population of Pregnant Women and Their Newborns from San Francisco," *Environmental Science & Technology* 50(22) (2016): 12464–12472, https://doi.org/10.1021/acs.est.6b03492.

2. Min-Ji Kim, Philippe Marchand, Corneliu Henegar, et al., "Fate and Complex Pathogenic Effects of Dioxins and Polychlorinated Biphenyls in Obese Subjects Before and After Drastic Weight Loss," *Environmental Health Perspectives* 119(3) (2011): 377–383, https://doi.org/10.1289/ehp.1002848.

3. Yong-Song Guan, Qing He, "Plants Consumption and Liver Health," *Evidence-Based Complementary and Alternative Medicine* 2015(824185) (2015), https://doi.org/10.1155/2015/824185.

4. Birgit M. Dietz, Atieh Hajirahimkhan, Tareisha L. Dunlap, et al., "Biotanicals and Their Bioactive Phytochemicals for Women's Health," *Pharmacological Reviews* 68(4) (2016): 1026–1073, https://doi.org/10.1124/pr.115.010843.

5. Ibid.

6. Ibid.

7. Ibid.

8. Mahmoud Rafieian-Kapaei and Mino Movahedi, "Systematic Review of Premenstrual, Postmenstrual and Infertility Disorders of Vitex Agnus Castus," *Electron Physician* 9(1) (2017): 3685–3689, https://doi.org/10.19082/3685.

9. Erin Jackson, Robin Shoemaker, Nika Larian, et al., "Adipose Tissue as a Site of Toxin Accumulation," *Comprehensive Physiology* 7(4) (2017): 1085–1135, https://www.ncbi.nlm.nih.gov/pmc/articles/PMC6101675/.

10. Learning and Developmental Disabilities Initiative, "Mental Health and Environmental Exposures," *Collaborative on Health and the Environment*, November 2008, https://www.healthandenvironment.org/uploads-old/MentalHealth.pdf.

11. Stephani Kim, Monica Arora, Cristina Fernandez, et al., "Lead, Mercury, and Cadmium Exposure and Attention Deficit Hyperactivity Disorder in Children," *Environmental Research* 126 (2013): 105–110, https://www.ncbi.nlm.nih.gov/pmc/articles/PMC3847899/; Joel T. Nigg, PhD, "Understanding the Link Between Lead Toxicity and ADHD," *Psychiatric Times*, September 30, 2016, https://www.psychiatrictimes.com/view/understanding-link-between-lead-toxicity-and-adhd.

12. "Baby teeth link autism and heavy metals, NIH study suggests," National Institutes of Health, News & Events, June 1, 2014, https://www.nih.gov/news-events/news-releases/baby-teeth-link-autism-heavy-metals-nih-study-suggests; Daniel A. Rossignol, MD, "Environmental Toxicants and Autism Spectrum Disorder," *Psychiatric Times*, September 30, 2016, https://www.psychiatrictimes.com/view/environmental-toxicants-and-autism-spectrum-disorder.

13. Montserrat González-Estecha, Elena M. Trasabares, Kazuhiro Tajima, et al., "Trace elements in bipolar disorder," *Journal of Trace Elements in Medicine and Biology* 25(1) (2011): S78–S83, https://doi.org/10.1016/j.jtemb.2010.10.015.

14. A Modabbernia, E Velthorst, C Gennings, et al., "Early-life metal exposure and schizophrenia: A proof-of-concept study using novel tooth-matrix biomarkers," *European Psychiatry* 36 (2016): 1–6, https://www.ncbi.nlm.nih.gov/pmc/articles/PMC5300790/; James S. Brown, "Introduction: An Update on Psychiatric Effects of Toxic Exposures," *Psychiatric Times*, September 30, 2016, https://www.psychiatrictimes.com/view/introduction-update-psychiatric-effects-toxic-exposures.

15. Ivy Shiue, "Urinary heavy metals, phthalates and polyaromatic hydrocarbons independent of health events are associated with adult depression: USA NHANES, 2011–2012," *Environmental Science and Pollution Research* 22 (2015): 17095–17103, https://doi.org/10.1007/s11356-015-4944-2; Michael Berk, Lana J. Williams, Ana C. Andreazza, et al., "Pop, heavy metal and the blues: secondary analysis of persistent organic pollutants (POP), heavy metals and depressive symptoms in the NHANES National Epidemiological Survey," *BMJ Open* 4 (2014), https://doi.org/10.1136/bmjopen-2014-005142.

16. M. Luisa Leret, Jose Antonio San Millán, M. Teresa Antonio, "Perinatal exposure to lead and cadmium affects anxiety-like behaviour," *Toxicology* 186(1–2) (2003): 125–130, https://doi.org/10.1016/S0300-483X(02)00728-X.

17. Hayriye Gonullu, Edip Gonullu, Sevdegul Karadas, et al., "The Levels of Trace Elements and Heavy Metals in Patients With Acute Migraine Headache," *Journal of the Pakistan Medical Association* 65(7) (2015): 694–697, https://pubmed.ncbi.nlm.nih.gov/26160074/.

18. Iowa State University, "Metal exposure and Parkinson's symptoms: Link explored," ScienceDaily, March 13, 2019, https://www.sciencedaily.com/releases/2019/03/190313143233.htm#:~:text=A%20new%20study%20describes%20the,and%20better%20outcomes%20for%20patients.

19. W. Michael Caudle, Thomas S. Guillot, Carlos R. Lazo, et al., "Industrial toxicants and Parkinson's disease," *Neurotoxicology* 33(2) (2012): 178–188, https://www.ncbi.nlm.nih.gov/pmc/articles/PMC3299826/.

20. Melanie D. Napier, Charles Poole, Glen A. Satten, et al., "Heavy metals, organic solvents and multiple sclerosis: an exploratory look at gene-environment interactions," *Archives of Environmental & Occupational Health* 71(1) (2016): 25–34, ncbi.nlm.nih.gov/pmc/articles/PMC4334728/.

21. Tee Jong Huat, Judith Camats-Perna, Estella A. Newcombe, et al., "Metal Toxicity Links to Alzheimer's Disease and Neuroinflammation," *Journal of Molecular Biology* 431(9) (2019): 1843–1868, https://pubmed.ncbi.nlm.nih.gov/30664867/; Gabriella Notarachille, Fabio Arnesano, Vincenza Calò, et al., "Heavy metals toxicity: effect of cadmium ions on amyloid beta protein 1-42. Possible implications for Alzheimer's disease," *BioMetals* 27 (2014): 371–388, https://doi.org/10.1007/s10534-014-9719-6.

22. P Schofield, "Dementia associated with toxic causes and autoimmune disease," *International Psychogeriatrics* 17(S1) (2005): S129–S147, https://doi.org/10.1017/S1041610205001997; Manjari Tripathi, Deepti Vibha, "Reversible dementias," *Indian Journal of Psychiatry* 51(1) (2009): S52–S55, https://www.ncbi.nlm.nih.gov/pmc/articles/PMC3038529/.

23. Yu-Ming Chang, Mohamad El-Zaatari, John Y Kao, "Does stress induce bowel dysfunction?" *Expert Review of Gastroenterology & Hepatology* 8(6) (2014): 583–585, https://doi.org/10.1586/17474124.2014.911659.

24. Vida Mokhtari, MSc, Parvaneh Afsharian, PhD, Maryam Shahhosein, PhD, et al., "A Review on Various Uses of N-Acetyl Cysteine," *Cell Journal* 19(1) (2017): 11–17, https://www.ncbi.nlm.nih.gov/pmc/articles/PMC5241507/.

25. Ezhilarasan Devaraj, "Hepatoprotective properties of Dandelion: Recent update," *Journal of Applied Pharmaceutical Science* 6(6)(04) (2016): 202–205, https://www.researchgate.net/publication/302959005_Hepatoprotective_properties_of_Dandelion_Recent_update.

26. Fonyuy E. Wirngo, Max N. Lambert, Per B. Jeppesen, "The Physiological Effects of Dandelion (Taraxacum Officinale) in Type 2 Diabetes," *Review of Diabetic Studies* 13(2-3) (2016): 113–131, https://doi.org/10.1900/RDS.2016.13.113.

27. Christine Tara Peterson, PhD, Kate Dennisto, BS, Deepak Chopra, MD, "Therapeutic Uses of Triphala in Ayurvedic Medicine," *Journal of Alternative Complementary Medicine* 23(8) (2017): 607–614, https://doi.org/10.1089/acm.2017.0083.

28. Romilly E. Hodges, Deanna M. Minich, "Modulation of Metabolic Detoxification Pathways Using Foods and Food-Derived Components: A Scientific Review with Clinical Application," *Journal of Nutrition and Metabolism* 2015(760689) (2015), https://doi.org/10.1155/2015/760689.

29. Joanna Kapusta-Duch, Aneta Kopeć, Ewa Piqtkowska, et al., "The beneficial effects of Brassica vegetables on human health," *Roczniki Państwowego Zakladu Higieny* 63(4) (2012): 389–395, https://www.researchgate.net/publication/236598046_The_beneficial_effects_of_Brassica_vegetables_on_human_health.

30. Paul B. Tchounwou, Clement G. Yedjou, Anita K. Patlolla, et al., "Heavy Metals Toxicity and the Environment," *Experientia Supplementum* 101 (2012): 133–164, https://www.ncbi.nlm.nih.gov/pmc/articles/PMC4144270/.

CHAPTER 9

1. Roma Pahwa, Amandeep Goyal, Pankaj Bansal, and Ishwarlal Jialal, *Chronic Inflammation* (Treasure Island, FL: StatPearls Publishing, 2020), https://www.ncbi.nlm.nih.gov/books/NBK493173/.

2. John Danesh, Peter Whincup, Mary Walker, et al., "Low grade inflammation and coronary heart disease: prospective study and updated meta-analyses," *BMJ* 321(7255) (2000): 199–204, https://doi.org/10.1136/bmj.321.7255.199.

3. Lisa M. Coussens, Zena Werb, "Inflammation and cancer," *Nature* 420(6917) (2002): 860–867, https://www.ncbi.nlm.nih.gov/pmc/articles/PMC2803035/.

4. R. Peila, L.J. Launer, "Inflammation and dementia: epidemiologic evidence," *Acta Neurologica Scandinavica* 114(s185) (2006): 102–106, https://doi.org/10.1111/j.1600-0404.2006.00693.x.

5. "Autoimmune Disease List," American Autoimmune Related Diseases Association, Education and Awareness, 2018, https://www.aarda.org/diseaselist/.

6. Jenny Amaya-Amaya, Juan Camila Sarmiento-Monroy, and Adriana Rojas-Villarraga, Chapter 38: Cardiovascular involvement in autoimmune diseases. In: JM Anaya, Y Shoenfeld, A Rojas-Villarraga, et al., editors, *Autoimmunity: From Bench to Bedside* (Bogota, Colombia: El Rosario University Press, 2013), https://www.ncbi.nlm.nih.gov/books/NBK459468/.

7. Tamara Bhandari, Washington University School of Medicine, "Link between autoimmune, heart disease explained in mice," ScienceDaily, November 8, 2018, https://www.sciencedaily.com/releases/2018/11/181108130543.htm.

8. "The cancer and autoimmune disease connection may increase disease risk, complicate treatments," *Cancer Treatment Centers of America* (blog), October 17, 2018, https://www.cancercenter.com/community/blog/2018/10/the-cancer-and-autoimmune-disease-connection.

9. Monica H. Carlsen, Bente L. Halvorsen, Kari Holte, et al., "The total antioxidant content of more than 3100 foods, beverages, spices, herbs and supplements used worldwide," *Nutrition Journal* 9(3) (2010), https://doi.org/10.1186/1475-2891-9-3.

10. Kelly L. Wolfe, Xinmei Kang, Xiangjiu He, et al., "Cellular Antioxidant Activity of Common Fruits," *Journal of Agricultural and Food Chemistry* 56(18) (2008): 8418–8426, https://doi.org/10.1021/jf801381y.

11. Emilio Ros, Isabel Núñez, Ana Pérez-Heras, et al., "A Walnut Diet Improves Endothelial Function in Hypercholesterolemic Subjects: A Randomized Crossover Trial," *Circulation* 109(13) (2004): 1609–1614, https://doi.org/10.1161/01.CIR.0000124477.91474.FF.

12. Monica H. Carlsen, Bente L. Halvorsen, Kari Holte, et al., "The total antioxidant content of more than 3100 foods, beverages, spices, herbs and supplements used worldwide," *Nutrition Journal* 9(3) (2010), https://doi.org/10.1186/1475-2891-9-3.https://www.ncbi.nlm.nih.gov/pmc/articles/PMC2841576/#B71.

13. Ibid.

14. Ibid.

15. Ibid.

16. Ibid.

17. Ibid.

18. Renan Corrêa-Oliveira, José Luís Fachi, Aline Vieira, et al., "Regulation of immune cell function by short-chain fatty acids," *Clinical & Translational Immunology* 5(4)(e73) (2016), https://doi.org/10.1038/cti.2016.17.

19. Ranil Jayawardena, Piumika Sooriyaarachchi, Michail Chourdakis, et al., "Enhancing immunity in viral infections, with special emphasis on COVID-19: A review," *Diabetes & Metabolic Syndrome* 14(4) (2020): 367–382, https://doi.org/10.1016/j.dsx.2020.04.015.

20. Ibid.

21. Evelin Tiralongo, Shirley S. Wae, Rodney A. Lea, "Elderberry Supplementation Reduces Cold Duration and Symptoms in Air-Travellers: A Randomized, Double-Blind Placebo-Controlled Clinical Trial," *Nutrients* 8(4)(182) (2016), https://doi.org/10.3390/nu8040182.

22. John P. Campbell, James E. Turner, "There Is Limited Existing Evidence to Support the Common Assumption That Strenuous Endurance Exercise Bouts Impair Immune Competency," *Expert Review of Clinical Immunology* 15(2) (2019): 105–109, https://doi.org/10.1080/1744666X.2019.1548933.

23. John P. Campbell, James E. Turner, "Debunking the Myth of Exercise-Induced Immune Suppression: Redefining the Impact of Exercise on Immunological Health Across the Lifespan," *Frontiers in Immunology* 9(648) (2018), https://doi.org/10.3389/fimmu.2018.00648.

24. Jennifer E. Graham, Lisa M. Christian, and Janice K. Kiecolt-Glaser, Chapter 36: Close Relationships and Immunity. In *Psychoneuroimmunology* (Burlington, MA: Elsevier, Inc., 2006), https://sites.psu.edu/stresshealth/wp-content/uploads/sites/54275/2016/06/close-relationships-and-immunity-2006.pdf.

INDEX

A

abusive relationships, 144–148
acupuncture, 52, 328
adaptive immune system, 216, 217, 219
adenosine triphosphate (ATP), 42, 46, 48
adrenal glands, 23, 35, 42, 54, 210. *see also* endocrine system
affirmations, 39
aging, 53, 65–70, 75–76, 125–126, 167
air quality, 201–203
ALA (alpha-linolenic acid), 33
alcohol, 58, 196
All-Day Elk Bolognese with Zucchini Noodles, 315
Alzheimer's disease. *see* neurodegenerative diseases
amla berry, 225
anti-aging medicine, 117, 330–331
anti-aging supplements, 73–74
antioxidants, 170, 172, 192, 225
anxiety. *see* mental health
aromatherapy, 330
ashwagandha, 175
astragalus, 60
atherosclerosis, 129, 207–208
Atkins, Robert, 91
autoimmune diseases, 24, 220–221
    as cause of death, 55
    and diet, 91
    and immune system, 217, 219
    labels for, 223
    and leaky gut, 97
    and weight, 129
autoimmunity, 219–221
avocado, 105
Ayurveda, 44, 48, 225, 328–329

B

bacopa monnieri, 175
basal metabolic rate (BMR), 118–120
beauty. *see* glow
Beauty Breathing, 79, 244
becoming vibrant, 15–39
diagnosing yourself, 18–25
    habit profile, 25–30
    having the power for, 35–38
    supplements for, 30–35
    wins for, 38–39
berries, 105, 171, 201, 224, 225

Berry Beautiful Parfaits, 274
beverages list, 110
biofeedback, 329
biotin, 74
black cohosh, 194
Bland, Jeffrey, 6
blood, 68
blood pressure, 2, 129
blood sugar, 2
    and chemical exposure, 191
    for energy, 51
    with exercise, 124, 125
    and food choices, 89
    and meal times, 178, 209, 210
    and polycystic ovary syndrome, 70
    stabilizing, 101
body awareness, 20–21, 39, 111, 239
body fat, 2, 119, 191
body mass index (BMI), 122–123, 129
body positivity movement, 129–130
brain, 167–189. *see also* nervous system
    de-stressing, 179–186
    eating for health of, 170–172
    exercise and function of, 173–174
    relationships and function of, 174
    sleep for repair of, 176–179
    supplements for health of, 174–176
    technology and, 186–187
    wins for, 188–189
brain-derived neurotrophic factor (BDNF), 124, 125, 132, 168, 173
brain training, 170
breakfast, 53, 264
breakfast recipes, 273–283. *see also* Vibrant Recipes
breathing, 79, 181–182, 244, 256
Bredesen, Dale, 176

C

caffeine, 58, 172
calcium, 32–33
calcium supplements, 95
calories, 118–119
cancers, 8–9, 100, 129. *see also* chronic diseases/conditions
    as cause of death, 8, 55
    and connection, 140
    and diet, 91–92

and exercise, 125–126
and immune system, 217
and leaky gut, 97
and weight, 129
carbohydrates, 16, 89
and cardiac risk, 91
for energy, 42
and gluten, 99 (*see also* gluten)
refined, as energy crutch, 58
in Vibrant Diet, 94–95
cardio, 132
cardiovascular fitness, 2
casein, 100, 228–229
Cast Iron Venison Steaks, 313
celiac disease, 68, 96–100
chakras, 44, 45
Chapman, Gary, 159–160
chelation therapy, 207–208
chi (ki), 44, 46, 49, 69–70. *see also* energy
Chicken Sausage Breakfast Skillet, 279
chiropractic care, 327
chocolate, 224
Chocolate Cherry Bomb Smoothie, 277
cholesterol levels, 2, 129
choline, 171, 175
chronic diseases/conditions, 9. *see also*
    individual diseases
    autoimmune (*see* autoimmune diseases)
    Big Six, 55, 217
    as causes of death, 55
    and definitions of disease, 221–223
    and diet, 89, 93
    and energy reserves, 57
    and exercise, 118, 125–126
    and immune system failure, 217
    and inflammation, 219
    labels for, 221, 222
    and lifestyle, 54–55
    supplements and risk of, 31
Clean Turmeric and Paprika Roasted Kale
    Chips, 300
coffee, 58, 172, 224
collagen, 73–74
connection (relationships), 139–162, 253,
    267, 322
    abusive relationships, 144–148
    and autoimmunity, 220
    and brain function, 174
    and empowerment for men, 156–159
    and immune system, 227
    and inflammation, 218
    loving for life, 150–156
    relationship resources, 159–160
    romance, love, and marriage, 141–143
    sex in, 151–153

wins for, 161–162
    with yourself, 148–150
connective tissue, 24
constipation, 198–201
conventional medicine, 4–9, 19–20,
    53–54, 326
cortisol, 142
and adrenal health, 54
    and deep breathing, 181
    and energy crutches, 57
    and fasting, 53, 210, 211
    as men age, 159
    and sleep, 177
Creamy Roasted Cauliflower Soup, 286
criticism, 253
cruciferous vegetables, 204

D
dairy, 16
    eliminating, 260
    food list for, 109
    and immune system, 228–229
    sensitivity to, 95–96
    and skin issues, 68
    and weight loss, 101–102
dandelion root, 200
dark chocolate, 105, 171, 224
Date and Pecan Power Truffles, 303
deer antler velvet, 60
dementia. *see* neurodegenerative diseases
dental fillings, 208
depression. *see* mental health
Desert Island Five, 31–32, 52
dessert recipes, 296–304. *see also* Vibrant
    Recipes
detoxification, 53, 191–213
    easing toxic burden, 196–206
    elimination for, 199–201
    and heavy metals, 207–208
    of hormones, menopause and, 193–194
    and intermittent fasting, 208–211
    liver in, 192–193
    reducing toxic exposure, 201–204
    timing of detoxes, 198–199
    and toxic load, 195–196
    wins for, 212–213
    yoga for, 205–206
Detox Salad with Kale, Pomegranate Seeds,
    and Forbidden Rice, 287
DHA (docosahexaenoic acid), 33, 78, 79, 175
diagnosing yourself, 18–25. *see also*
    self-assessment
diaphragmatic breathing, 181–182, 256
diet. *see also* food
    and autoimmunity, 220

and glow, 66
and hair condition, 70–71
and inflammation, 216, 218
and nails, 73
to support detoxification, 193
diets, 16, 90–94. *see also* Vibrant Diet;
Vibrant Recipes
digestion, 2, 53
digestive system, 23, 90
digital detox, 187, 258
Dijon-Encrusted Lamb Loin Chops with
Cauliflower Smash, 314–315
dinner recipes, 307–317. *see also* Vibrant
Recipes
diseas(es). *see also individual diseases*
autoimmune (*see* autoimmune disease)
and brain function, 168–169
as cause of death, 55
chronic (*see* chronic diseases/conditions)
and connection, 140, 227
and diet, 91–92
doctors' view of, 1, 5
and energy reserves, 57
and inflammation, 219
as labels, 221–223
and nail condition, 73
and weight, 129–130
disease diets, 91–94
doctors, 8–9, 19–20, 53–54
dopamine, 142
drugs, 8, 204, 220. *see also* medications

E

earlobe crease, 68–69
Easy 30-Minute Roasted Chicken and Kale
Soup with Bone Broth, 293
Easy Apples with Cinnamon Raisin
Almond Butter, 302
eggs, 71, 171, 175
elderberry, 227
elimination, 192, 199–201
emotions, 2, 77. *see also* connection
(relationships)
endocrine system, 23–24, 50–51, 89,
141–142, 165, 168
The End of Alzheimer's (Bredesen), 176
energy, 41–63
assessing/rating level of, 21, 29–30,
56–57, 236, 320
brain's use of, 170
and energy boosters, 59–60
and energy crutches, 57–59
integrative medicine perspective on, 43–46
lack of, as cause versus as symptom, 53–56
maximizing flow of, 47–50

organ reserves, 52–53
sources of, 42, 44
and stress, 50–52
wins for, 62–63
energy boosters, 59–60
energy crutches, 57–59, 241
environmental medicine, 329
EPA (eicosapentaenoic acid), 33, 78, 79, 175
exercise. *see* movement (exercise)
expression, 66, 74, 75
eyes, 21, 74–75

F

facial hair, 70
facial yoga, 75–76
Fasano, Alessio, 97–98
fasting, 53, 208–211
fats, dietary, 78–79, 89
and cardiac risk, 91
for energy, 42
food list for, 108
for healthy brain, 170
in Vibrant Diet, 94–95
feedback mechanisms, 23–24
Ferraro, Jay, 146–150, 153–156
50-year challenge, 319–322
fish, 71, 105, 106, 171
The Five Love Languages (Chapman), 159–160
flexibility training, 132–133
food(s), 85–115. *see also specific foods or
nutrients*
anti-inflammatory, 224–226
as both problem and intervention, 16–17
carbs and saturated fats, 94–95
dairy, 95–96, 99–102
detoxifying, 203
and disease diets versus wellness diets,
91–94
gluten, 95–99, 101–102
for healthy brain, 170–172
for immune system, 224–226
importance of, 87–89
and microbiome, 90
at night, 178
protein shakes, 102–103
sugar, 95–96, 101–102
superfoods, 105
in Vibrant Diet, 93–105 (*see also* Vibrant
Recipes)
vibrant food list, 106–110
vibrant meal plan, 111–113
wins with, 114–115
free radicals, 172
Frozen Banana "Nice Cream" with
Madagascar Vanilla, 298

Frozen Berry Beauty "Nice Cream," 299
fruits, 90, 101, 108, 170–171, 200, 224
functional medicine, 6, 326–327

G
gallbladder disease, 129
garlic, 105
Gingery Sesame Tuna Poke Bowls, 289
glow (beauty), 1, 65–80. *see also* becoming
  vibrant
  anatomy of, 67–77
  eyes and expression, 74–75
  factors in, 77–79
  hair, 69–71
  movement, 76–77
  nails, 73
  psychology of, 77
  skin, 67–69
  supplements for, 73–74
  and thyroid function, 71–72
  wins for, 80
  yoga for your face, 75–76
gluten, 16, 68, 95–99, 101–102, 228–229, 249
Gluten Freedom (Fasano), 97
Gottman, John, 150, 151, 160
Gottman, Julie Schwartz, 160
Gottman Institute, 160
grains, 58, 96, 109, 249, 264
Greek Roasted Salmon Power Bowl, 291
greens, 105
Ground Turkey Taco Salad Bowls, 285
guided visualization, 185–186
gums, 21

H
habit profile, 25–30
habits, 36, 59, 168, 319. *see also* Vibrant
  Habits Makeover Plan
hair, 69–71, 77–78
health. *see also* mental health
  in current climate, 4
  defining, 1
  diagnosing yourself, 18–25
  doctors' lack of training in, 5
  empowering men for, 156–159
  external indicators of (*see* glow [beauty])
  how you feel as indicator of, 2–3
  making choices for, 9
  power for achieving, 35–38
  spectrum of, 222–223
  turning around your, 10
health data, privacy of, 134
heart disease, 9. *see also* chronic diseases/
  conditions
  as cause of death, 8, 55, 158
  and connection, 140

and diet, 91
and earlobe crease, 68–69
and exercise, 125–126, 128
and heavy metals, 207–208
and immune system, 217
and weight, 129
heavy metals, 207–208
herbal medicine, 48, 329
herbs, 53, 60, 109–110, 194–195, 225–226
HIIT (high-intensity interval training), 133
Hippocrates, 117
holistic healing methodologies, 326–331
homeopathy, 330
hormones, 70, 141–142, 165, 176, 193–194
hormone therapy, 194
Huntington's disease. *see* neurodegenerative
  diseases
hydration, 73, 74, 78, 193, 243

I
immune system, 215–229
  adaptive, 216, 217, 219
  and autoimmunity, 219–221
  and connection, 227
  and diseases as labels, 221–223
  and exercise, 227
  foods for, 224–226
  and inflammation, 217–219
  innate, 216–217
  restoring natural ability of, 223–227
  supplements for, 226–227
  wins for, 228–229
inflammation, 2, 89, 91, 129, 216–221,
  224–226
innate immune system, 216–217
integrative medicine, 6–7, 18, 43–46, 54,
  326–331
intermittent fasting, 53, 208–211
intuition, 20–21, 23
intuitive eating, 210–211
iron supplements, 95

J
joints, 76

K
kale, 105
ketogenic diet, 92
kidney disease, 9, 55. *see also* chronic
  diseases/conditions
kidneys, 53

L
leaky gut, 97–98
learning, brain and, 173–174
licorice root, 195

lifestyle, 36–38, 54–55, 61, 167–168, 216, 218. *see also* connection (relationships); food(s); movement (exercise); Vibrant Habits Makeover Plan
Liu, Jing, 60, 158, 176, 194, 195
liver, 53, 192–196, 200–201, 203–208, 272. *see also* detoxification
liver disease, 55, 129, 196
longevity, 53, 118, 121, 123, 125–126
love, 141–143, 150–156
lunch recipes, 284–295. *see also* Vibrant Recipes
lung disease, 9, 55. *see also* chronic diseases/conditions
lymphatic system, 24, 68, 206–207

M

Mackerel with Zucchini Wrapped in Parchment, 308
magnesium, 32–33
magnesium citrate, 200
mantra meditation, 184–185
marriage(s), 141–143
   author's experiences with, 144–148
   and loving for life, 150–156
   signs of problems in, 150–151
massage therapy, 206, 330
meal plan, 111–113
meaning, 321
medical errors, 8
medical training, 5–6
medications, 8, 9, 34, 196, 204, 262
meditation, 183–186, 257
Mediterranean Ahi Steaks with Roasted Red Pepper Compote, 311
Mediterranean Crustless Quiche, 281
Mediterranean diet, 16
melatonin, 175–176
men, personal empowerment for, 156–159
menopause, 193–194
mental health, 3
and body's feedback systems, 23–24
   and brain function, 168–170
   and causes of death, 55
   and connection, 140, 141, 143, 174 (*see also* connection [relationships])
   and diet, 172
   and energy level, 51
   and expression in eyes, 19, 21, 75
   and glow, 77
   and gluten intake, 97
   and meditation, 183, 184
   and movement, 76, 128, 173
   and sex, 152
   and stress, 180
   supplements for, 33

and technology, 186
and thyroid, 71
and toxins, 197–198
and weight, 129
meridians, 44
Mermaid Bowl with Blue Butterfly Pea Powder, 275
microbiome, 89, 90, 168, 170–171
mind, 2
mindfulness, 61, 180–181
mirror assessment, 21–25, 38–39, 238, 320
mitochondria, 42
mocktail recipes, 296, 305–306
movement (exercise), 117–137, 250, 266
   and autoimmunity, 220
   and basal metabolic rate, 118–120
   and body positivity movement, 129–130
   and brain health/function, 168, 173–174, 178, 180
   calories, 118–119
   cultural differences in, 49
   excuses to avoid, 126–127
   finding your "why" for, 123–125
   and glow, 66
   as health indicator, 76–77
   and immune system, 227
   to increase energy, 47–48
   and inflammation, 216
   for men, 157
   personalization of, 49
   primary types of, 131–133
   reasons for lack of, 120–122
   self-assessment of, 22
   starting where you are with, 128–131
   and wearable technology, 133–134
   wins with, 136–137
movement therapies, 330
multivitamins, 34–35
muscle tone, 2, 76–77
mushrooms, 105
Myers' cocktail, 208

N

N-acetyl cysteine, 200
nadis, 44, 45. *see also* energy
nails, 21, 73
naps, 59
naturopathy, 327
nervous system, 23, 50–51, 172, 174, 175, 181. *see also* brain
netherspace energy, 45–46, 50
neurodegenerative diseases, 9, 168–169
   as cause of death, 55
   and connection, 174
   and diet, 91, 92, 171, 172

and exercise, 125–126, 173
and immune system, 217
supplements to prevent, 33, 175
and toxicity, 198
nicotine, 58
Non-Celiac Gluten Sensitivity (NCGS), 96
nutrition. *see* diet; food(s)
nutrition therapy, 327–328
nuts, 105, 109, 224

O
obesity, 129–130
and autoimmunity, 220
BMI for, 123
as cause of death, 55
and diet, 92
and exercise, 124
and immune system, 217
and inflammation, 218
in men, 158
and menopause, 194
oils, 78–79, 108
organ reserves, 52–53
Ornish, Dean, 91
orthomolecular medicine, 331
osteoarthritis, 129
osteopathy, 327
osteoporosis, 125–126
oxidative stress, 172
oxytocin, 142

P
pain, 2
panax ginseng, 60
Parkinson's disease. *see* neurodegenerative
    diseases
passion, 79, 321
personalized medicine, 13, 92
polycystic ovary syndrome (PCOS), 70
positive outlook, 2
positive psychology, 331
postbiotics, 226
posture, 22, 76
prebiotics, 226
probiotics, 226, 261
prostate health, 158
protein food lists, 106–107
proteins, 89, 170
protein shakes, 102–103, 248
psychology of glow, 77
purpose, 321

Q
qi gong, 49
Quinoa Breakfast Bowl with Sautéed
    Apples, 278

R
recipes. *see* Vibrant Recipes
red clover, 194–195
Refreshing Sliced Cucumber with Hand-
    Smashed Guacamole, 304
regenerative medicine, 331
Reiki, 329
relationship coaching, 143, 146, 160
relationships. *see* connection
resistance training, 132
rest, 53
retreats, 160
Roasted Athenian Chicken Cobb Salad,
    294–295
Roasted Beets Over Leafy Greens, 288
Roasted Butternut Squash and Kale Hash, 316
Roasted Salmon with Blueberry
    Compote, 309
romantic partnership, 141–143. *see also*
    marriage(s)
Rosemary Release Mocktail, 305
Ruby-Throated Dragon Mocktail, 306
Rule of Halves, 59, 187

S
Sapolsky, Robert, 179
saturated fats, 94–95
schizophrenia. *see* mental health
Schuyler, Quenby, 271
seaweed, 71, 105
seaweed mask, 72
seeds, 105
seeds food list, 109
selenium supplements, 95, 226
self-assessments
    of energy, 21, 29–30, 56–57, 236
    of habits, 25–30, 268
    mirror assessment, 21–25
self-care, 252, 322
self-love, 238
senses, feedback from, 23
serotonin, 142
*The Seven Principles for Making Marriage
    Work* (Gottman and Gottman), 160
sex, 151–153, 157–158
shamanic healing, 331
shrimp, 71
silhouette, 22, 66
Simple Family Fun Chocolate Stackers, 301
Simple Massaged Kale Caesar Salad with
    Protein-Packed Anchovy Dressing, 290
skin, 21, 67–69, 204
sleep, 2, 53, 168, 176–179, 242, 255
Sliced Blood Oranges with Shaved Dark
    Chocolate, 297

Slow Cooker Bison Stew, 312
Smoked Salmon and Veggie Breakfast
  Platter with Chive-Yogurt Sauce, 282
Smoked Salmon Niçoise Salad with Dijon
  Tarragon Dressing, 292
snack recipes, 296–304. *see also* Vibrant
  Recipes
somatic therapies, 330
spices, 109–110, 225–226
spiritual energy, 45–46, 50
stimulants, 58
stress
  and autoimmunity, 220
  and brain, 168, 179–186
  and energy, 50–52
  and inflammation, 216, 218
  in men, 158
  relationship-related, 139–140
stress management, 51–52, 153
stroke, 129
sugar, 58, 95–96, 101–102, 263
Summer Patty Pan Egg Cups, 280
Summer Turmeric Chicken Over Sautéed
  Purple Kale and Mushrooms, 310
superfoods, 105
supplements, 262
  antioxidant, 225
  for becoming vibrant, 30–35
  for brain health, 174–176
  for de-mineralized diet, 95
  for detoxification, 200–201
  for glow, 73–74
  for immune system, 226–227
  for organ reserves, 52–53
  quality of, 33–34
  for quick energy, 60
sweeteners, 110, 263. *see also* sugar

T
tai chi, 49
teas, 58, 105, 224–226
technology, 133–134, 186–187, 258
telemedicine, 20
Tempeh Taco Lettuce Cups, 317
testosterone, 159
thyroid, 23, 35, 71–72. *see also* endocrine
  system
  and autoimmune diseases, 220
  dysfunction of, 54
  and energy level, 42, 55
  and toxins, 196
tongue, 21
toxins. *see also* detoxification
  and autoimmunity, 220
  and brain, 168, 170

easing load/burden of, 196–206
  exposure to, 191–192
  and glow, 66
  heavy metals, 207–208
  liver's handling of, 195–196
  and neurological conditions, 197–198
  and skin, 67
Traditional Chinese Medicine (TCM), 44,
  48–50, 60, 69–70, 328
triphala, 200, 225
Triple Oil Treatment, 78–79, 245
Tropic Green Smoothie, 276
Turmeric Tofu Scramble, 283
tu si zi, 194
type 2 diabetes, 9, 55, 125–126, 129, 217. *see
  also* chronic diseases/conditions

V
vegan diet, 92
vegetables, 246–247
  for brain health, 171–172
  cruciferous, 203
  for detoxification, 203
  fiber from, 90, 200
  food lists for, 107–108
  sea vegetables, 71
  as superfoods, 105
vibrancy, 1–3, 10, 13, 65, 234. *see also*
  becoming vibrant; glow (beauty)
Vibrant Diet
  for brain function, 170
  food list for, 106–110
  foods in, 93–105
  meal plan for, 111–113
VibrantDoc, 3–4, 7
vibrant food, 103–105
Vibrant Habits Makeover Plan, 235–269
  daily actions and thoughts for, 238–268
  overview of, 235–236
  printable version of, 269
  and rating your energy, 236
Vibrant Recipes, 104, 271–272
  All-Day Elk Bolognese with Zucchini
    Noodles, 315
  Berry Beautiful Parfaits, 274
  breakfasts, 273–283
  Cast Iron Venison Steaks, 313
  Chicken Sausage Breakfast Skillet, 279
  Chocolate Cherry Bomb Smoothie, 277
  Clean Turmeric and Paprika Roasted
    Kale Chips, 300
  Creamy Roasted Cauliflower Soup, 286
  Date and Pecan Power Truffles, 303
  Detox Salad with Kale, Pomegranate
    Seeds, and Forbidden Rice, 287

Dijon-Encrusted Lamb Loin Chops with Cauliflower Smash, 314–315
dinners, 307–317
Easy 30-Minute Roasted Chicken and Kale Soup with Bone Broth, 293
Easy Apples with Cinnamon Raisin Almond Butter, 302
Frozen Banana "Nice Cream" with Madagascar Vanilla, 298
Frozen Berry Beauty "Nice Cream," 299
Gingery Sesame Tuna Poke Bowls, 289
Greek Roasted Salmon Power Bowl, 291
Ground Turkey Taco Salad Bowls, 285
lunches, 284–295
Mackerel with Zucchini Wrapped in Parchment, 308
Mediterranean Ahi Steaks with Roasted Red Pepper Compote, 311
Mediterranean Crustless Quiche, 281
Mermaid Bowl with Blue Butterfly Pea Powder, 275
mocktails, 296, 305–306
Quinoa Breakfast Bowl with Sautéed Apples, 278
Refreshing Sliced Cucumber with Hand-Smashed Guacamole, 304
Roasted Athenian Chicken Cobb Salad, 294–295
Roasted Beets Over Leafy Greens, 288
Roasted Butternut Squash and Kale Hash, 316
Roasted Salmon with Blueberry Compote, 309
Rosemary Release Mocktail, 305
Ruby-Throated Dragon Mocktail, 306
Simple Family Fun Chocolate Stackers, 301
Simple Massaged Kale Caesar Salad with Protein-Packed Anchovy Dressing, 290
Sliced Blood Oranges with Shaved Dark Chocolate, 297
Slow Cooker Bison Stew, 312
Smoked Salmon and Veggie Breakfast Platter with Chive-Yogurt Sauce, 282
Smoked Salmon Niçoise Salad with Dijon Tarragon Dressing, 292
snacks and desserts, 296–304

Summer Patty Pan Egg Cups, 280
Summer Turmeric Chicken Over Sautéed Purple Kale and Mushrooms, 310
Tempeh Taco Lettuce Cups, 317
Tropic Green Smoothie, 276
Turmeric Tofu Scramble, 283
in Vibrant meal plan, 111–113
Vibrant Triad, 52, 83, 165, 234, 320, 321. *see also* connection (relationships); food(s); movement (exercise)
vitamin B complex, 32, 226
vitamin C, 31, 226, 258
vitamin D3, 31–32, 226
vitamin E, 74
vitex, 195
voice, 22

W

walking, 59, 117, 120–121, 132, 240
water, 202
water consumption, 243. *see also* hydration
wearable technology, 133–134
weight loss, 71, 101–102, 158–159, 173, 211
wellness, power to achieve, 35–38. *see also* health
wellness diets, 91–94. *see also* Vibrant Diet
whole-food day, 265
whole foods, 88, 122, 203, 265
Why Zebras Don't Get Ulcers (Sapolsky), 179
wins. *see also* Vibrant Habits Makeover Plan
for becoming vibrant, 38–39
for brain and nervous system, 188–189
for connection, 161–162
for detoxification, 212–213
for energy, 62–63
with food, 114–115
for glow (beauty), 80
for immune system, 228–229
with movement, 136–137

Y

yoga, 49, 59–60, 75–76, 182–183, 205–206
yogurt, 105
yourself, relationship with, 148–150

Z

zinc supplements, 95, 226

ACKNOWLEDGMENTS

If I were to go back in time and start at the moment when a seed was planted that would eventually become this book, I would have to go back decades and thank more people than I could possibly name here. I have to start somewhere, so I'll start by going back to childhood and thanking my parents for instilling health values in me at a very young age. My mother rarely let me eat sugar or have dessert. I thought it was draconian at the time, but I'm grateful now. We were not a household where food and emotion had any sort of codependent relationship, and that has helped me keep food in perspective ever since. My father instilled in me an appreciation for athletics, a curiosity about the power of food (he was always trying some new diet), and a holistic perspective on health. So thank you, Mom and Dad, for inspiring me to think about these things as far back as I can remember!

I had many influential and important mentors when I was a "baby doctor," just coming up in the world of lifestyle medicine, but specifically I want to thank my functional medicine mentors, Dr. Jeffrey Bland, who first showed me there was a different way to practice medicine, and Dr. Jeff Brist, my Minnesota Internship Supervisor, whose trial-by-fire methods taught me more than I ever thought I could learn in such a short time. I thought he hated me, but later found out he often mentioned me in lectures and referred to me as his favorite intern, "My Stacie." I was thrilled when he showed up later in my life in the audience, when I was the lecturer.

Thank you to my naturopathic mentors, Joe and Lara Pizzorno, who have been huge supporters of my journey over the years, especially when I was on the lecture circuit.

Thanks also to all those doctors along the way who didn't think I could do it—they compelled me to prove them wrong!

In my life now, I must thank the delightful Dr. Jing Liu, whose passion for Traditional Chinese Medicine matches my passion for lifestyle medicine. She has been my Eastern medicine mentor, and our friendship has become one of the most collegial relationships in my life.

On a broader scale, thank you to Cancer Treatment Centers of America—little did I know, when I was in practice during the early years, that there was a legitimate and truly holistic cancer care center out there providing top-quality care. I never would have imagined that, 15 years later, I would land there to implement a functional medicine model. Thanks also to the American Nutrition Association and the American Heart Association for working with me to change policy and perspectives at the national level.

Thanks to Natalie Hood, for telling me not to write a book. I see now that it wasn't time yet. Thanks to Christine Avante Fisher, a fellow author who offered me meaningful encouragement. Thank you to my dear friends Michael and Cassandra Ravenhill, for support and enthusiasm.

Thanks to Charles Harris, for reviewing every imaginable contract, and Terri Ucci, for figuring out the finances behind it all.

A huge and heartfelt thanks to my internal team: Lauren Stigben, you have kept all the parts moving and you never drop any balls. You are a generous and meticulous wonder! Livanga Saxon, you keep it all organized and keep me on track and on schedule, which is not easy by any means! Sara Ponte, you always know what I need, and that means a lot. The three of you never let me down.

Thank you to Annie, Carolyn, and Kamela at Rubenstein PR, for helping guide my public persona in a fruitful way and for being such lovely and caring people.

Thanks to the dynamic and creative team at Commune Communications: Jimmy, Ryan, Caleb, DJ, and Nicole, you brought VibrantDoc to life and gave it movement, color, and personality.

To all those who worked behind the scenes on creating the beautiful insert in this book—thank you, Rishi, Markus, Patric, Rosie, and Olivia! You made a work of art.

Thank you to Bob and Dawn Davis and Michael Franco for the gorgeous photography. You know how to capture me, and the beauty of the world.

Thank you to Dr. Jay Ferraro, for his relationship insights—I hope his words help my readers a fraction of the amount he has helped my husband and me over the years.

Thank you to Chef Quenby Schuyler (Chef Q) for the amazing and delicious recipes. I'm no chef, so I'm glad you are!

Thank you to my writing partner, Eve Adamson. You are in my head and know what I'm going to say before I say it, and that is a rare and surprising thing. I foresee a long and fruitful partnership.

Thank you to my agent, Alex Glass, for seeing the value in my vision and giving me the confidence to take what was in my head out into the world.

Thank you to the wonderful, supportive, and truly collaborative team at BenBella, especially Glenn, Alexa, Sarah, Lindsay, and Laurel.

My most precious and penultimate thanks go to my husband, who has supported me, cheered me on, read my drafts, edited my typos, and provided support of every kind and at every level for me to make this dream come true. I love you dearly!

Finally, I want to thank every woman out there who has ever captured me after a meeting, over a cocktail, while doing my hair, while serving me food, in a boardroom, in a car, on an airplane, at a party, or in an elevator, to ask me their burning health questions. Every doctor experiences that "Hey, Doc, may I ask you a quick question?" phenomenon, but when they find out they are talking to an integrative practitioner, people ask what they would never dare to ask their "regular" doctors.

I love these conversations, and I want every one of you to know that I heard you. I wrote down what you said. I put it all in my quiver because I knew I would need it someday. I paid attention to the repeated questions and the patterns, and I assimilated the information. Yes, you made an impression, and I know you still have questions, and always will, because health is ever-changing and you want it to change for the better. I wrote this book for you because I want to share more than I could share in all the elevators in the world. I tried to incorporate the most pressing questions and concerns I've heard over the years, and that I continue to hear every day. This book is about foundations, and those foundations underlie all your questions, but I will keep sending information out into the world for you, because you deserve to know how to take care of yourself. I hope *Vibrant* helps to set you on that path.

ABOUT THE AUTHOR

DR. STACIE STEPHENSON is a recognized leader in functional medicine focused on integrative, regenerative, anti-aging, and natural medicine modalities. She is the founder and CEO of VibrantDoc, a health and wellness media enterprise dedicated to making integrative medicine concepts and optimal wellness accessible to all. She serves as the Chair of Functional Medicine at Cancer Treatment Centers of America (CTCA), is a board member for the American Nutritional Association, an ambassador for the American Heart Association, and the Vice Chair of Gateway for Cancer Research, a nonprofit organization dedicated to funding breakthrough cancer research and early stage clinical trials.

Dr. Stephenson was in the first group of advance practice module-certified functional medicine practitioners trained by the renowned Institute for Functional Medicine, and went on to be one of the first female practitioners to offer functional medicine care to patients in the Midwest. She graduated magna cum laude from Northwestern Health Sciences University with a Doctor of Chiropractic, studied cognitive and behavioral assessment at Adler Graduate School of Clinical Psychology, is a Certified Nutrition Specialist with the American College of Nutrition, and is a Diplomate of the American Board of Anti-Aging Health Practitioners.

Dr. Stephenson spent close to 15 years in private practice before she was named Chair of Functional Medicine for Cancer Treatment Centers of America. She has always championed a whole-person approach to disease prevention and healing, with an emphasis on healthy lifestyle and natural medicine to augment and improve outcomes from those conventional medicine treatments that remain necessary. She continues to share her knowledge, expertise, and integrative perspective with hospitals and health advocacy groups across the country, giving talks on subjects ranging from innovations in genomics and personalized cancer therapies to nutritional strategies that support recovery and long-term management of chronic and other diseases.

Today, Dr. Stephenson devotes a large share of her time and energy to improving cancer treatment and care, both through her advisory work for CTCA as well as through her work as Vice Chair of Gateway for Cancer Research. Dr. Stacie spearheads the organization's annual Cures

Gala in Chicago and is the founder and chairwoman of Gateway's second marquis fundraising event, Vino con Stelle.

Together with her husband, Richard, Dr. Stephenson is a passionate philanthropist, committed to funding high-impact organizations in the areas of children's health and wellness, poverty, and education. Driving positive change on a global scale is simply a part of the couple's mission. Dr. and Mr. Stephenson are also focused on grassroots advocacy, supporting local and regional causes in Illinois, Arizona, Michigan, the U.S. Virgin Islands, and beyond.

The end of the book.
The beginning of your journey.

Visit vibrantdoc.com for bonus content and tips to help you ignite your glow every day.

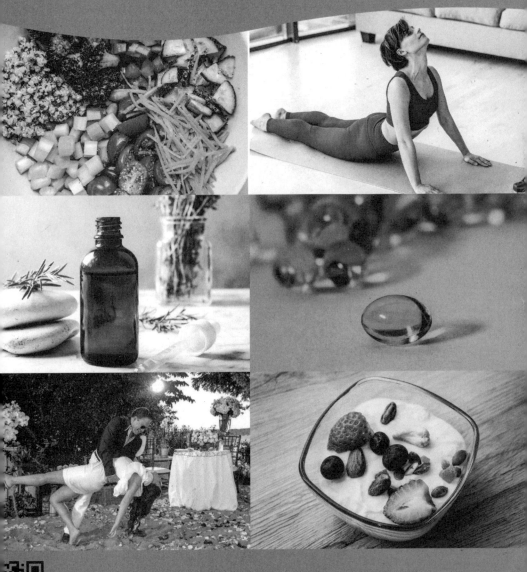